Legal Epide

Legal Epidemiology

Theory and Methods

Second Edition

Alexander C. Wagenaar
Rosalie Liccardo Pacula
Scott Burris

EDITORS

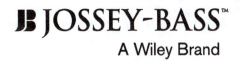

JB JOSSEY-BASS™
A Wiley Brand

Published by John Wiley & Sons, Inc., Hoboken, New Jersey.
Published simultaneously in Canada.

For general information on our other products and services or for technical support, please contact our Customer Care Department within the United States at (800) 762-2974, outside the United States at (317) 572-3993 or fax (317) 572-4002.

Wiley also publishes its books in a variety of electronic formats. Some content that appears in print may not be available in electronic formats. For more information about Wiley products, visit our web site at www.wiley.com.

Library of Congress Cataloging-in-Publication Data
Names: Wagenaar, Alexander C., editor. | Pacula, Rosalie Liccardo, 1968– editor. | Burris, Scott, editor.
Title: Legal epidemiology : theory and methods / Alexander C. Wagenaar, Rosalie Liccardo Pacula, Scott Burris, editors.
Other titles: Public health law research.
Description: Second edition. | San Francisco : Jossey-Bass, [2023] | Preceded by Public health law research / Alexander C. Wagenaar, Scott Burris, editors. c2013. | Includes bibliographical references and indexes.
Identifiers: LCCN 2023012962 (print) | LCCN 2023012963 (ebook) | ISBN 9781119906520 (paperback) | ISBN 9781119906544 (adobe pdf) | ISBN 9781119906537 (epub)
Subjects: MESH: Legal Epidemiology
Classification: LCC RA651 (print) | LCC RA651 (ebook) | NLM WA 100 | DDC 614.4–dc23/eng/20230621
LC record available at https://lccn.loc.gov/2023012962
LC ebook record available at https://lccn.loc.gov/2023012963

Cover Design: Wiley
Cover Image: © mmelnikoff/Adobe Stock Photos; itestro/Adobe Stock Photos

SKY10051490_071823

Contents

PART ONE
Frameworks for Legal Epidemiology

PART TWO
Understanding How Law Influences Environments and Behavior

Figures and Tables

Tables

Foreword to the First Edition

This book represents a major milestone in the development of public health law research, both as a field of study and as a tool for using law and policy to improve health. A vibrant community of innovative scientists engaged in rigorous public health law research is essential for making informed decisions on the laws and policies that will lead to better health.

For the Robert Wood Johnson Foundation, this book represents a unique and lasting contribution to the field of public health law. The Foundation conceived and funded a national program for public health law research to make the case for laws that improve health. At this writing, the Public Health Law Research program has funded 60 studies in its first 4 years. Many of those studies have already had an impact at the local, state, and national levels. For example, a program study has shown how local laws in Rochester, New York, have made a difference in children's exposure to lead. Another program study on New Jersey's graduated driver licensing laws has shown how the law reduced teen car crashes and saved lives. And yet another program study on drug patent laws and their impact on public health has already been cited by the United States Solicitor General in documents filed before the US Supreme Court.

Some of the studies funded by the Public Health Law Research program raised new questions. Others provided new insights. Collectively, they point to a need for a critical review of the basic concepts, theories, mechanisms, and measurement techniques of public health law research. That this need has been recognized and acted on is a tribute to the leadership of the Public Health Law Research program and the authors who have contributed to this book.

The intersection of law, policy, advocacy, and health is complex. Applied at the right time, in the right places, with the right partners, laws, and policies have the potential to create lasting positive changes in the lives of people. I am confident that this book will enhance the quality of public health law research. It will strengthen the role of research in policy deliberations. And that will heighten the ability of policy makers, advocates, and leaders to craft and implement effective laws and policies to improve health for years to come.

I want to express my gratitude to the authors, editors, and all who have made this book possible. To the reader, I invite you to take full advantage of the insights and wisdom herein and apply them to your work to improve health.

Michelle A. Larkin, JD, MS, RN
Assistant Vice President, Health Group
Robert Wood Johnson Foundation
April 2013

Foreword to the Second Edition: The Case for Legal Epidemiology

What is epidemiology? The field has had several definitions over the decades, but my favorite definition has always been that epidemiology is the science that aims to identify the causes of disease, so that we may do something about them (Keyes & Galea, 2014). I think this definition usefully clarifies what epidemiology should be doing and sharpens our thinking about why legal epidemiology represents such an important development toward our shared ends of creating a better, healthier world. My brief prefatory remarks to this volume use three elements of this definition to illustrate the contribution that I think legal epidemiology can make.

The first part of the definition places epidemiology as a science. Acknowledging that epidemiology is a science insists that epidemiology is committed to the scientific method, to the articulation of hypotheses informed by prior knowledge, to the development of experiments to test—and attempt to falsify—those hypotheses, to the careful and honest analysis of data from these experiments, and to drawing judicious inference that can guide subsequent study and inform policy formation. This scientific framework should apply to any post-Enlightenment human endeavor that is tasked with a better understanding of the world. Insofar as the legal system puts in place the legal framework within which we all live, the study of that system should similarly be based on the norms of science, aiming to apply as rigorous as possible a framework to ensure that our system emerges from the data and is free of the biases and superstitions that otherwise might lead us to incorrect inference.

Second, epidemiology is concerned with identifying causes of disease. The use of the word "cause" in this context matters (Hernán, 2018). It says that we are interested in identifying what results in health and disease—conditions or behaviors that then might be manipulated to change the occurrence of disease. Causal thinking in epidemiology emerged at the dawn of the microbial era. In 1884, for example, Robert Koch and Friedrich Loeffler articulated postulates to suggest how it is that we may know if a particular pathogen caused a disease (Evans, 1978). These included that a particular microorganism must be found in all organisms suffering from disease, but not in those that are not. These postulates have long since become outdated and have been supplanted by a rich scholarship around causal thinking. However, the spirit on which they rested remains reasonable to this day: causes are things that make disease happen. This is where the evolution of our causal thinking becomes so important. The infectious disease dawn of epidemiology soon gave way to the chronic disease era in epidemiology where we broadened our conception of cause from the individual microorganism to individual behavior, including for example smoking, or drinking alcohol. Over the past few decades, as our thinking about what is a cause has continued to evolve: social-ecological frameworks of thought have largely taken center stage, helping us organize our recognition that microorganisms and behaviors can be causes, and so also can be the conditions of neighborhoods where we live, the quality of our cities, and the characteristics of our countries (Kaplan, 2004). Given that law establishes the framework for the world within which we live, law is a quintessential cause of disease and should be studied within the same causal framework as we study other causes. I recognize that a skeptic may say that law is somewhat more complicated than a bacterium, but of course in the mid-nineteenth century bacteria were plenty complicated, and we have come far (although not far enough) in our understanding of infectious disease epidemiology. If we are here at a comparable dawn of an era of legal epidemiology, that is a public good and I look forward to seeing where that scholarship evolves over the coming decades.

The third part of the definition of epidemiology is also relevant. Epidemiology aims to identify causes of disease so that we may intervene. Defining epidemiology in this way suggests a very particular, and not uncontroversial (Rothman, Adami, & Trichopoulos, 1998), view of the field and its role. It is a pragmatic vision, one that says that we should pursue the best possible science, with an eye to creating change (Galea, 2013; Susser, 1991). This does not mean that science should not have the latitude to pursue questions that advance our understanding without immediate practicability. The history of science is replete with examples of discoveries that did not have immediate applicability, only to emerge as quite useful much later. This approach rather says that epidemiology is a science with an explicit public purpose. It is a discipline that is committed to the health of the public and as such aims to identify causes to guide how we can manipulate those causes because the end in question— health—matters to us, quite a bit. Seen through this lens, legal epidemiology is quintessentially in line with this definition. We want to understand how laws and legal practices may cause health and disease, and certainly the inquiry is of interest. But fundamentally, laws exist to be implemented, and there is an easy argument to be made that we want to understand laws so that we can have better laws that generate our health. Legal epidemiology then is very much a pragmatic field of inquiry, one that should be committed to the most rigorous norms of inquiry, to the end of understanding how we can have better laws that generate health and reduce disease.

All this suggests that the time for legal epidemiology as a robust field of inquiry has arrived. For those of us who are outside the legal profession, it often comes as a cold surprise whenever we read about or encounter the legal system and recognize how much the way our laws are made and implemented rests on history and precedent and how little rests on a systematic inquiry into which laws produce better outcomes for populations. In the context of health, it is reassuring to see the evolution of legal epidemiology, committed to a better scientific understanding of how laws cause health and disease, so that we can have better laws, and a healthier world.

Sandro Galea, MD, MPH, DrPH
Dean and Robert A. Knox Professor
Boston University School of Public Health
May 2022

Preface

"Each individual in society has a right to be protected in the enjoyment of his life. ... And it is the duty of the State to extend over the people its guardian care, that those who cannot or will not protect themselves, may nevertheless be protected; and that those who can and desire to do it, may have the means of doing it more easily. This right and authority should be exercised by wise laws, wisely administered; and when this is neglected the State should be held answerable for the consequences of this neglect. If legislators and public officers knew the number of lives unnecessarily destroyed, and the suffering unnecessarily occasioned by a wrong movement or by no movement at all, this great matter would be more carefully studied, and errors would not be so frequently committed."

—Lemuel Shattuck, Report of a General Plan for the
Promotion of Public and Personal Health (1850, p. 304).

Modern public health practice began with counting. The idea that disease and injury could be prevented started with what became the science of epidemiology—counting cases and documenting their distribution. The idea of preventable disease led directly to the idea that society has the opportunity and indeed the obligation to take a strong hand in doing the preventing. When we take collective action, we usually do it through government, acting on behalf of the community. Once government is in the picture, law is there, too.

Law matters to public health. It is a tool for intervention to promote healthier places and people. It sets the powers, duties, and limitations of health agencies. Sometimes laws and legal practices with no deliberate relation to health have positive or negative effects on our health. Yet if we go back to the roots of modern public health practice—to epidemiology—and we look at public health as it is practiced today, we can see why it is not enough to assert the important roles of law in public health. Science is the lifeblood of public health, the source of much of its effectiveness and legitimacy. Effective public health work begins with understanding the nature, effects, and distribution of the threats to our health and the facilitators of our well-being and extends to carefully evaluating the interventions designed to support our thriving. So it must also be with law.

If law matters to public health, we have to be able to show how, under what circumstances, to what degree. We have to produce *evidence*. Legal Epidemiology is the field devoted to creating, disseminating, and deploying that evidence. It is also an important tool for addressing the special challenges law poses in public health practice. Law is made by politicians and by officials who report to politicians. Politicians respond to advocacy, lobbying, money, and public opinion. The legal data and evidence produced by legal epidemiology research helps shape understanding of problems and possible solutions, and can create some level of accountability for success and failure in meeting social needs. Evidence and theory about law and health are also crucial to the proper design and effective implementation of legal interventions for public health. "Following the science" in public health cannot just be launching whatever interventions might seem to be apt from the point of view of epidemiology's understanding of the causes of morbidity and mortality. Rules that in the abstract seem to address a vulnerable link in a causal chain of pathogenesis are not ipso facto effective in actual practice; the rules have to be such that humans are disposed to follow them, and enforcers can enforce them. Legal epidemiology is part of a transdisciplinary approach to public health law that draws on the full range of social, psychological, sociological, and sociolegal disciplines to better understand, measure—and predict—how and to what extent laws will influence health-relevant behaviors and environments.

This book describes scientific theory and methods for investigating the development, implementation, and effects of public health law. The empirical study of law deploys normal scientific methods. There is no special science of legal epidemiology. Epidemiology, economics, physiology, and sociology do not change when law is the topic of investigation. That said, there are unique challenges to studying law, and a set of theory, measurement, and research design tools that specifically help to meet those challenges. This book is not a general primer on scientific research methods. Its focus is on the problems that arise in legal epidemiology—and their solutions. And so it is intended for many kinds of readers: experienced social science researchers who are interested in adding public health law research to their repertoire; experienced health scientists who wish to expand their research from interventions at the individual or small-group levels to community or society-wide "treatments" operating through law; legal scholars interested in how social scientists approach the study of law; policy analysts seeking to enhance their toolkit to include empirical evaluations of public health laws and policies; students and novice scientists who can hone their general skills through the study of public health law; and nonscientists who are seeking a general orientation to legal epidemiology.

The book is presented in four parts, each beginning with an introduction delineating the topics to be covered. Part One is an introduction to the basic concepts of the field. Part Two presents a rich collection of theories that researchers have used to study *how* law influences behavior—the mechanisms or processes through which a rule manages to have measurable effects on what people do, the cultural and institutional structures and environments they experience, and how they fare. Part Three is devoted to special questions of measurement that arise when law is the independent variable. Finally, with this grounding in how law works and how it can be measured, Part Four considers the various study designs for legal epidemiology.

We are grateful to Bethany Saxon and Hope Holroyd at the Center for Public Health Law Research for their meticulous work in editing and formatting the manuscript of this edition for publication. The editors would also like to acknowledge invaluable support from the Robert Wood Johnson Foundation, the National Institutes of Health, and the Centers for Disease Control and Prevention, which have enabled the research and thinking that now constitutes a field of legal epidemiology. Most importantly, we acknowledge the fundamental contributions of lawyers, scientists, and lawyer-scientists who have laid the foundations of legal epidemiology and transdisciplinary public health law. We owe a great intellectual debt not only to those pioneers in the field included as authors in this volume but also to our long-term collaborators in transdisciplinary public health law including Marice Ashe, Micah Berman, Doug Blanke, Jamie Chriqui, Laura Hitchcock, Tara Ramanathan Holiday, Martha Katz, Michelle Larkin, Donna Levin, Gene Matthews, and Matthew Penn.

Lemuel Shattuck's words were true when he wrote them of Massachusetts in 1850, and they are true of every state today. We all lose when preventable ills cause death or injury. None of us can, alone, create the conditions in which we can be healthy. Effective, well-designed collective action is required. Through careful scientific study, researchers can help policy makers achieve "wise laws, wisely administered," and can enable the polity to hold government answerable for neglect, waste and error in the deployment of law for public health.

Alexander C. Wagenaar
Rosalie Liccardo Pacula
Scott Burris

The Editors

Scott Burris, JD, is professor of Law and Public Health at Temple University, where he directs the Center for Public Health Law Research. His work focuses on how law influences public health, and what interventions can make laws and law enforcement practices healthier in their effects. He is the author of over 200 books, book chapters, articles, and reports on issues including urban health, HIV/AIDS, research ethics, and the health effects of criminal law. He founded and directed the Public Health Law Research and Policies for Action programs for the Robert Wood Johnson Foundation, and his work has been supported by organizations including the Open Society Institute, the National Institutes of Health, the Bill and Melinda Gates Foundation, the UK Department for International Development, and the CDC. He has served as a consultant to numerous US and international organizations including WHO, UNODC, and UNDP. He has been a visiting scholar at RegNet at the Australian National University, the Center for Health Law at the University of Neuchatel, the Department of Transboundary Legal Studies at the Royal University of Groningen, and the University of Amsterdam. He was a Fulbright Fellow at the University of Cape Town Law School. He has been the recipient of the American Public Health Law Association Health Law Section Lifetime Achievement Award and the Jay Healey Health Law Teachers Award from the American Society of Law, Medicine and Ethics. He is a fellow of the College of Physicians of Philadelphia and the UK Faculty of Public Health (honorary). Professor Burris is a graduate of Washington University in St. Louis (AB) and Yale Law School (JD).

Rosalie Liccardo Pacula, PhD, holds the Elizabeth Garrett Chair in Health Policy, Economics & Law in the Sol Price School of Public Policy at the University of Southern California. Her research focuses on issues related to the market for intoxicating substances, examining factors influencing demand and supply for both licit and illicit intoxicating substances, as well as treatment for substance abuse and mental health conditions. She has been the lead investigator on several NIH studies examining the impact of state marijuana liberalization policies (decriminalization, medicalization, and legalization), opioid policies (those targeting treatment, supply reduction, and harm reduction), and insurance mandates (parity benefits for mental health and/or addiction, coverage requirements related to treatment). Her groundbreaking work in these areas has led to her invitation to serve on NIDA's National Advisory Council Cannabis Policy Workgroup (2017), the World Health Organization's Technical Expert Committee on Cannabis Use and Cannabis Policy (December 2019), the CDC's National

Injury Prevention's Board of Scholarly Counsellors (2021–present), and the National Academy of Science, Engineering and Medicine (NASEM) Committee on the Review of Specific Programs in the Comprehensive Addiction and Recovery Act (CARA). She served as president of the *International Society for the Study of Drug Policy* but remains a research associate at the National Bureau of Economic Research, and sits on several journal editorial boards.

Alexander C. Wagenaar, PhD is a research professor at the Emory University Rollins School of Public Health and professor emeritus at the University of Florida College of Medicine. He has published 2 books and 200 scientific papers on social and behavioral epidemiology, public health policy; legal evaluations; community intervention trials; drug, alcohol and tobacco studies; traffic safety; and injury control. His research papers are widely cited—over 17,000 citations to date.

In 1987, Professor Wagenaar received the Exceptional Leadership Award from the American Public Health Association. In 1999, he received the Jellinek Award for lifetime achievement in research on alcohol. In 2001, he received the Innovator's Award from the Robert Wood Johnson Foundation, and in 2004 was named by the Institute for Scientific Information as a Highly Cited Researcher, an honor limited to less than one-half of one percent of published scientists worldwide. In 2009, he received the Prevention Science Award, in 2016 the Nan Tobler Award, and in 2018 he was inducted as fellow of the Society for Prevention Research, all in recognition of his decades of work investigating and advancing the methods and outcomes of prevention research.

The Contributors

Evan D. Anderson, JD, PhD is an advanced senior lecturer in the Public Health program and in the School of Nursing at the University of Pennsylvania. He was formerly the senior legal fellow at the Robert Wood Johnson's Public Health Law Research program. His work focuses on empirical legal studies, with an emphasis on the measurement of law for policy evaluation. Prior to joining the Public Health Law Research program, Mr. Anderson was a research associate at the Johns Hopkins Bloomberg School of Public Health and a fellow at the Center for Law and the Public's Health: A Collaborative at Johns Hopkins and Georgetown Universities.

Alida Bouris, PhD, MSW is an associate professor at the University of Chicago Crown Family School of Social Work, Policy and Practice, where she co-directs the Chicago Center for HIV Elimination, the Behavioral, Social, and Implementation Sciences Core of the Third Coast Center for AIDS Research, and the Transmedia Lab at the Center for Interdisciplinary Inquiry and Innovation in Sexual and Reproductive Health. Her research addresses the relationship between social context and health, with a particular emphasis on understanding how social inequalities, social networks, and social support shape inequities in HIV/AIDS, mental health, and substance abuse among marginalized populations. Her work has been funded by the National Institutes of Health, Ford Foundation, and the Centers for Disease Control and Prevention. She received a BA in Women's Studies from the University of California at Berkeley and a MSW, MPhil, and PhD in Social Work from the Columbia University School of Social work.

Frank J. Chaloupka, PhD recently retired from the University of Illinois at Chicago, after nearly 33 years on the faculty and after nearly 20 years as director of the UIC Health Policy Center. He is a research associate in the National Bureau of Economic Research's Health Economics Program and Children's Program. Dr. Chaloupka's research focuses on the economics of health behaviors, including cigarette smoking and other tobacco use, alcohol use and abuse, illicit drug use, diet, and physical activity, as well as on various outcomes related to substance use and abuse. Dr. Chaloupka co-directed the Bridging the Gap: Research Informing Policy and Practice for Healthy Youth Behavior research program for 20 years and was director of BTG's ImpacTeen Project. Dr. Chaloupka also founded the Tobacconomics: Economic Research Informing Tobacco Control Policy program and was director of the program for over a decade.

Scott Cunningham, PhD is a professor of economics at Baylor University. He is the author of the book, *Causal inference: The mixtape*, and has published in journals throughout economics such as *Review of Economic Studies*, *Journal of Human Resources*, *Journal of Public Economics*, and others. He lives in Waco, Texas.

Kazi Faria Islam, MPH, has cutting edge research experience with a range of vulnerable communities, including breast cancer patients and sexually exploited survivors. Her research interests are community-based approaches to enhancing mental health and psychosocial well-being. Ms. Islam is now obtaining her doctoral degree in Indigenous and Rural Health with a focus on mental health at Montana State University while working as a graduate research assistant. She believes that pursuing a doctoral degree grounded on the mental health aspect will help her develop the necessary skills and mindset to thrive and sustain in the role of a public health professional.

Brian R. Flay, PhD (1947–2021), was a social psychologist internationally recognized for his research on health promotion and the prevention of disease, smoking, drug abuse, and violence. He established the Theory of Triadic Influence to further understanding of the core factors driving behaviors affecting human health. Brian had a distinguished career at the University of Southern California, University of Illinois-Chicago, Oregon State University, and Boise State University as faculty and center director. His life work will continue to have a long-lasting and meaningful impact on public health research and practice.

Mark Hall, JD is one of the nation's leading scholars of health care law and public policy. He is the author or editor of 20 books and has published scholarship in leading journals of law, medicine, and health policy. At Wake Forest University, Prof. Hall is on the faculty of both the Division of Public Health Sciences and the Law School, and he is a member of the National Academy of Medicine.

Jennifer K. Ibrahim, PhD, MPH is an associate professor and associate dean for Academic Affairs in the College of Public Health at Temple University. She earned a BS degree from Boston College in 1997; an MPH degree from the University of Massachusetts Amherst in 1999; a PhD degree in health services and policy analysis and an MA in political science from the University of California, Berkeley, in 2002; and MEd degree in higher education from Temple University. Prior to joining the faculty at Temple University in 2005, she was an American Legacy Foundation postdoctoral fellow at the University of California, San Francisco. Ibrahim's area of research interest is in health policy development and implementation, particularly at the state and local levels. Most recently, she has been investigating means to address tobacco use through policy modifications and integration within existing public health systems, domestically and internationally.

Wesley G. Jennings, PhD is Gillespie Distinguished Scholar, chair, professor, and director of the Center for Evidence-Based Policing & Reform (CEBPR) in the Department of Criminal Justice & Legal Studies in the School of Applied Sciences and a faculty affiliate at the School of Law at the University of Mississippi. He has over 275 publications, his h-index is 62 (i-index of 170), and he has over 127,500 citations to his published work. He has been recognized as the #1 criminologist in the world in previous publications based on his peer-reviewed publication productivity. His major research interests are quantitative methods, longitudinal data analysis, and experimental and quasi-experimental designs. He is a member of the American Bar Association, the International Association of Chiefs of Police, the National Sheriffs' Association, the American Society of Criminology, the American Society of Evidence-Based Policing, and a Lifetime Member of both the Academy of Criminal Justice Sciences and the Southern Criminal Justice Association. He is also a fellow of the Academy of Criminal Justice Sciences. He is a past president of the Southern Criminal Justice Association.

Kelli A. Komro, PhD, MPH is a professor of behavioral, social, and health education sciences in the Rollins School of Public Health at Emory University in Atlanta, Georgia. Dr. Komro is a child health epidemiologist and has led and contributed to NIH, CDC, and foundation-funded legal epidemiology research to study health effects of state laws related to family economic security. Dr. Komro has also partnered with numerous communities in the conduct of community randomized trials to test effectiveness of preventive interventions, most recently with the Cherokee Nation. She has published over 130 peer-reviewed scientific papers in leading public health, prevention science, preventive medicine, addiction, and health behavior journals and her research has been highlighted by the National Institutes of Health and National Academies of Sciences. Dr. Komro served as director of Graduate Studies from 2016 to 2019 and has been recognized for her teaching and mentoring as recipient of awards from the American Public Health Association; Society for Prevention Research; Department of Behavioral, Social, and Health Education Sciences at Emory University; and the College of Medicine at the University of Florida. She is a member of Delta Omega Society, the honorary public health society. She has held academic positions at the University of Minnesota and the University of Florida, where she served as associate director of the Institute for Child Health Policy. She is a graduate of the Division of Epidemiology, School of Public Health, University of Minnesota.

Glen P. Mays, PhD, MPH serves as professor and chair of the Department of Health Systems, Management and Policy at the University of Colorado School of Public Health. Dr. Mays's research focuses on strategies for organizing and financing public health services, preventive care, and social services for underserved populations. Currently, he directs the Systems for Action Research Program funded by the Robert Wood Johnson Foundation, which studies strategies for aligning the delivery and financing systems that support health and social services. Mays also directs the National Health Security Preparedness Index Program funded by the Robert Wood Johnson Foundation and the US Centers for Disease Control and Prevention, which studies health system readiness for large-scale hazardous events. Mays earned an undergraduate degree in political science from Brown University, earned MPH and PhD degrees in health policy and administration from UNC-Chapel Hill, and completed a postdoctoral fellowship in health economics at Harvard Medical School.

Michelle M. Mello, JD, PhD is professor of law and public health in the Department of Health Policy and Management at the Harvard School of Public Health. Dr. Mello conducts empirical research into issues at the intersection of law, ethics, and health policy. She is the author of more than a hundred articles and book chapters on the medical malpractice system, medical errors and patient safety, research ethics, the obesity epidemic, pharmaceuticals, clinical ethics, and other topics. Among other current projects, Dr. Mello is studying disclosure and compensation of medical injuries as the recipient of a Robert Wood Johnson Foundation (RWJF) Investigator Award in Health Policy Research. In 2006, she received the Alice S. Hersh New Investigator Award from Academy Health for exceptional promise for contributions to the field of health services research. Dr. Mello is director of the Program in Law and Public Health at the Harvard School of Public Health and chair of the school's Institutional Review Board. She teaches courses in public health law and public health ethics. Dr. Mello served as a key consultant to the National Program Office of RWJF's Public Health Law Research program and a member of the Institute of Medicine's Committee on Ethical and Scientific Issues in Studying the Safety of Approved Drugs. She holds a JD degree from the Yale Law School; a PhD degree in health policy and administration from the University of North Carolina at Chapel Hill; an MPhil degree from Oxford University, where she was a Marshall Scholar; and a BA degree from Stanford University.

Avital Mentovich, PhD received BA degrees in psychology, philosophy, and law, and practiced law for several years as a criminal and constitutional lawyer. She is pursuing a PhD degree in social psychology at New York University.

Tom Mieczkowski, PhD is professor and chair of the Department of Criminology in the College of Behavioral and Community Sciences at the University of South Florida. He is a researcher and academic whose interests have included drug smuggling, theories of syndicated crime organizations, street gangs, drug distribution organizations and methods, drug epidemiology, validation of various drug detection technologies, and estimation of drug prevalence and incidence using bioassays and survey methods. Dr. Mieczkowski has published over a hundred scholarly articles and book chapters, and three books. Since receiving his PhD degree from Detroit's Wayne State University in 1985, he has received more than $1 million in research funding. He is a member of the International Association of Forensic Toxicology, The British Academy of Forensic Sciences, The European Hair Research Society, and The American Society of Criminology.

Harold Pollack, PhD is the Helen Ross Professor at the Crown Family School of Social Work, Policy, and Practice. Co-director of the University of Chicago Health Lab, he is an affiliate professor in the Biological Sciences Collegiate Division and the Department of Public Health Sciences. His current research concerns improved services for individuals at the boundaries of the behavioral health, disability, and criminal justice systems. His journalism regularly appears in the Washington Post and other popular publications.

Marc B. Schure, PhD holds a doctoral degree in public health, master's degrees in adult education and health promotion, and bachelor's degree in cultural anthropology. He is currently associate professor of community health and Montana State University and serves as Principal Investigator for several mental health-related projects. He teaches a graduate course entitled Theories and Models in Health.

F. Douglas Scutchfield, MD, ScD (1942–2022) received his MD degree from the University of Kentucky, where he was selected as a member of Alpha Omega Alpha. He completed internship and residency training at Northwestern University, the US Centers for Disease Control and Prevention, and the University of Kentucky. At the University of Kentucky, Dr. Scutchfield held administrative responsibilities of founding director of the School of Public Health and founding director of the Center for Health Services Research and Management. Prior to his death, he held faculty appointments in the Department of Preventive Medicine and Environmental Health, the Department of Family Practice, the Department of Health Services, and the Martin School of Public Policy and Administration. Dr. Scutchfield was also the founder of the Graduate School of Public Health at San Diego State University. His research focused on community health, public health organization and delivery, quality of care issues, and democracy in health care decision-making. He also served as editor of the *American Journal of Preventive Medicine*.

Robin Stryker, JD is professor of sociology and an affiliated professor of law at the University of Arizona. She has two interrelated research programs, one in American regulatory law and politics, the other in cross-national study of the welfare state and labor markets. She has written on sociological theory and methods, and on a variety of substantive topics, including organizations and institutional change, law's legitimacy, globalization and the welfare state; cross-national family policy and gendered labor markets; law, science, and public policy; the political economy and culture of labor, antitrust, and employment regulation; affirmative action and pay equity; and US political culture and welfare reform. Supported by National Science Foundation grants (2005–2009; 2010–2012) and a John Simon Guggenheim Foundation Fellowship (2008–2009), she is writing a book on the role of economic, sociological, psychological, and statistical expertise in equal employment opportunity law and politics, 1965 to the present, and she is coediting a book on domestic and global legal rights and their translation into practice.

Jeffrey W. Swanson, PhD is professor in psychiatry and behavioral sciences at Duke University School of Medicine. He is a faculty affiliate of the Wilson Center for Science and Justice at Duke Law School, the Center for Firearms Law at Duke Law School, and the Center for Child and Family Policy at Duke Sanford School of Public Policy. Swanson holds a PhD in sociology from Yale University. He is a social scientist researcher who collaborates across disciplines to build evidence for interventions, policies and laws to improve outcomes for adults with serious mental illnesses in the community, and to reduce firearm-related violence and suicide in the population. Swanson and his colleagues have published benchmark research studies on the epidemiology of violent behavior in connection to psychiatric disorders, effectiveness of involuntary outpatient civil commitment, psychiatric advance directives, and extreme risk protection orders. Swanson received the 2020 Isaac Ray Award from the American Psychiatric Association and the American Academy of Psychiatry and Law for outstanding contributions to the psychiatric aspects of jurisprudence. He received the 2011 Carl Taube Award from the American Public Health Association for outstanding contributions to mental health services research. Swanson served as a member of the John D. and Catherine T. MacArthur Foundation Research Network on Mandated Community Treatment and the Methods Core of the Robert Wood Johnson Foundation Public Health Law Research Program. He has frequently commented on gun violence in the national media and served as a consultant to policymakers at the national and state level.

Sue Thomas, PhD a political scientist, is senior research scientist at the Pacific Institute for Research and Evaluation (PIRE) and director of PIRE-Santa Cruz, which specializes in the intersection of social science and law as applied to public health legal policy research. In addition to PIRE projects and publications, she has published seven books and dozens of journal articles, books chapters, encyclopedia entries, and book reviews on women, politics, and policy and American government. In 2020, she was the recipient of the Malcolm Jewell Enduring Contribution Book Award from the State Politics and Policy Section of the American Political Science Association for her book *How Women Legislate* published by Oxford University Press.

Ryan D. Treffers, JD is a Research Scientist at the Pacific Institute for Research and Evaluation (PIRE). For over fifteen years, he has contributed work to a range of public health policies, strategies, and projects focused on issues including alcohol, cannabis, healthy retail, and the impacts of preemption on policy implementation. In addition to having extensive expertise in researching and tracking legislation, laws, and policies at all levels of government, he has worked with advocates, community organizations, and governmental officials throughout the country to identify and implement policies and strategies that promote public health. Prior to joining PIRE, he received his JD from Northeastern University School of Law in 2005 and his legal background includes regulatory and advocacy work involving housing and employment issues.

Tom R. Tyler, PhD is the Macklin Fleming Professor of Law and professor of Psychology at Yale Law School. Dr. Tyler's research explores the role of justice in shaping people's relationships with groups, organizations, communities, and societies. In particular, he examines the role of judgments about the justice or injustice of group procedures in shaping legitimacy, compliance, and cooperation. He is the author of several books, including *Why People Cooperate* (2011), *Legitimacy and Criminal Justice* (2007), *Why People Obey the Law* (2006), *Trust in the Law* (2002), and *Cooperation in Groups* (2000). He was awarded the Harry Kalven prize for "paradigm shifting scholarship in the study of law and society" by the Law and Society Association in 2000, and in 2012 was honored by the International Society for Justice Research with its Lifetime Achievement Award for innovative research on social justice. He holds a BA degree in psychology from Columbia and MA and PhD degrees in social psychology from the University of California at Los Angeles.

Jennifer Wood, PhD is a professor of criminal justice at Temple University. Dr. Wood is a criminologist with expertise in policing and regulation. Her research focuses on the many intersections between policing and public health, including developments in first response models for assisting people with social and medical vulnerabilities including mental illness.

Part One

Frameworks for Legal Epidemiology

Part One focuses on the position of legal epidemiology in the broader context of public health science and the study of law. Chapter 1 defines legal epidemiology as the scientific study and deployment of law as a factor in population health and presents a framework for understanding this emerging field. Law is broadly defined, including both "law on the books"—constitutions, statutes, regulations—and "law on the streets"—the rules as put into action by administrative and enforcement agents and people and organizations subject to law. Legal epidemiology is a fundamentally transdisciplinary field, combining legal scholarship with theory and methods from numerous social science disciplines to better understand how law affects population health. The field spans the whole range of research, from qualitative studies of how health policies are made, through implementation research, to society-wide studies of natural experiments with policy implementations at scale. Chapter 1 defines three categories of public health law: interventional public health law (in which the objective is to address a public health problem), incidental public health law (law without public health aims but with public health effects), and infrastructural public health law (which shapes public health agencies and systems). The third category, infrastructural law, is a point of intersection between legal epidemiology and public health

Legal Epidemiology: Theory and Methods, Second Edition. Edited by Alexander C. Wagenaar, Rosalie Liccardo Pacula, and Scott Burris.
© 2023 John Wiley & Sons, Inc. Published 2023 by John Wiley & Sons, Inc.

systems and services research; Chapter 2 explores this relationship and the need for research at this intersection. The breath of law with possible public health effects, combined with the breath of health problems of concern to public health scientists and practitioners, highlights the size and scope of the field and the tremendous untapped opportunities for scientific research to advance the effective use of law to promote the health of the population.

Chapter 1

A Framework for Research in Legal Epidemiology

Scott Burris   Alexander C. Wagenaar   Jeffrey W. Swanson

Jennifer K. Ibrahim   Jennifer Wood   Michelle M. Mello

Learning Objectives

- Describe the field of legal epidemiology.
- Differentiate three types of public health law.
- Identify principal types of legal epidemiology research.

Law is an important discipline within public health (Gostin, Burris, & Lazzarini, 1999). Legal "powers, duties and restraints" structure the mission of public health agencies and shape how it is carried out (Gostin & Wiley, 2016). Law is a prominent intervention tool to achieve particular public health goals. Laws and their implementation also have important unintended effects, both positive and negative, on population health. Law is so important a part of public health that it cannot be seen as solely the business of lawyers: legal epidemiology—*the scientific study and deployment of law as a factor in population health*—is part of an emerging "transdisciplinary model of public health law" that aims to better integrate legal and scientific disciplines in public health generally (Burris, Ashe, Levin et al., 2016).

Evidence produced by empirical research has an important role in public health law practice and scholarship. It constitutes the "facts" justifying regulatory action and supporting normative arguments about which policies are most desirable, most effective, or most consistent with human rights or other legal standards. To be sure, law legitimately serves as a site for the articulation and clash of values, and lawmaking often necessitates decisions that cannot await full information. Not all law is or can be "evidence-based," even in public

---

Legal Epidemiology: Theory and Methods, Second Edition. Edited by Alexander C. Wagenaar, Rosalie Liccardo Pacula, and Scott Burris.

health. At the same time, empirical research is not just an armory for adversarial legal battle. The responsible use of law as a tool for improving public health requires a commitment to the pursuit and consideration of scientific evidence when possible. In public health, just as in health care (Sox & Greenfield, 2009), evidence should inform the investment in and implementation of policy, and a consciousness of data and the scientific method can improve the decisions of policy makers and practitioners even in the absence of data. This is the promise of legal epidemiology.

Legal Epidemiology Within a Transdisciplinary Model of Public Health Law

Lawrence Gostin's widely cited definition of public health law is "the study of the legal powers and duties of the state to ensure the conditions for people to be healthy (for example, to identify, prevent, and ameliorate risks to health and safety in the population), and the limitations on the power of the state to constrain the autonomy, privacy, liberty, proprietary, or other legally protected interests of individuals for protection or promotion of community health" (Gostin, 2000). Using this power-duty-restraint formula, Gostin succeeds in focusing the field on the state's role in managing collective action to protect population health while still encompassing a diverse range of cooperating actors and related functions, including private actors and the health care system. Broad in its vision of what law can do for health, Gostin's definition still rests on traditional understanding of law as a practice of lawyers, whose job centers on building and applying normative frameworks; providing representation in legal matters; and advising nonlawyers on policy development, implementation, and advocacy (Burris, Ashe, Blanke et al., 2016).

In contrast with more traditional conceptions of public health law, legal epidemiology is concerned not with what is right, proper, or legitimate but with whether law can empirically be shown to affect the health of the population. It builds on more than half a century of rigorous scientific research on the health effects of laws and their implementation (Burris & Anderson, 2013). Commentators might disagree upon whether equality, for example, ought to be considered a public health issue, but that is a different question from whether it is possible to empirically identify ways in which law affects health inequalities. Empirical data can be highly salient to disputes about normative concepts and positions but do not in and of themselves resolve disputes about the legitimate scope of public health or public health law or the extent to which health promotion should be traded off against other social goods, such as civil liberties. Traditional public health law practice is as important as ever, but legal epidemiology enriches public health law by naming and highlighting the important legal roles of nonlawyers in creating, enacting, implementing, and evaluating law for better health.

Legal Epidemiology and Legal Scholarship

Legal epidemiology entails the use of systematic methods within explicit theoretical frameworks to collect and analyze data. Legal epidemiology includes both qualitative and quantitative studies using experimental, quasi-experimental, observational, and participatory designs. It ranges from health impact assessments gathering limited data on legal effects in order to inform policy making in real time, on the one hand, to complex experiments and quasi-experiments studying the effects of law on health over extended periods of time, on the other. Formal decision analyses; simulations; econometric analyses; laboratory and field experiments; survey, interview, and focus group studies; systematic reviews; and meta-analyses are included, as is legal research to systematically and reproducibly collect, classify, and quantify laws and judicial decisions for analytic purposes (Hall & Wright, 2008; Tremper, Thomas, & Wagenaar, 2010).

Theory and methods may be drawn from a variety of disciplines in the social sciences, including epidemiology, biostatistics, law, sociology, history, political science, economics, anthropology, and psychology. From the natural sciences, legal epidemiology imports the scientific method, approaching research questions with a theory-based hypothesis to be tested rather than a position to be defended, gathering data for the purpose of testing whether the world is actually consistent or inconsistent with the hypothesis, and reaching conclusions on the basis of a careful and restrained analysis and interpretation of relevant data.

Legal epidemiology research as we define it is thus distinguishable from public health law scholarship. *Scholarship* embraces a range of nonempirical work about public health law, from work grounded in philosophy or ethics (Ruger, 2006) to doctrinal exegesis (Lazzarini & Rosales, 2002) to the crafting of model laws to legal analysis arguing how the law ought to be applied in various situations (Ruhl, Stephens, & Locke, 2003). What we call legal epidemiology does not exhaust all forms of knowledge gathering or analysis concerning public health law. Public health law scholarship includes many outstanding and influential works that have shaped the field of public health law, but do not fall within our definition of legal epidemiology.

Law and Public Health

A key challenge in defining legal epidemiology for public health arises from the potential breadth of the definitions of *law* and *public health* (Magnusson, 2007). In linking the two in legal epidemiology, we take a broad sociological stance, encompassing not simply written laws on one side and morbidity and mortality on the other, but the whole range of institutions, practices, and beliefs through which laws influence health and the determinants of health. This is particularly important given that the timelines for law to influence health may be long and data on key outcome variables scarce; it may be important to examine effects of law on mediating factors such as organizational practices or health behaviors. The key aspect of such a study, from the perspective of whether it is properly classified as legal epidemiology, is that it examines the relationship between a law variable and a health variable.

Theory is central to studying the health effects of law. Social epidemiology, the branch of epidemiology aimed at understanding social determinants of health (Berkman & Kawachi, 2000), provides one example of a theoretical framework into which legal epidemiology can readily fit (Burris, Kawachi, & Sarat, 2002). Most things human beings do, and most characteristics of our environments, have some effect on the level and distribution of health in a population. Whether styled as health inequities or health disparities, differences in health among identifiable subpopulations have become a major concern in health and policy (Commission on Social Determinants of Health, 2008). Health law scholars, too, increasingly recognize the need to examine individual interests and choices through the lens of population health, recognizing that "the choices individuals exercise and the health risks they face are determined, to a large degree, by the environments they experience and the populations they comprise" (Parmet, 2009, p. 268; see also Sage, 2008).

Our conception of *law* is not confined to "law on the books"—constitutions, statutes, judicial opinions, and so on. The mainstream of empirical legal research over the past 30 years has acknowledged the salience of law as it is implemented in practice and experienced by those it targets. Studies of legality or legal consciousness (Ewick & Silbey, 1998), behavioral law and economics research (Jolls, 2006), scholarship on compliance theory (Tyler, 1990), scholarship on deterrence theory and tort law (Mello & Brennan, 2002), and regulation and governance studies (Braithwaite, Coglianese, & Levi-Faur, 2007) all explore this theme. Legal epidemiology is necessarily interested in the psychosocial mechanisms through which compliance is achieved (Tyler, 1990), the range of regulatory techniques that may be deployed (Braithwaite et al., 2007), and how law "operates through social life as persons and groups deliberately interpret and invoke law's language, authority and procedures to organize their lives and manage their relationships" (Ewick & Silbey, 1998, p. 20). Law is fundamentally a social practice embedded in institutions and implemented by agents. It is part of, not distinct from, the social environment whose influence on health is the focus of social epidemiology.

Legal epidemiology also properly encompasses both laws that were intended to affect population health or public health practice and laws that have unintended health effects. "Interventional public health law" is law or legal practices that are intended to influence health outcomes or health-related mediators directly. "Infrastructural public health law" establishes the powers, duties, and institutions of public health (Moulton et al., 2009). But much of the law that influences population health was not adopted for that purpose and may on its face seem to have no connection to health at all. For example, criminal laws aimed at controlling illicit drug use may increase the risk of users acquiring HIV (Friedman et al., 2006). Research that investigates the relationship of law and legal practices to population health falls within legal epidemiology when it investigates health effects or otherwise deploys an explicit population health framework, whether or not the law itself is health-oriented on its face. We label this important category "incidental public health law."

Finally, legal epidemiology is distinguishable from other kinds of public health research in that it evaluates not merely the effectiveness of a public health intervention but the effectiveness of *law* as the tool used to implement the intervention at scale (Burris, 2017). For example, research on whether abstinence-only education reduces teenage pregnancy is not legal epidemiology merely because abstinence-only education happens to be required by law; a study would only be legal epidemiology if it also encompassed research on the implementation or health effects of the abstinence-only education laws themselves (Sonfield & Gold, 2001).

Health Services Research and Public Health Systems and Services Research

Access to health care is an important determinant of population health, and health care is widely acknowledged to be a key component of the public health system (Institute of Medicine, 2002). The study of how law affects population health through the mediating structure of the health care system falls squarely within the definition of legal epidemiology. Legal epidemiology therefore overlaps with the field of health services research, "the multidisciplinary field of scientific investigation that studies how social factors, financing systems, organizational structures and processes, health technologies, and personal behaviors affect access to health care, the quality and cost of health care, and ultimately our health and well-being" (AcademyHealth, 2009). Effects of law on racial disparities in cardiac care outcomes, for example, is an important subject for both health services research and legal epidemiology.

The area of overlap, however, is limited to research that focuses on *law* as an independent variable and population health (or an intermediate outcome with a well-demonstrated relationship to population health) as the outcome of interest. Research is not legal epidemiology if it merely examines effects of some element of health care organization, financing, or delivery on health, without an important connection to law—for example, a study of the effect of capitated reimbursement in private managed care plans on utilization of branded drugs. However, law that applies to the access to, benefit structure, payment method, and efficiency of public health insurance (e.g., Medicaid, Medicare, and so on) is certainly within its scope.

Public health systems and services research "examines the organization, financing, and delivery of public health services within communities and the impact of those services on public health" (Scutchfield, 2009). Its relationship with legal epidemiology is discussed in Chapter 2.

A Causal Diagram for Legal Epidemiology

A wide range of laws and legal practices affects the health of the population in cities, counties, states, and nations. Cataloging all possible effects of law is impossible, and any schema for organizing such effects is characterized by tradeoffs and simplifications. Nevertheless, the field of legal epidemiology is

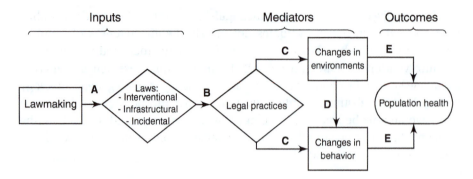

Figure 1.1. Logic Model of Public Health Law Research.

advanced by a shared understanding of the range of possible effects of laws, and potential mechanisms for such effects, encompassed within the field.

The way that law influences population health at the most general level is illustrated in Figure 1.1. The independent variable in legal epidemiology will be some aspect of lawmaking, laws, or the activities of legal agents. These will be studied in relation to dependent variables that can be arrayed along the presumed causal chain that includes key mediators as well as the distal or ultimate outcomes of interest—population morbidity and mortality.

First are studies of policy making—the factors that influence which laws are enacted and that shape the specific characteristics of the statutes and regulations adopted (path A in Figure 1.1). In these studies, public health laws (or judicial decisions) themselves are the outcome variable, and political and other jurisdictional characteristics are often the key explanatory variables tested.

Paths B and C examine key mediators in the causal chain linking laws and health outcomes. Studies of how law affects legal practices (path B) focus on the implementation or enforcement of the law on the books, including how the law affects the structure or operation of various regulatory systems. Laws may vary considerably in the degree to which they are effectively implemented; for example, whether a legal mandate for health education in schools translates into all pupils receiving the education that legislators envisioned may depend critically on the appropriation attached to the bill. There are opportunities and resources for litigation in some matters and not others. Unfunded mandates, unclear statutory provisions, failure to identify an administrative agency responsible for issuing implementing guidelines and overseeing rollout of the new legal provisions, lack of political commitment, and many other factors may undermine implementation. Similarly, laws may induce varying levels of compliance on the part of the regulated entities or population, depending on the degree of political resistance, the extent to which the administering agency is armed with effective enforcement mechanisms, the litigation environment, and many other factors. Completeness of implementation and effectiveness of mechanisms for ensuring compliance with the law are critical elements influencing the law's effect on health outcomes. Legal practices studies explore these influences as mediators of the statute or regulation's effect on health.

Paths C and D involve studying the effect of law (as implemented through legal practices) on environments and health behaviors. We use the term *environment* broadly to refer not only to the physical environment but also to the social structures and institutions. Even private institutions, such as corporations or the family, are influenced by law. Laws and their implementation affect social institutions and environments by creating or reducing opportunities, increasing or decreasing available resources, expanding or reducing rights and obligations, and creating incentives and penalties. Research in this area examines these mechanisms of influence and how they shape the conditions for people to be healthy.

Law may affect health behaviors both directly (path D) and by shifting the environmental conditions that make particular behavioral choices more or less attractive (paths C–E). For example, land use laws may influence where supermarkets and restaurants are located, affecting the availability of healthy food options and the healthfulness of the diet of local residents. Ultimately, changes in environments and behaviors lead to changes in population-level morbidity and mortality (paths F and G).

Legal epidemiology examines health outcomes directly or may use mediating environmental and behavioral changes as proxy outcome variables. While directly measuring health effects generally is desirable because it provides more information to policy makers about the public health returns to lawmaking, a focus on intermediate outcomes is often appropriate. For example, laws designed to improve rates of immunization with the human papillomavirus vaccine might best be evaluated in terms of their effects on the prevalence and burden of cervical cancer, but the time horizon for observing such effects is on the order of decades. Consequently, measuring rates of vaccinations is a reasonable intermediate measure.

Legal Epidemiology in Practice

Table 1.1 offers a typology of the principal forms of legal epidemiology studies. In this section, we describe the primary methods for studying each of the paths described earlier.

Policy-Making Studies

Studies of policy-making processes are a mainstay of political science and sociology. They explore issues such as the determinants of legislative, administrative, and judicial lawmaking (Law, 2005; McDougall, 1997; Waters & Moore, 1990); lawmaking processes (Rosenberg, 1991; van der Heijden, Kuhlmann, Lindquist, & Wellstead, 2021); and stakeholders' use of law to achieve their goals (McCann, 1994). Although in broad terms the policy process does not vary by topic area, health policy making has generated a substantial research literature focusing on how generic policy-making processes unfold in a health context. This literature treats policy-making processes as among the legal practices that affect the potential for law to promote health.

Table 1.1. Typology of Legal Epidemiology Studies.

Study Type	Purpose	Methods Examples
Policy-making studies	Identify factors influencing the likelihood that public health laws will be adopted, the nature of laws adopted, and the process through which they are adopted	• Multivariate regression • Key informant interviews • Content analysis of transcripts, rulemaking notices, memos, and other policy materials • Surveys of policy makers
Mapping studies	Analyze the state of the law or the legal terrain currently or over time and the application of laws surrounding a particular public health topic	• Content analysis of statutes, administrative regulations, and formal policy statements • Key informant interviews • Surveys of state and local policy makers
Implementation studies	Examine how and to what extent the "law on the books" is implemented and enforced through legal practices	• Content analysis of administrative agency documents, including public communications • Key informant interviews • Direct observation of enforcement actions • Examination of business records of regulated entities • Surveys of regulators, regulated entities, and the public
Intervention studies	Assess the effect of a legal intervention on health outcomes or mediating factors that influence health outcomes	• Descriptive analysis of outcomes data • Multivariate regression • Case-control designs • Controlled experiments; natural experiments • Simulations • Surveys of persons targeted by the law
Mechanism studies	Examine the specific mechanisms through which the law affects environments, behaviors, or health outcomes	• Controlled experiments • Surveys, focus groups, or interviews of persons targeted by the law

Advocacy groups traditionally have been crucial instigators of health law, and researchers of "legal mobilization" have studied how advocates have integrated legislation and litigation into their strategies (Ashe, Jernigan, Kline, & Galaz, 2003; Mamudu & Glantz, 2009). The relative advantages of litigation versus legislative approaches have been investigated empirically and debated in public health law scholarship (Jacobson & Soliman, 2002; Jacobson & Warner, 1999; Parmet & Daynard, 2000; Wagenaar, 2007), as have the factors influencing legislative outcomes and the legislative process (Backstrom & Robins, 1995; Corrigan et al., 2005). Of particular interest for legal epidemiology are studies that examine how research evidence influences policy makers (Chalkidou et al., 2009; Cochrane Collaboration, 2009; Innvaer, Vist, Trommald, & Oxman, 2002; Jewell & Bero, 2008; Lavis, Oxman, Moynihan, & Paulsen, 2008). Other works have examined the behavior and strategies of policy actors; for example, how they use devices such as preemption and litigation to shift policy battles into fora where they have a greater expectation of success (Jacobson & Wasserman, 1999), how community organizations may be brought more effectively into the lawmaking or law enforcement process (Tyler & Markell, 2008), or how consulting can be used to more effectively translate research knowledge for policy makers (Jacobson, Butterill, & Goering, 2005). There has been interest in the question of how model laws are developed for public health purposes, and whether and under what circumstances model legislation is more likely than other proposals to be enacted (Hartsfield, Moulton, & McKie, 2007).

Both quantitative and qualitative methods are appropriate for policy-making studies. Statistical analyses are useful for examining the extent to which various observable characteristics of a state or local government—such as the political party in control of the legislature or past legislative output—predict the likelihood that a particular kind of law will pass. For example, researchers have used multivariate regression to examine predictors of state legislative action on childhood obesity (Boehmer, Luke, Haire-Joshu, Bates, & Brownson, 2008; Cawley & Liu, 2008). Macinko and Silver used event-history analysis to identify determinants of state adoption of impaired driving laws (Macinko & Silver, 2015). Such research may make important contributions by identifying "friendly" venues for experimentation with new public health law approaches and suggesting strategies for spreading successful strategies to other jurisdictions.

Qualitative methods are appropriate for obtaining a rich understanding of the policy-making process. (Chapter 15 in this volume describes qualitative methods.) Interviews are commonly and effectively used to understand the factors that lead policy makers to take or fail to take particular actions. Researchers have, for instance, conducted key informant interviews with state legislators and their staff to examine factors enabling and inhibiting the passage of obesity prevention laws (Dodson et al., 2009). Content analysis is another useful method of exploring political deliberations that occur "on the record"—for example, legislative hearings and debate concerning public health issues or legislation and the notice-and-comment process of administrative agency rule-making. Researchers have used content analysis to explore, for example, the use of evidence and argumentation in debates over workplace smoking legislation (Apollonio & Bero, 2009; Bero, Montini, Bryan-Jones, & Mangurian, 2001). Although it may be difficult to generalize the results of qualitative studies across jurisdictions, the high-resolution picture of the policy-making environment that they provide can inform strategies for advancing evidence-based public health law.

Mapping Studies

Legal epidemiology includes studies that gather purely legal data for empirical purposes: information about the prevalence and distribution of specific laws (Gostin, Lazzarini, Neslund, & Osterholm, 1996; Hodge, Pulver, Hogben, Bhattacharya, & Brown, 2008), what levels of government have relevant authority (Horlick, Beeler, & Linkins, 2001), and variation in characteristics of the law across jurisdictions and over time (Centers for Disease Control and Prevention, 1999f; Chriqui et al., 2008; Shaw, McKie, Liveoak, & Goodman, 2007; Wells, Williams, & Fields, 1989). Methods may include content analysis of legal texts (laws, regulations, court decisions, and so on), qualitative research designed to elicit information from officials and others who are knowledgeable about the state of the law, or a combination of the two approaches (Horlick et al., 2001). Although no independent–dependent variable relationship is studied, these studies can be scientific—and therefore fall within the field of legal epidemiology—if they involve the systematic collection and analysis of data using transparent, replicable methods. Methods for mapping law are the focus of two chapters in this volume (Chapters 11 and 12).

Mapping studies often contribute information that is useful in its own right—state and local policy makers are keen to know what other jurisdictions are doing and what they might consider borrowing or learning from policy experiments in other jurisdictions. Mapping studies facilitate "policy surveillance," the "ongoing, systematic collection, analysis, interpretation, and dissemination of data" about law (Burris, Hitchcock et al., 2016; Chriqui, O'Connor, & Chaloupka, 2011, p. 21). However, mapping studies are typically an early phase of larger projects designed to evaluate the magnitude and nature of effects of laws on health. Properly conducted, they provide reliable and valid measures of the key explanatory variable(s) in such studies. Thus, a rigorously conducted mapping study requires consistent implementation of a clearly defined protocol for identifying and classifying laws. It will specify a definition of the type of law being investigated, with explicit inclusion and exclusion criteria; search methods that acknowledge strengths and weaknesses of extant databases; and a coding scheme identifying key features of the laws, such as population covered and enforcement mechanisms specified (Tremper et al., 2010). Mapping studies are also the starting point for the development of instruments that characterize laws according to some overall scale of stringency, scope, or strength through transparent and reproducible means. For example, a mapping study of state laws regulating sales of sugar-sweetened beverages in schools coded laws according to seven substantive features and eight process features and then grouped laws into "strong," "moderate," and "weak" categories (Mello, Pomeranz, & Moran, 2008). Mapping data can also be used to create scales that encompass multiple laws constituting a "policy environment," such as an alcohol policy scale comprised of 29 different alcohol policies aimed at binge drinking (Naimi et al., 2014).

Implementation Studies

For a law to be effective, its implementation must be such that it actually influences the behavior of its targets. As in any other aspect of health policy or program implementation (Estabrooks, Brownson, & Pronk, 2018), the process of putting a law into practice can be understood in terms of a series of mediating factors, including attitudes, management methods, capacities, and resources of implementing agencies and their agents; methods and extent of enforcement; the relationship between legal rules and broader community norms; and attitudes and other relevant characteristics of the population whose behavior is targeted for influence (Pawson, Greenhalgh, Harvey, & Walshe, 2005). Text of the law and resources appropriated for its enforcement constrain, but do not eliminate, discretion of bureaucratic entities to reshape rules to fit their existing culture and mission (Deflem, 2004).

Implementation research in law classically starts with investigating the "transformation process" that occurs along path B in Figure 1.1, the differences between the goals and methods of the law as explicitly or implicitly contemplated in the "law on the books" and the "law on the streets" actually put into practice by legal agents charged with enforcing the law (Percy, 1989). Case studies or other analyses of how health agencies organize their mission or perform in a given mission are a common form of implementation research (Buehler, Whitney, & Berkelman, 2006) and often look at the question of what legal powers an agency has or how it uses them (Lawson & Xu, 2007). Creative compliance and outright resistance on the part of targets of regulation are also studied (Nakkash & Lee, 2009). Implementation research in legal epidemiology includes studies of the relationship between "legal infrastructure," legal or other competencies, and agency function (Kimball et al., 2008). Such studies may examine effects of law on private agencies operating under a legal authorization, such as the effect of legal authorization on syringe exchange programs (Bluthenthal, Heinzerling, Anderson, Flynn, & Kral, 2007). Implementation researchers also measure proximate outcomes of new rules that may provide an early indication of health-relevant effects—for instance, the actual speeds observed on highways after a change in the nominal speed limit (Retting & Cheung, 2008). Implementation research also demands, and provides an opportunity for, investigating how facially neutral laws can have more or less dramatic inequitable effects (Brownson, Kumanyika, Kreuter, & Haire-Joshu, 2021).

Research on legal practices in legal epidemiology may investigate the means through which systems can be better governed or regulation better designed to achieve their goals. Although it has yet had little influence specifically on legal epidemiology, the study of techniques of regulation and governance has become an important part of broader empirical legal research and scholarship (Ayres & Braithwaite, 1995; Croley, 2008; Moran, 2002; Rhodes, 1997). For nearly three decades, regulation in the United States and many other developed countries has exhibited an increasing pluralism, not just in spreading of regulatory functions beyond government to private parties and public–private hybrids (Burris, Kempa, & Shearing, 2008; Lobel, 2004; Osborne & Gaebler, 1993) but also in the use of a wide range of strategies beyond detailed rules backed by carrots and sticks (Parker & Braithwaite, 2003). Contemporary regulators use cooperation, deliberation, education, competition, and other "soft" strategies that can be more effective than traditional command-and-control bureaucracy (Lobel, 2004). Theory and research in governance have highlighted the importance of actors outside of government—such as advocacy groups, corporations, and gangs—in managing the course of events in social systems and have investigated how these actors regulate governments and each other (Buse & Lee, 2005; Scott, 2002).

New regulatory and governance approaches have raised a fascinating range of empirical questions, from the role of audit as a compliance tool (Power, 1997) to the design and effectiveness of public–private and self-governing regulatory structures (Gunningham, 2009a; Ostrom, 2005). This work resonates with research in behavioral law and economics, captured in Sunstein and Thaler's book *Nudge*, which describes how regulators can creatively structure options to systematically influence behavior by means other than simple legal rules (Thaler & Sunstein, 2009).

Because so much regulation is now conducted outside of traditional bureaucratic frameworks (and indeed outside of the government), scholars working in this area begin with a generic definition of regulation and its constituent elements. *Regulation* is the "sustained and focused attempt to alter the behavior of others according to defined standards or purposes in order to address a collective issue or resolve a collective problem" (Black, 2008, p. 139). It uses a combination of basic strategies of control, including standard setting, monitoring, and enforcement (Scott, 2001). The use of these strategies can be studied regardless of the particular mode through which the regulatory task is accomplished and without regard to what sort of entity is performing it (Braithwaite & Drahos, 2000; Drahos, 2017). This analytic approach allows researchers both to better capture the regulatory role of actors outside of traditional regulatory agencies—for example, the role of Mothers Against Drunk Driving in fostering stronger social norms condemning drunk driving—and to offer more creative approaches to regulation, as exemplified by *Nudge* and other works in behavioral law and economics (Lobel & Amir, 2009).

Although research in regulation and governance has been limited (van der Heijden, 2019a, 2019b, 2020a, 2020b), its applicability to public health law is plain (Biradavolu, Burris, George, Jena, & Blankenship, 2009; Burris, 2008; Magnusson, 2009; Trubek, 2006). Public health services are provided by a diversity of public and private actors (Institute of Medicine, 2002). It is widely recognized that complex systems such as health care cannot be managed solely or even primarily by top-down rules but require use of a range of flexible tools, such as professional self-regulation, ethics, accreditation, collaborative and deliberative decision-making, continuous quality improvement, and market incentives (Berwick & Brennan, 1995; Braithwaite, Healy, & Dwan, 2005;

Lobel, 2004; Trubek, 2006). Internationally, health governance has been dramatically altered by the rise of new public–private hybrid institutions, such as the Global Fund to Fight AIDS, Tuberculosis, and Malaria; the enormous wealth of the Gates Foundation; and the consolidation of authority over national health, safety, and intellectual property law in the World Trade Organization (Hein, Burris, & Shearing, 2009; McCoy & Hilson, 2009). The Framework Convention on Tobacco Control is a typical instance of the "soft law" approach, setting broad goals for national action but minimizing binding rules in favor of deliberation and flexibility. Legal scholarship has explored the "constitutional" implications of these structural changes (Fidler, 2004), and legal epidemiologists have studied their impact (Hoffman et al., 2019).

Intervention Studies

Intervention studies evaluate the intended and incidental effects of legal interventions on health outcomes or key mediating factors that drive health outcomes. They may focus on "law on the books"—for example, examining the effect of states' passage of graduated driver's license statutes on rates of injury-causing crashes (Foss, Feaganes, & Rodgman, 2001)—or on legal practices, such as the effect of issuing restraining orders against perpetrators of domestic violence on future victimization (Harrell & Smith, 1996). Intervention studies can be deployed to evaluate interventional health law but also to investigate the health effects of public health's legal infrastructure and the unplanned effects of what we have called incidental public health law. Intervention studies lie at the heart of legal epidemiology, as they most directly address the core question of the field: When it comes to using legal tools to promote health, what works?

Intervention studies can draw from an extensive methodological toolkit (Table 1.1). The strongest are experimental or quasi-experimental designs employing careful controls and comparisons. These designs are discussed in two chapters in this volume (Chapters 13 and 14). Variation in how and when laws are implemented from jurisdiction to jurisdiction provides a rich set of opportunities for quasi-experimental studies, although sophisticated methods may be required to account for other ways in which jurisdictions differ from one another, and extensive longitudinal data are required. Useful study designs and analytical methods can be borrowed from the fields of econometrics and epidemiology (Abadie & Cattaneo, 2018; Ludwig & Cook, 2000). Real-world, randomized experiments are rare but have been employed to study judicial-branch reforms such as specialized courts (Gottfredson, Najaka, & Kearley, 2003). Experimental studies can also be carried out using simulations, such as tabletop exercises (Dausey, Buehler, & Lurie, 2007; Hodge, Lant, Arias, & Jehn, 2011; Hupert, Mushlin, & Callahan, 2002; Lurie et al., 2004).

There is already a substantial evidence base on the effectiveness of interventional public health law, ranging from single studies through literature reviews to meta-analyses and systematic reviews conducted by entities such as the Campbell Collaboration (2009) and the US Task Force on Community

Preventive Services (The Community Guide, 2009). There is also a rich, if less-well-organized, research literature on incidental public health law. For example, researchers have studied the unintended consequences of HIV reporting laws on attitudes toward testing, time of testing, and willingness to be tested (Hecht et al., 2000; Tesoriero et al., 2008) or the unintended effects of opioid supply reduction policies (Alpert, Powell, & Pacula, 2018; Powell & Pacula, 2021). Research on the health effects of infrastructural health law has been more limited.

Consistent with ecological models in public health, intervention studies may investigate how laws influence health by changing environments. For example, zoning rules, clean indoor air laws, and laws regulating the condition of rental properties can directly shape residents' exposures to noise, environmental toxins, and stress, as well as their activity patterns, social connections, collective efficacy, and many other factors that appear to influence population health outcomes (Browning & Cagney, 2002; Maantay, 2002; Schilling & Linton, 2005). Occupational health and safety laws affect workers' exposure to hazardous conditions on the job. Product regulations protect consumers from a range of hazards arising from the use of products, from herbal supplements to firearms (Larsen & Berry, 2003; Robson, 2007; Vernick & Teret, 2000).

Interventional research focuses not only on how the law changes physical environments but also on how it may change social environments in ways that affect health or health behaviors. Law may shape people's health knowledge and attitudes, the way they perceive risks and benefits of different choices, frames through which they view particular choices, and social norms against which their health decisions are set. Legal epidemiology can measure any or all of these dependent variables, as well as changes in health behaviors. There are many examples: research on the effects of indoor smoking prohibitions on social expectations about exposure to secondhand smoke in public (Kagan & Skolnick, 1993), the effect of laws requiring disclosure of calorie information on restaurant menus on consumers' awareness of calorie content and attitudes about the role of calorie information in food-purchasing decisions (Bassett et al., 2008), and the effect of punitive laws concerning substance abuse during pregnancy on the prenatal-care-seeking behavior of pregnant women (Faherty et al., 2019), to name a few.

Finally, intervention research can illuminate policy choices under conditions of uncertainty. When problems or policy responses are new, there, naturally, will be little or no intervention research directly on point. Policy making can still be informed by established theory on mechanisms of legal effects, understandings of how law typically works to influence environments and behaviors, and evidence about analogous policies, although all analogies are, of course, imperfect proxies for the situation at hand. An example is the area of legal restrictions on cell phone use by drivers (Ibrahim, Anderson, Burris, & Wagenaar, 2011). Although public health research recently has provided good evidence of the injury risk associated with this behavior, comprehensive evidence about the relative effectiveness of different legal and policy approaches to the problem is not yet available. Until it is, lawmakers seeking to respond to what is clearly a significant health risk might be guided by the lessons learned about the design and enforcement of laws requiring safety belt and helmet use and prohibiting driving under the influence of alcohol. Health impact assessment has also emerged as a useful way to use mixed methods to develop and inform policy decisions with reliable data on possible effects, intended and unintended (Collins & Koplan, 2009; Lee, Ingram, Lock, & McInnes, 2007; Mindell, Sheridan, Joffe, Samson-Barry, & Atkinson, 2004). Monte Carlo simulations, widely in use in the field of decision science but rarely used in legal epidemiology (Studdert, Mello, Gawande, Brennan, & Wang, 2007), offer an intriguing method for accounting for uncertainty about multiple parameters of importance to evaluating the likely effect of law. Economic evaluation that systematically explores the costs and benefits of policy options (or enacted policies) can and generally should influence policy choices. Methods for cost-effectiveness and cost-benefit studies of public health law are described in Chapter 16.

Mechanism Studies

To advance the field, we need to have not only more evidence of law's health effects but a greater understanding of *how* law has the effects it has. There are a number of reasons this is important. Evidence of mechanisms strengthens specific causal claims. Understanding how a particular intervention influences environments and behavior facilitates identification of further interventions, or of alternatives to eliminate superfluous requirements or unintended side effects and strengthen the mechanisms that are working. The better we understand how law works, the better we can deploy it, replicate its successes across jurisdictions, and extend its approach to other kinds of health risks. Informed by theories of health behavior, legal epidemiology can develop and test models to explain the manner in which public health law effects change in health behaviors and ultimately health outcomes.

At a simple level, laws encourage healthy, safe, and socially beneficial behaviors and discourage unhealthy, dangerous, and socially deleterious ones by shaping incentives (rewards) and deterrents (punishments). Though the theory may be simple, the process is not. There are myriad levers and tactics that regulators can use to influence behavior directly or through manipulation of the environment, and each choice in a regulatory system can and should be studied for its effectiveness, both in absolute terms and relative to less burdensome alternatives. The many mechanisms through which law exerts its influence are the focus of Part II of this volume.

With respect to laws imposing outright prohibitions on particular behaviors, many of the key research questions relate to mechanisms of implementation and enforcement: What penalties are applied to violators of legal rules? What processes are used to detect violators? With what degree of certainty and swiftness will sanctions ensue from a violation? Sociolegal research drawing on disciplines such as psychology, criminology, and sociology has a great deal to contribute to mechanism studies in legal epidemiology. The psychological literature has explored contingencies of reinforcement, criminologists have fleshed out the factors influencing deterrence, and sociological research has plumbed the normative effects of standard setting. Tom Tyler's influential work, for example, has shown the importance of experiences of procedural fairness to compliance with law (Tyler, 1990).

A classic example of compliance research in public health law is investigation of primary versus secondary enforcement of safety belt laws. Primary enforcement laws permit police to pull over motorists for not wearing a safety belt, while secondary enforcement laws permit police to issue a ticket for not wearing a belt only when the motorist has been pulled over for another reason. Because secondary enforcement relies primarily on social norms to enforce safety belt use, with the threat of a ticket serving a greatly subordinate role, studies comparing these approaches to enforcement are essentially a test of the relative effectiveness of punishment versus social norms as a means of encouraging compliance (Dinh-Zarr et al., 2001). Among the most interesting findings of this legal epidemiology is that the relative benefits of primary enforcement laws varied across population subgroups, with the greatest marginal benefit observed for groups that tend to have lower rates of safety belt use, including males, young people, African Americans, and American Indians (Beck, Shults, Mack, & Ryan, 2007).

These and other studies make clear that deterrence is a complex phenomenon. The deterrent effect of law often seems to be assumed, without appreciation of the factors that will influence whether a person's behavior will be influenced by a fear of detection or punishment. Threat of fines may have a different effect than threat of jail (Wagenaar, Maldonado-Molina, Erickson et al., 2007). Deterrence may be weak or incomplete because people are ill-informed about what the law requires, because they do not believe violation will result in a sanction, because they are insulated from the adverse effects of a sanction (for instance, by insurance coverage), or because the sanction is not strong enough to outweigh the perceived benefits of noncompliance with the law (Mello & Brennan, 2002). Uncertainty about legal standards can also have the opposite effect, fostering overcompliance in an attempt to avoid sanctions (Mello, Powlowski, Nañagas, & Bossert, 2006). Mechanism studies can examine all these phenomena. Survey methods, interviews, focus groups, and formal decision analysis can be used to deconstruct how people think through the costs and benefits of different actions. Analysis of administrative data on enforcement actions can shed light on the degree to which popular perceptions reflect what actually happens when a law is transgressed.

Another variable of interest in mechanism studies that focus on compliance with legal rules is the perceived legitimacy of the body imposing the legal rule. Weber classically tied obedience to law to the acceptance of the legitimacy of the system. Even people who are aware of the law may not trust the system or may see strategies other than compliance as more useful to them in achieving their goals (Burris, 1998b). Studies of the perceived legitimacy of public health lawmakers and law enforcers may be particularly useful in understanding differences in compliance across population groups whose historical experience in the United States has led to different levels of trust in government.

Mechanism studies may also focus on understanding how law shapes behavior in ways more subtle than outright prohibitions. How do regulatory tools such as taxes and subsidies, mandated disclosure or receipt of information, default rules, accreditation and certification, and delegations of authority to private institutions shape how individuals and organizations behave? When are these alternatives more effective and desirable than traditional, command-and-control regulation utilizing rigid rules and penalties? For many of these forms of regulation, understanding the cognitive biases and heuristics that affect individual decision-making about risk is critical (Kahnemann, Slovic, & Tversky, 1982) and empirical research can examine how these biases operate to influence compliance and health outcomes.

Mechanism studies are at the core of legal epidemiology because they explore the generic drivers of legal effect. In Chapter 13 Pollack and colleagues discuss a related type of study that is relevant to legal epidemiology even though no actual law is involved: experimental studies of "policy candidates." Such studies test the effects of interventions that, if effective, could be generalized via legislation or regulation. For example, researchers might evaluate the effectiveness of an educational intervention on underage drinking using a rigorous randomized controlled trial (RCT). If the intervention appears to be effective, the legislature might make it a required part of the high school curriculum. The RCT of the intervention would be research on a behavior, standard, or program that might be mandated by law, but would not in itself be a study of a policy or law. By contrast, research on the implementation of the law and the effectiveness of the intervention as a legal mandate would fall within the scope of legal epidemiology.

Legal epidemiology takes a number of forms, each utilizing diverse methods (Table 1.1). By illuminating the paths we have delineated in our causal model, these forms each play important roles in establishing how law is being deployed to promote population health, and how and to what extent it is achieving its intended purpose.

Conclusion

Lawyers have long proclaimed the maxim that "the health of the people is the supreme law," but in practice, making law work for public health is a constant challenge that requires a diverse set of disciplines and perspectives to achieve. Through policy-making studies, legal epidemiology can identify forces that shape public health policy and strategies for effecting policy change. Through mapping studies, it can measure what has been put into law and thus what kind of action it is possible for various government units to take. Through implementation studies, it can provide information about how best to ensure that "law on the books" becomes effective "law on the streets." Through intervention studies, it can determine which legal approaches are most efficacious in improving health environments, behaviors, and outcomes, and identify harmful side effects. Finally, through mechanism studies, it can tell us why laws have the effects they do and what mechanisms are at our disposal for improving the effectiveness of legal interventions addressing the entire range of public health concerns. Through the production of knowledge and conscientious efforts to translate research findings for decision makers, legal epidemiology can make the case for laws that improve health.

Summary

Legal epidemiology may be defined as the scientific study and deployment of law as a factor in population health. It encompasses policy making; mapping types and distributions of law across jurisdictions and over time, implementation; and effects of all these on physical and social environments, behaviors, and, ultimately, population health. Research on the content and prevalence of public health laws; processes of adopting and implementing laws; and the extent to which and mechanisms through which law affects health outcomes can be pursued using theory and methods drawn from epidemiology, economics, sociology, and other disciplines. Public health law research is a growing field that holds great promise for supporting evidence-based policy making that will improve population health.

Further Reading

Burris, S., Ashe, M., Blanke, D., Ibrahim, J., Levin, D. E., Matthews, G., ... Katz, M. (2016). Better health faster: The 5 essential public health law services. *Public Health Reports, 131*(6), 747–753.

Burris, S., Ashe, M., Levin, D., Penn, M., & Larkin, M. (2016). A transdisciplinary approach to public health law: The emerging practice of legal epidemiology. *Annual Review of Public Health, 37*(1), 135–148.

Drahos, P. (Ed.) (2017). *Regulatory theory: Foundations and applications*. Canberra, Australia: ANU Press.

Gostin, L. O., & Wiley, L. F. (2016). *Public health law: Power, duty, restraint* (3rd ed.). Berkeley, CA: University of California Press.

Moulton, A. D., Mercer, S. L., Popovic, T., et al. (2009). The scientific basis for law as a public health tool. *American Journal of Public Health, 99*(1), 17–24.

Note: This chapter is an updated version of the article "Making the case for laws that improve health: A framework for public health law research," published in *The Milbank Quarterly, 88*(2), 169–210. Used with permission.

Chapter 2

Law in Public Health Systems and Services Research

Scott Burris   Glen P. Mays   F. Douglas Scutchfield

Jennifer K. Ibrahim

Learning Objectives

- Differentiate public health law research from public health systems and services research.
- Identify key research questions at the intersection of the two fields.
- Assess quality and coverage of existing infrastructural public health law research.

The role of law in establishing, empowering, and constraining public health agencies has long been a matter of interest to legal scholars and health practitioners (Gostin, 2008; Gostin, Burris, & Lazzarini, 1999; Tobey, 1939). The importance of "legal infrastructure" to public health and the need to review and possibly update statutes that define the authority of health agencies at the federal, state, and local levels have now been emphasized in three major Institute of Medicine (IOM) reports since 1988 (Institute of Medicine, 1988, 2002, 2011). Other commentaries have identified "essential public health law services" (Burris, Ashe, Blanke et al., 2016) and stressed the importance of the public health workforce exhibiting competency in the use of legal authority and the appreciation of its boundaries (Center for Law and the Public's Health, 2001; Gebbie, Rosenstock, & Hernandez, 2003; Moulton, Gottfried, Goodman, Murphy, & Rawson, 2003). *Healthy People 2010's* chapter "Public Health Infrastructure" included as an objective "Increas[ing] the proportion of Federal, Tribal, State, and local jurisdictions that review and evaluate the extent to which their statutes, ordinances, and bylaws ensure the delivery

Legal Epidemiology: Theory and Methods, Second Edition. Edited by Alexander C. Wagenaar, Rosalie Liccardo Pacula, and Scott Burris.

of essential public health services" (Office of Disease Prevention and Health Promotion & US Department of Health and Human Services, 2010). *Healthy People 2020* likewise encouraged the use of public health law research and public health systems and services research to measure and understand improvements in public health system outcomes (Office of Disease Prevention and Health Promotion & US Department of Health and Human Services, 2011). While *Healthy People 2030* does not specifically address the intersection of public health law and public health systems (Office of Disease Prevention and Health Promotion & US Department of Health and Human Services, 2020), there is a focus on public health department accreditation and the use of core competencies for training the public health workforce, both of which have requirements related to public health law (Council on Linkages Between Academia and Public Health Practice, 2021).

The importance of law to the effective operation of public health agencies and systems, often and plausibly asserted, has infrequently been the subject of academic research or practice-based evaluations. While there has been a modest increase in research in this space over the last decade, most work examining the relationship between law and public health system performance has not been informed by an explicit, shared conceptual framework, or research agenda. The development of much-needed research and evaluation requires an intentional integration of legal epidemiology and public health systems and services research (PHSSR). In the wake of the COVID-19 pandemic, Supreme Court decisions and a high level of state legislative activity altering state and local public health authorities make this line of research an even more important field of study (Gostin, Parmet, & Rosenbaum, 2022; Network for Public Health Law, 2021).

PHSSR is a "field of study that examines the organization, financing, and delivery of public health services within communities and the impact of those services on public health" (Scutchfield & Patrick, 2007, p. 173; see also Mays, Halverson, & Scutchfield, 2004). Growing from the field of health services research, which focuses on the delivery and financing of medical care, PHSSR is concentrated on parallel concerns within the realm of public health service delivery (Scutchfield, Marks, Perez, & Mays, 2007). The 1998 Institute of Medicine report called for research focused on the solution of "real-world problems," including research questions actively derived from public health practice (Institute of Medicine, 1988). Both the 2002 Institute of Medicine report and *Healthy People 2010* noted the need for more research to inform policymaking, with a focus on workforce, infrastructure, and financial investments (Institute of Medicine, 2002), as well as better information on the performance and nature of local health departments (Office of Disease Prevention and Health Promotion & US Department of Health and Human Services, 2010). The federal Patient Protection and Affordable Care Act of 2010 (42. US Code § 300u-15) called attention to the need for PHSSR by authorizing an ongoing, federally funded program of research aimed at optimizing public health services delivery (Mays & Scutchfield, 2012). There is a more recent focus on accreditation and proper training of the workforce to strengthen public health infrastructure moving forward (Council on Linkages Between Academia and Public Health Practice, 2021; Office of Disease Prevention and Health Promotion & US Department of Health and Human Services, 2020).

The field of PHSSR focuses on six categories of investigation surrounding public health services: (1) organization and structure of public health agencies, (2) finance, (3) access to services for defined populations, (4) infrastructure and workforce, (5) quality and performance improvement, and (6) evaluation (Scutchfield, Mays, & Lurie, 2009). The causal model for research efforts in each domain considers the context in which a local public health department functions; its resources, processes, and services; and the health outcomes achieved. PHSSR recognizes that a health department operates within a larger system of agencies and organizations in communities that contribute to the mission of public health, "assuring conditions in which people can be healthy" (Institute of Medicine, 1988). PHSSR has begun to focus attention on the mechanisms through which public health agencies interact with and influence other system actors, including medical and social service providers, to assess their collective impact on health outcomes (Hamer and Mays 2020).

Across each of these areas, there is a range of legal considerations, including the authority to act or create policies, regulations on routine functions, and even agency composition. The perception of law and its utility among individuals within a health agency and other members of the public health system may have a powerful effect on the effective use of legal powers and tools. While such legal factors have been assumed or implicitly included in previous research, more research is needed to draw out these factors and carefully examine their role in public health systems and the delivery of public health services.

The framework offered in this chapter identifies three broad areas of inquiry at the intersection of PHSSR and legal epidemiology that deserve closer attention:

- The structural role of law in shaping the organization, powers, prerogatives, duties, and limitations of public health agencies, and thereby their functioning and ultimately their impact on public health ("infrastructure")

- How public health system characteristics influence the implementation of interventional public health laws ("implementation")

- Individual and system characteristics that influence the ability of public health systems and their community partners to develop and secure enactment of legal initiatives to advance public health ("innovation")

We present a causal diagram illustrating the main domains of interest, which is used to frame a critical discussion of research to date (Figure 2.1). Our analysis demonstrates opportunities for integrating legal epidemiology and PHSSR through common methods drawing upon both health services and empirical legal research traditions and points the way to a common research

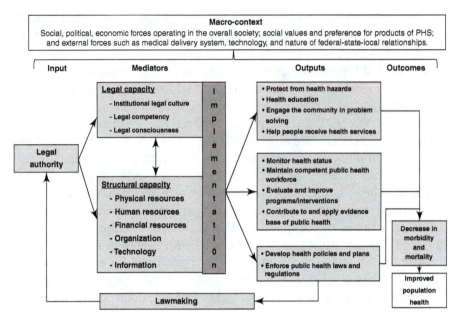

Figure 2.1. Effects of Law and Legal Practices on Public Health System Performance.

agenda. We conclude with examples of research addressing infrastructure, implementation, and innovation in this important area of health research.

Integrating Legal Epidemiology and PHSSR

PHSSR and legal epidemiology both had early support from the CDC (Burris, Cloud, & Penn, 2020; Horton et al., 2002; Scutchfield et al., 2007) and were nurtured by the Robert Wood Johnson Foundation (Larkin & McGowan, 2008; Pérez & Larkin, 2009; Scutchfield et al., 2009), but the two fields have nevertheless developed independently. Meeting at the intersection of law and public health services, PHSSR and legal epidemiology draw on different research traditions, theories, and perspectives. To address this challenge, we offer a causal diagram of the relationship among public health law, public health system characteristics, system outputs, and public health outcomes (see Chapter 10 for more on the utility of causal diagrams). We start with the input of law and move to the factors that mediate the performance of public health agencies, including legal culture and legal capacity, authority to act, structural capacity, and implementation of the law. Important outputs include a variety of regulatory and health activities and the development of new health policy tools (Figure 2.1). The main focus of the causal diagram is on the mechanism by which law and legal authority affect public health agencies and system performance. We also recognize that public health agencies operate within a larger context that includes social, political, and economic forces, as well as the system of medical care delivery. The following sections provide detailed explanations of each component of the model.

Law on the Books as a Structural Factor in Public Health System Performance

Is "legal infrastructure," the law that establishes the powers, duties, organization, and jurisdiction of public health agencies, a significant factor in agency performance? The hypothesis that legal infrastructure matters has been repeatedly stated (Gostin et al., 1999) and put into intervention practice in the form of widely circulated and adopted "model law" provisions (Hartsfield, Moulton, & McKie, 2007). The starting point in Figure 2.1 is, therefore, legal authority. Public health agencies are established by constitutions and laws that set their powers, geographic and topical jurisdiction, procedures, and management structures. Public health departments are organized on state, county, or local levels, or in a variety of combinations; they are established as stand-alone entities or as units within larger health and human services agencies (Beitsch, Brooks, Grigg, & Menachemi, 2006; Beitsch, Grigg, Menachemi, & Brooks, 2006). There may or may not be a board of health, and the powers of boards of health vary from giving advice when asked, to formal rulemaking to exercising emergency powers in times of crisis (National Association of Local Boards of Health, 2011). And not all agencies that regulate important public health matters such as education, transportation, and land use planning have "public health"—or even "health"—in their name (Institute of Medicine, 2011).

Although the federal government has used its authority to spend money, levy taxes, and regulate interstate commerce to become a powerful force in public health over the past century, the Constitution places the authority for core public health activities in the hands of the states (Grad, 2005). The heterogeneous legal architecture of public health systems across the states amounts to a long-term natural experiment in public health management, but one that has not been extensively evaluated. Even in recent textbooks, discussion of law in public health administration is limited to the functions of the agency in the context of the larger governmental bureaucracy (Novick, Morrow, & Mays, 2008), as opposed to a more thorough examination of the internal processes by which the law shapes public health agency performance.

Legal Implementation and Public Health System Performance

The exercise of legal authority—implementation—is mediated by two sets of variables in Figure 2.1: legal capacity and structural capacity. Health administration during the COVID-19 pandemic demonstrated, and empirical research over decades has documented, the decisive effect of implementation factors on how law on the books is expressed in practice (Nilsen, Ståhl, Roback, & Cairney, 2013; Parmet et al., 2021). The rich tradition in legal and policy implementation research has not been widely drawn upon in public health, nor has the newer field of implementation science turned its attention to infrastructural public health law. How actors in public health systems understand and apply the law, and the resources they have to do so, are likely to be powerful mediators of the effect of legal infrastructure on public health system outputs and outcomes (Bullock, Lavis, Wilson, Mulvale, & Miatello, 2021).

Perhaps the largest deficit in existing research on the role of law in public health agency performance is its thin conception of legal capacity. There is a small literature that defines "legal competencies" (Center for Law and the Public's Health, 2001; Gebbie et al., 2008; Lichtveld, Hodge, Gebbie, Thompson, & Loos, 2002). More recently, scholars have elaborated five essential public health law services, with the aim of making the range of necessary legal functions of public health professionals more explicit, measurable, and improvable (Burris, Ashe, Blanke et al., 2016). These services include developing policy concepts, putting them into effective legal form, getting laws enacted, implementing laws, tracking their diffusion, and evaluating their implementation and impact. Despite this progress, the field has not yet drawn on the theoretically richer sociolegal literature on "legal consciousness" and "legality" of individuals and organizations (Chapter 4). In this approach, the law is not treated simply as a "tool" or "rule" that agents wield or consciously or subconsciously obey, but also as a set of individual beliefs and organizational norms about what the legal system is, how it works, and whether and why people should obey its commands. It encompasses what people consciously believe about law but also a range of unconsciously accepted norms and assumptions. Sociolegal theory moves beyond how people "use law," or their explicit legal knowledge, allowing researchers to bring critical empirical attention to bear on how the rule of law is socially constructed, contested, and perpetuated in social fields (Cooper, 1995). At both the individual and the institutional levels, we cannot get a strong grasp on why the law is used to advance public health goals without understanding "when and by whom it is not used" (Silbey, 2005, p. 326). It is as important to study why some health departments avoid law as a tool as it is to identify the determinants of creative and effective regulatory behavior. The sociolegal literature provides powerful theoretical concepts and research methods for getting at how health system agents understand their legal roles and authority to implement laws, their ability to act within a legal framework, and indeed the nature of that legal framework itself (Yngvesson, 1988).

Both objective legal competency—explicit knowledge of the law and one's legal role—and the individual's ideas about law ("legal consciousness") are important determinants of an individual and agency's capacity to use legal authority effectively. Figure 2.1 illustrates that these can be understood both as individual-level attributes and as characteristics of an agency or other organizational unit, and that individual legal consciousness and competencies influence and are influenced by the institution's legal culture. The effect of law on organizations, particularly in terms of compliance, traditionally has been a core concern of empirical legal research and has produced a distinguished body of theory and evidence (Ayres & Braithwaite, 1995; Braithwaite & Drahos, 2000; Chriqui, O'Connor, & Chaloupka, 2011; Gunningham, 2009b; Power, 1997). Work on law in organizations has shown the value of understanding the construction of law at an organizational level and the processes through which legal decisions are made (Edelman & Suchman, 1997). Organizations are not simply passive recipients of outside legal commands but are actively engaged in interpreting and reshaping law to make it consistent with organizational imperatives, norms, and beliefs (Edelman, 2005; Teubner, 1987). Strategies of law enforcement and regulation are shaped by politics and even a version of fashion, not just evidence and experience (Power, 1997; Wood, 2004). Understanding the institutional culture and its determinants is essential to a proper assessment of the work of a regulatory agency.

This leads to the second set of mediating variables—the structural capacity of the health department and the public health system in which it operates. In the health services tradition, PHSSR posits that a set of basic structural capacities can be measured and assessed for their effect on the performance of public health systems (Bhandari, Scutchfield, Charnigo, Riddell, & Mays, 2010). These include human, physical, and financial resources; organization and relationships; agency information; and technology. From the capacity of agency leaders to use their legal authority to the implementation skills of front-line sanitarians, capacities mediated by resources and networks influence the implementation of the system's legally established mission (Anderson & Burris, Forthcoming). For example, environmental work such as inspection and citation are dependent on agency budgets, and as the budget drops, so does environmental work at the health department (Arnett, 2011). Similarly, routine disease surveillance and information sharing across departments or between public health agencies are contingent upon the organization and technology within the system (van Panhuis et al., 2014). Finally, the capacity of agency leaders also includes their leadership. It is not sufficient to just manage the resources of an agency, but it is critical to have a vision and lead, which includes maximizing the use of given legal authority among all members of the agency to advance the objectives of the agency (Fraser, Castrucci, & Harper, 2017; Kaufman et al., 2014).

Structural capacity interacts with legal capacity and the larger social context. If there are constraints in human or financial resources, there may not be time to think about law or funds available for public health staff to collaborate with legal counsel. If public health imperatives like mask-wearing or vaccination become politicized, health officers may be deterred or even legally barred from issuing mandates. If self-regulation and small government are the current fashion, advancing new command-and-control rules enforced by a bureaucracy will be difficult. Health departments *are* bureaucratic regulatory agencies. They operate within a larger administrative system and may be constrained by competition for rewards or resources, or jurisdictional confusion. Authority may be conferred to other departments or divisions within the bureaucracy (for example, environmental, public safety, or transportation) or the authority to act may be shared. Sharing health surveillance data is a good example of the interaction between structural and legal authority, because while a health department may have the technological abilities to share information if the staff are not aware of limits or powers granted under privacy laws, they may not share data in practice (van Panhuis et al., 2014).

Public Health System Outputs and Outcomes

Figure 2.1 depicts the outputs of the public health system as 10 essential public health services. This typology is now at the center of efforts within PHSSR to develop robust measures of public health agency performance. Their origin is the 1988 IOM report (Institute of Medicine, 1988), which defined public health governmental responsibility as assessment, policy development, and assurance. These were seen as specifically governmental activities to be carried out by governmental public health agencies in partnership with other organizations that contribute to public health. The IOM report called attention to the unique roles played by governmental public health agencies in mobilizing, coordinating, and monitoring the contributions of other organizations that operate within the larger public health system. Later work elaborated those 3 governmental responsibilities into the 10 essential public health services shown in the figure. The 10 essential public health services have become a touchstone for public health activities involving performance and drafting public-health-related documents describing the role of local health departments and their system partners (Erwin, 2008). Updated in 2020, the revised version of the 10 essential services integrates equity as a central tenant in the work of health departments (Public Health National Center for Innovation & Public Health Accreditation Board, 2020). There have also been proposals to expand the two services related to policy development and policy enforcement (Public Health National Center for Innovation & Public Health Accreditation Board, 2020) by defining five essential public health services, including access to evidence and expertise, designing legal solutions, collaboration with communities to build political will, support for enforcing and defending against legal challenges, and surveillance and evaluation of policies.

Work with the 3 core responsibilities and the 10 essential public health services derived from them has led to a new understanding of the mechanisms by which public health infrastructure and inputs influence performance. For example, the services have been used to develop an evidence-based typology of local public health systems that allows classification and comparison of systems according to the scope of public health activities performed, the array of organizations involved in performing these activities, and the distribution of effort between the governmental public health agency and other system partners (Mays, Scutchfield, Bhandari, & Smith, 2010). The instruments developed by the National Public Health Performance Standards Program have become vital to the establishment of the Public Health Accreditation Board, which began its initial accreditation efforts in the fall of 2011 (Martin et al., 2010; Mays, Beitsch, Corso, Chang, & Brewer, 2007; Public Health Accreditation Board, 2009).

Public Health Policy Innovation

Health policy is an important *output* as well as an input for public health systems (Anderson & Burris, 2014). The practice, experience, and knowledge acquired by actors within the public health system can drive the development of new public health laws, regulations, and enforcement strategies to improve system performance and public health outcomes. Health agencies often have substantial regulatory authority themselves and can partner with other stakeholders to advance legislative and regulatory initiatives before other policy-making bodies and, in some instances, be involved in litigation. The extent to which individual staff and particular health agencies have an appetite for understanding and using the law, and under what circumstances this occurs, is a gap in the existing literature on policy innovation within health departments.

Existing Research

Research related to incidental and interventional legal epidemiology has answered important questions of legal effect in several health domains, but there are few studies addressing infrastructural legal questions (Burris & Anderson, 2013; Hyde & Shortell, 2012). Such research as has been carried out at the intersection of PHSSR and legal epidemiology has to date clustered in the lower reaches of the evidence hierarchy (Harris, Helfand, & Woolf, 2001). Research at the intersection of PHSSR and legal epidemiology has also to date clustered in the lower reaches of this hierarchy. In this respect, the intersection of PHSSR and legal epidemiology is consistent with other areas of empirical health law (Mello & Zeiler, 2008). While the conceptual connections between PHSSR and legal epidemiology are apparent when one looks for them, the research has not fully engaged both disciplines. The limited literature offers instances of ambitious design and rigorous execution, but also weaknesses. Law, in general, is insufficiently theorized or measured, or a thorough legal analysis is used in a study that does not adequately account for the influence of the public health department or system's organizational characteristics (Bullock et al., 2021). Strong qualitative findings are not followed up with quantitative research that could yield generalizable results. We will draw on examples from the existing literature addressing infrastructural law in PHSSR to illustrate these weaknesses and suggest topical and methodological directions for integrating the two fields.

Infrastructure Research

The important implications for the practice of rigorous infrastructural research at the intersection of legal epidemiology and PHSSR can be seen in studies that have taken on one of the most widely held assumptions in public health law. For quite some time, influential scholars in public health law have pointed to antiquated or technologically superannuated statutes as a barrier to effective public health agency performance (Gostin et al., 1999). The work in PHSSR to develop measures of public health system performance makes it possible now to investigate that issue empirically, and a few studies have attempted to do so. McCann (2009), for example, examined the core question of how the type and extent of discretion granted by a statute to a public health agency influenced the agency's success in implementing the statute. Using a quasi-experimental time-series design, the study defined three forms of discretion in setting standards for newborn screening: to decide which conditions to include in the screening panel; to set the charges assessed on hospitals, and to develop the criteria for including conditions in the panel. The study tested the hypothesis that each of these forms of discretion would be associated with fewer implementation problems. Fiscal discretion and authority to choose what conditions to include were associated with successful implementation, while, interestingly, the discretion to set criteria slowed implementation. The study, as the author puts it, "only scratches the surface of public health law's importance for public health practice" (McCann, 2009). Discretion is well theorized and has a robust impact, but the contradictory findings suggest that key mediating factors are missing from the theoretical framework.

One widely promoted cure for laws that are out of date or inconsistent with best practices has been the "model law." Model laws are intended to set out clearer requirements in keeping with current technologies, health practices, and legal norms (Erickson, Gostin, Street, & Mills, 2002). Hartsfield et al. (2007) asked a deceptively simple question: To what extent did the sponsors of model laws provide information on the procedures—and the evidence—used to develop them? Such information was, it turned out, provided for only 7 of 107 model public health laws published between 1907 and 2004. Model laws can embody evidence-based best practices, but there is no evidence that they do. Simple in design and narrow in scope, the study illustrates valuable insights that can be gleaned from systematic legal research and straightforward content analysis.

Using performance data from the National Public Health Performance Standards (Centers for Disease Control and Prevention, 2011a), Merrill and colleagues examined the congruence among state enabling statutes, the mission and essential services of public health as defined in *Public Health in America* (Public Health Functions Steering Committee Office of Disease Prevention and Health Promotion, 1994), and self-reported delivery of at least some essential services in 207 localities (Merrill, Keeling, Meier, Gebbie, & Jia, 2009). The data in this cross-sectional, observational study were analyzed using binary logistic regression. In most local public health systems, the agency mission and essential services were rated congruent or highly congruent with the state statutory language constituting the agencies' legal infrastructure. The association between congruence and agency performance varied from positive to negative across the ten essential services. As the authors themselves observe, the challenge for future research is to integrate legal variables with the wider range of structural capacity and other factors depicted in Figure 2.1 in a design that will support causal inference.

Jacobson et al. (2012) investigated how federal and state laws influence the preparedness of public health systems as reflected in the knowledge and attitudes of 144 agency staff, their legal counselors, and legislative staffers in nine states. Explicit criteria were used to select sites that varied by key characteristics (per capita health expenditure, geographic region, organization of the public health system, and level of emergency preparedness). Semi-structured interviews were used to elicit which laws respondents thought were influencing preparedness and how. Although the study did not explicitly deploy sociolegal theories of individual or organizational legal consciousness, the researchers took it as given that there are "gaps between the objective and perceived legal environments" (Jacobson, Wasserman, Botoseneanu, Silverstein, & Wu, 2012, p. 299), and that much of the explanation of how law influences preparedness would be found in such gaps. The study found that local public health agency practitioners are ill-informed and poorly advised about legal requirements influencing preparedness. Though not statistically generalizable, the study is richly informative of the kinds of legal conundrums health officials worry about, how they try to resolve them, and the types of effects law has on preparedness. The study exemplifies the potential for qualitative research to address important questions in rigorous ways—and the need for follow-up quantitative research to investigate specific hypotheses emerging from a qualitative study.

A comprehensive review of state laws that grant legal authority for injury prevention practice in state health departments was conducted in 2012 (Stier, Thombley, Kohn, & Jesada, 2012). The authors collected the laws in the 50 states governing injury surveillance and prevention between March 2007 and April 2008. The result was a table of states listing the scope of legal authority to act related to specific locations (workplace, public place, healthcare facility, motor vehicle, etc.) and injury type (brain, spinal cord, dental, motor-vehicle, violence-related, etc.). The benefit is the exploration of the authority for state health agencies to act. The limitation is that the study was cross-sectional and resulted in a table rather than an empirical legal data set that could be linked with injury-related data to evaluate the effects of these laws governing the agencies' ability to act.

A similar study examining legal authority for reporting infectious disease was conducted in 2011–2012 following the 2009 H1N1 pandemic (Danila et al., 2015). Using mixed methods, the team collected the text of the laws in place in the 50 states, Washington, DC, and New York City at the time of the H1N1 pandemic. The laws were coded for key features such as the type of disease to be reported, who was required to do the reporting, inclusion of suspected or only confirmed cases, and requirements for biological materials to be submitted to a public health laboratory; a subscale was created for similar variables but with a specific focus on influenza only. Beyond examining the laws, the team surveyed epidemiologists or key informants in each jurisdiction to understand the obstacles to collecting and using data on influenza, and semi-structured telephone interviews with a subset of survey respondents regarding their perceptions of how the reporting laws functioned during the H1N1 pandemic. The team found that while laws did exist and respondents were aware of the laws, they were not robust enough. For example, 38% of agencies did not have the legal authority to immediately require reporting of a new disease without going through the formal rulemaking process (Danila et al., 2015).

More recently, in 2017, Shah and colleagues created a taxonomy to describe local health departments based on a model composed of six domains, including policy development, resource stewardship, legal authority, partner engagement, continuous improvement, and oversight (Shah, Sotnikov, Leep, Ye, & Van Wave, 2017). Using data from the 2015 survey of local boards of health, the research team created an index scale to document the responsibilities and functions of each health department. The study did not only measure what the local boards of health did but measured the legal authority of the board to act, thereby creating a framework in which to evaluate performance and the gaps between what can be done within their legal authority and what has been done. A similar study was conducted in 2020 using data from the 2016 National Profile of Local Health Departments survey to examine factors contributing to engagement in obesity policymaking (Feng & Martin, 2020). Feng and Martin found that higher levels of obesity-related policymaking were associated with local boards of health having advisory and governance roles, larger workforces, accreditation, higher obesity rates, and being more politically liberal. They did not explore legal authority or access to counsel, and the study was a cross-sectional study, thereby limiting the ability to speak to causation. Despite limitations, these are examples of research that can easily be modified to better evaluate the effect of infrastructure on policymaking.

One of the major challenges to pursuing work at the intersection of PHSSR and legal epidemiology is data. The collection of legal data using standardized transparent and reproducible methods required by science is relatively rare, especially at the local level. McCann's (2009) study included the collection of data on newborn screening statutes in all 50 states over a period of 16 years. And Meier, Merrill, & Gebbie (2009) collected basic public health enabling statutes from all the states. In neither case, however, was there a detailed description of the legal data set or how it was created information on whether inter-coder reliability was assessed or any indication that the data are available to other researchers to build upon. Methods, tools, and recognition of scientific legal mapping and policy surveillance have improved (see Chapters 11 and 12), but the number of sub-state jurisdictions and difficulties in accessing local law mean that creating systematic open-source legal data capturing local health authority remains a challenge (Sanner, Grant, Walter-McCabe, & Silverman, 2021) to what would be an indispensable tool: a comprehensive, consistent, continually updated data set on infrastructural public health law.

Implementation and Enforcement Research

McCann examined the association between discretion and outcomes, but did not study the process of implementation itself, work that perhaps would have helped explain why discretion appears to have varying effects on outputs. Merrill and colleagues found associations between statutory language that matched public health mission and service standards and the delivery of services but likewise did not examine the processes through which that occurred. Moreover, they used a research design that could not illuminate whether more expansive statutes produce higher-functioning agencies or higher-functioning agencies earn more expansive powers. The study of how legal authority or other legal factors influence the day-to-day practices of health agencies is in its infancy. There are, as far as we know, no studies other than that of Jacobson et al. (2012) that observe and assess the actual day-to-day exercise of general legal authority within health agencies, let alone any that draw upon (and test) the elements posited as important in Figure 2.1.

Evaluations of particular interventional health laws are the most fully developed topic area of legal epidemiology. The depth of the literature is captured in reviews of such important interventions as safety belt laws (Houston & Richardson, 2005), alcohol taxes (Wagenaar, Tobler, & Komro, 2010), workplace smoking bans (Fichtenberg & Glantz, 2002), and school vaccination requirements (Briss et al., 2000). Some evaluations of interventional health laws include data on implementation, but by no means do all. Few studies consider in-depth the effect of health department activities or health system characteristics on implementation. An exception is the rich body of qualitative work that has looked at how power, values, and politics have played out in the enforcement by health and other agencies of smoking restrictions (Ashley, Northrup, & Ferrence, 1998; Howard, Ribisl, Howard-Pitney, Norman, & Rohrbach, 2001; Montini & Bero, 2008).

An excellent example of research on tobacco law implementation is Jacobson and Wasserman's (1999) report of case studies in 7 states and 19 local jurisdictions. They found a sharp divergence in enforcement practice between clean indoor air laws and youth access restrictions. The former was seen by health officials as largely self-enforcing, so most agencies only acted when there was a complaint. Laws that restrict youth access to tobacco, by contrast, were deemed by most agencies to require more active enforcement, though strategies and intensity varied. The authors identified several legal and structural capacity issues retarding enforcement, including lack of resources, concerns on the part of counsel that enforcement would not withstand legal challenge, and fragmented enforcement authority. Moreover, the mere threat of litigation connects back to legal consciousness and institutional legal culture and the question of whether and under what circumstances a health department will engage in work despite the threat of litigation (Bialous, Fox, & Glantz, 2001; Ibrahim & Glantz, 2006). This work illustrates the practical value of research illuminating determinants of effective enforcement. Like McCann's work, though, it offers only tantalizing glimpses of topics that could use much greater systematic attention, such as the nature and quality of the relationship between health officials and their legal advisers, or the gap between counsel's beliefs about litigation success and the actual outcomes (Nixon, Mahmoud, & Glantz, 2004). Like the preparedness work of Jacobson and colleagues, the Jacobson and Wasserman tobacco law implementation case studies invite follow-on confirmatory quantitative research.

Research on Innovation in Policy Making

Preemption of local health authority has been recognized as a major political issue with measurable population health effects (Pomeranz, Zellers, Bare, Sullivan, & Pertschuk, 2019; Wolf, Monnat, & Montez, 2021). Nevertheless, the role of state and local health agencies in the development of and advocacy for new health laws is another area in which there is a high level of interest and a low level of research. Again, the exception has to be made for anti-smoking policymaking, which has been the subject of many useful case studies that identify strategies and mediating factors influencing the success of health agencies in promoting new health laws (Dearlove & Glantz, 2002; Givel, 2005; Ibrahim, Tsoukalas, & Glantz, 2004; Macdonald & Glantz, 1997; Tsoukalas & Glantz, 2003). The HIV epidemic also produced some strong policy-making research, perhaps most notably the work of political scientist Ronald Bayer (1989). The ongoing political fight over local health authority, and the intense interest in public health law arising from COVID-19, may produce a burst of new empirical research over the next few years.

Putting aside their value as embodiments of best practices, model laws have received attention as a mechanism to "galvanize" lawmaker interest in public health. To test this effect, Meier and colleagues undertook a comparative case study of the process and impact of considering the Turning Point Model Public Health Act in four states (Meier, Hodge, & Gebbie, 2009). The Turning Point model law embodied a comprehensive set of recommendations regarding agency mission and function, infrastructure, collaborations and partnerships, and authorities and powers. The study conceptualized the use of the model law in three stages—use of the act to develop or focus support for reform, drafting of actual state legislation, and enactment—and identified barriers and facilitators at each stage. In two of the states, the model law process did in itself help set the agenda for change; in a third, it failed to generate momentum to the second stage, while in the fourth the model law added some impetus to reform efforts that were already underway. The study's careful, qualitative research gives us insight into questions no one has tried to answer before. The next step is to build on the formative findings in more robust, generalizable studies. It will be useful to take a broader view of health policymaking and its determinants, for example looking for patterns in the breadth of health issues states choose to regulate and the depth or intensity of their regulations on particular topics.

Policy development outside of legislatures—litigation, administrative rule-making, executive orders, and enforcement strategies—has been almost entirely neglected except for recent work examining policy responses to the COVID-19 pandemic. The public health work of attorneys general, which has led to such important results as the 1998 Master Settlement Agreement for tobacco, has not been studied by PHSSR or legal epidemiology researchers (Jacobson & Wasserman, 1999; Rutkow & Teret, 2010). What Kromm et al. (2009) call "public health advocacy in the courts" encompasses a wide range of "actions by public health professionals that inform and affect how courts approach matters that affect the public's health" (p. 889). These include not only filing suits but also providing expertise as witnesses, submitting amicus briefs, educating the judiciary, influencing the judicial selection, and monitoring and evaluating court outcomes. The production of administrative law, arguably the most important vehicle for regulation under the control of public health agencies

(Kinney, 2002), has likewise not been touched by empirical research in legal epidemiology or PHSSR. Recent COVID-19 research has focused primarily on the health and economic affects attributable to the adoption of state and local public health emergency policies by executive order, including shelter-in-place orders (Agrawal, Cantor, Sood, & Whaley, 2021), indoor dining restrictions (Schnake-Mahl et al., 2022), and masking requirements (Huang et al., 2022).

Conclusion

There can be no disputing that law is an important force at work in public health systems and that it requires the same careful study and attention as other drivers of public health agency characteristics, performance, and outcomes. Integration of legal epidemiology and PHSSR is essential because law, for all its importance, is a force that works in interaction with other factors—resources, training, community values—and the effects of law are likely to vary over time, topic, and place.

More and better research is needed—but research remains a means, not the end. Law has enormous potential to improve the delivery of public health services, in terms of both effectiveness and efficiency. In the face of demands for austerity, resistance to a "nanny state," and continuing ideological attacks on the effectiveness of government regulation of any kind, policymakers, and public health practitioners must be able to demonstrate what they are doing works and works cost-effectively. Reorganization of health departments, redrafting of enabling statutes, accreditation, and the development of new legal health interventions have no inherent value: they are justified by results. And so, it should be. PHSSR and legal epidemiology must work in partnership with practice to wisely use, credibly justify, and (in so doing) properly increase public funding and political support for further improvements in the health of the population.

Further Reading

Hyde, J. K., & Shortell, S. M. (2012). The structure and organization of local and state public health agencies in the U.S.: A systematic review. *American Journal of Preventive Medicine, 42*(5 Suppl. 1), S29–S41.

Institute of Medicine (2011). *For the public's health: Revitalizing law and policy to meet new challenges*. Washington, DC: The National Academies Press.

Silbey, S. S. (2005). After legal consciousness. *Annual Review of Law and Social Science, 1*(1), 323–368.

Note: This chapter is an amended version of the article "Moving from intersection to integration: Public health law research and public health systems and services research," published in *The Milbank Quarterly, 90*(2), 375–408. Used with permission.

Part Two

Understanding How Law Influences Environments and Behavior

Many evaluations of public health laws proceed without articulating a theory on how the law is expected to affect health. While such "black box" studies directly assessing the correlation between existence of a particular law and a health outcome often make useful contributions, both the quality of a study and causal inference are substantially enhanced by a clear articulation of *how* a particular law is expected to have an effect on health. Hypothesized mechanisms of legal effect directly influence many processes and decisions of the study. The investigator's theory of how a law affects health (1) shapes selection of specific statutes, regulations, or court cases to study and indicates which are similar enough to group together and which are so distinct as to represent a different type of law; (2) determines which specific provisions in a law are relevant and which may be ignored; (3) determines how to code and score dimensions of the law; (4) points to key measures of implementation that are most relevant; (5) suggests specific features of the physical, organizational, and social environment to observe for reactions to the law; (6) indicates high-priority response behaviors for measurement in

Legal Epidemiology: Theory and Methods, Second Edition. Edited by Alexander C. Wagenaar, Rosalie Liccardo Pacula, and Scott Burris.
© 2023 John Wiley & Sons, Inc. Published 2023 by John Wiley & Sons, Inc.

the population exposed to the law; and (7) affects specific health outcome variables to collect and analyze. Theory on how a law affects population health points to the expected timing, patterns, and diffusion of its effects, directly shaping decisions on the best research design to use. Theory helps the investigators understand the number and types of intermediate steps that must occur before an effect on health outcomes is expected. It shapes the statistical models analyzed by presenting hypothesized distributions of effects across groups, time, and space. The ability to identify plausible mechanisms through which a law might produce an effect is helpful in assessing causal claims and identifying practical steps to enhance implementation and effectiveness. The maxim "there is nothing so practical as a good theory" (Lewin, 1952, p. 169) holds for legal epidemiology as for all areas of scientific inquiry.

Part Two discusses the many mechanisms through which law works to affect the public's health. The diversity and breadth of possible ways law can operate to affect population health are exciting, and illustrate the many opportunities available for important research waiting to be conducted. The chapters that follow suggest hundreds of specific causal paths or links between law and health, links that warrant study across the whole range of contemporary public health problems. In this section, we are focused on theory, not in the "legal theory" sense in which the objective is to articulate how a given law might apply to a particular case, but scientific theory, in which the objective is to specify chains and systems of causal links that are supported by a body of scientific research. The theories and perspectives come from many disciplines and fields of scholarship, but all are highly relevant for legal epidemiology. A law can have multiple routes of effect, and understanding the whole range of mechanisms and how they operate in particular contexts is necessary to maximize beneficial public health effects while minimizing deleterious ones. Many theories overlap, with similar underlying mechanisms of action described using quite different terms across disciplines. Other times, differing terms suggest subtle but important differences in understanding how a law works to affect health. Taken together, they provide a rich menu of theoretical options and practical tools for the public health law researcher.

The section starts with Komro and Wagenaar presenting perspectives from the field of public health. Public health traditionally focuses on the production of health and illness through the interaction of behavior and environment, each of which can be manipulated to produce healthier outcomes. Major achievements in public health over the past century used law to dramatically reduce the burden of infectious diseases, motor vehicle injuries, dental caries, and chronic disease. Chapter 3 includes discussion of ways in which law affects the fundamental social determinants of health, a pressing issue for public health in the twenty-first century.

The public health perspective emphasizes explaining law's links to health outcomes in the population—what law "does" to influence pathways to health and disease. What law "means" is also important to health, as explained in Stryker's chapter about how scholars in the law and society tradition approach the question of how law affects health. In Chapter 4, she offers a view of law as more than just specific rules regulating particular behaviors; law also works by shaping culture and shared meanings in a society, with important consequences for population health. Thus, perhaps pollution laws reduce exposure to toxic chemicals, but also over time create the notion of a human right to clean air and water not subject to the vagaries and uncertainties of the market.

Jennings and Mieczkowski review key concepts from the field of criminology in Chapter 5, describing how laws deter unhealthy or unsafe behaviors and how law's role in labeling particular individuals or groups as dangerous can affect their behavior. Tyler and Mentovich, presenting procedural justice theory in Chapter 6, draw on research emerging from social psychology to suggest that deterrence is not always the best way to explain obedience to law. They describe how the public's perception of a law as legitimate, and the perceived fairness of procedures attendant to its implementation, have powerful effects on people's willingness to comply. Together the chapters highlight how complex a phenomenon obedience to law actually is and how important it is for government agents to be consistent, fair, and effective in their enforcement efforts.

Chaloupka and Pacula describe in Chapter 7 how economic theory applies to public health law research, beginning with the assumption of a rational individual maximizing their own well-being, and analyzing the need for and use of law in relation to the concept of market failure. Schure, Islam, and Flay follow in Chapter 8, building from a base in social psychology to present an ambitious theory that integrates concepts from many social science disciplines. The theory of triadic influence facilitates a coherent understanding of many ways laws operate to affect population health. Part Two concludes with Burris and Wagenaar drawing together the ideas from all these perspectives and illustrating how readily they can be applied to specific public health issues.

Careful attention to testing particular theory-based mechanisms of legal effect advances the field of legal epidemiology as well as science more broadly. When we not only demonstrate through carefully designed scientific research that a particular law affected a particular population health outcome, but in addition discover the causal pathways by which that effect was achieved, we create more general knowledge that can be applied to ameliorating the entire range of public health problems. We are also then effectively using the real-world laboratory of public health law across local, state, and national levels to contribute improved theory back to the basic science disciplines from which we draw.

Chapter 3

Perspectives from Public Health

Kelli A. Komro   Alexander C. Wagenaar

Learning Objectives

- Identify the central processes through which law can influence population health outcomes from a public health perspective.
- Illustrate the influence of law on economic, social, and physical environments, and, in turn, effects on population-level risks and protections.
- Formulate study hypotheses on specific causal pathways by which law affects population health outcomes.

The advent of public health as a discipline can be traced back to the late eighteenth century, when the first organized attempts were made to confront disease collectively. With the rise of industrialism and globalization, people shifted to urban centers and seaports, producing dense populations living and working in unsanitary conditions ideal for spreading infectious diseases. As incidences of typhoid, smallpox, influenza, cholera, tuberculosis, and other diseases reached unacceptable levels, the first boards of health were formed in urban centers to respond to the epidemics (McNeill, 1977). The formation of boards of health illustrated the start of infrastructural public health law, and their actions in quarantining ill persons illustrate early use of police powers on behalf of public health. Right from the start, law was central to public health action.

Public health pioneer John Snow implemented corrective environmental actions long before science determined that microorganisms were the causes of widespread infectious diseases. In 1854, Snow traced a cholera outbreak in London to well water drawn from the Broad Street pump. By simply removing

Legal Epidemiology: Theory and Methods, Second Edition. Edited by Alexander C. Wagenaar, Rosalie Liccardo Pacula, and Scott Burris.

the pump handle, he prevented perhaps thousands of additional cases (Brody, Rip, Vinten-Johansen, Paneth, & Rachman, 2000). Snow's action illustrates the practical orientation of the field—preventive action need not wait until all the detailed mechanisms and mediators are understood. More important, Snow's action illustrates the simplicity and effectiveness of changing the physical environment to improve the public's health, in contrast to attempts to change the behavior of thousands or millions of individuals, in the cholera case by boiling water thoroughly every time before drinking.

During the twentieth century, major public health achievements were realized through law. Vaccination laws resulted in the control of many preventable diseases, including smallpox and polio. Smallpox and polio were eliminated, and morbidity associated with seven other vaccine-preventable diseases reduced by nearly 100% (Centers for Disease Control and Prevention, 1999b). Annual death rates per vehicle miles traveled declined 90% as a result of mandated improvements in vehicle and road design and laws shaping driver behavior, such as safety belt use and drinking and driving (Centers for Disease Control and Prevention, 1999c).

As public health, safety, and medical breakthroughs of the early- to mid-twentieth century controlled infectious disease epidemics, increased safety, and expanded life expectancy (Centers for Disease Control and Prevention, 1999e), public health shifted attention to chronic disease prevention (Omran, 1971). Epidemiological studies of chronic disease showed that most cases in the population do not occur among those at high risk but rather among those at moderate risk, because there are more people with moderate risk levels than there are with very high risk levels (Epstein, 1996; Rose, 1985). Recognition of the widespread distribution of risk might have led to a return to addressing the environmental and social conditions that elevated risks in so much of the population, but in the second half of the twentieth century, chronic disease prevention efforts focused primarily on individual-level strategies designed to alter specific risk factors that are proximal causes of disease, such as education, screening, and use of antihypertensive and lipid-lowering drugs (Centers for Disease Control and Prevention, 1999a). In the late twentieth century, population-level strategies using law to prevent chronic diseases emerged, with particularly notable achievements in tobacco control (Centers for Disease Control and Prevention, 1999d, 2011b).

A limitation of the focus on proximal risk factors is the de-emphasis of "fundamental," structural or antecedent determinants of population health (such as broader political and economic conditions and one's social class position in society) that influence multiple proximal risks and maintain an association with disease even when specific proximal risks change (Link & Phelan, 1995; Solar & Irwin, 2010). Although an intervention may temporarily reduce proximal risk factors for those individuals exposed to a particular intervention (for example health education, screening), populations continue to be at-risk if the intervention fails to intervene on forces in society and communities that cause the problems in the first place (Solar & Irwin, 2010; Syme, 2004).

The field of social epidemiology (Berkman & Kawachi, 2000) and the growing recognition of "social determinants of health" (Marmot, 2005;

Solar & Irwin, 2010), structural racism (Pérez-Stable & Webb Hooper, 2021; Yearby & Mohapatra, 2020), and "structural interventions" (Blackenship, Friedman, Dworkin, & Mantell, 2006; Brown et al., 2019) signify that public health increasingly is returning to its classic emphasis on environmental and social conditions. Structural racism, income inequality, the climate crisis, and emerging infectious diseases/pathogens (e.g. the COVID-19 pandemic) lay bare the importance of structural determinants of health, and law as a fundamental tool to promote health and prevent ill health and loss of life (Atwoli et al., 2021; Komro, 2020; Perez-Stable & Webb Hooper, 2021; Siegler, Komro, & Wagenaar, 2020; Yearby & Mohapatra, 2020). Because law is such an important influence on environmental and social conditions, a return to classic public health action is also elevating empirical research on law's public health effects as an increasingly recognizable and critical field of study.

How Laws Affect Population Health

Figure 3.1, showing the Legal Determinants of Population Health Model, illustrates the central processes through which law can influence population health outcomes from a public health perspective. The causal diagram highlights the central public health focus on altering the economic, social, and physical environments in ways that reduce toxic exposures and increase protective opportunities, and ways that facilitate healthy behaviors and impede unhealthy behaviors. These many dimensions of the environment drive exposures, opportunities, and behaviors that, moderated by individual-level factors, ultimately affect aggregate levels of population health.

Law shapes environmental conditions through its effects on institutions, organizations, and other implementation structures and processes. Obviously, law can also have direct effects on individual behavior, as illustrated in the many other chapters in this volume. This chapter highlights the centrality of enhancing environmental conditions as a key role for law in improving population health. For simplicity, the many possible interactions across dimensions of environmental conditions, and the cybernetic nature of this causal system, are not depicted. Our goal is much more modest than a complete depiction of how law affects health. Because history shows most public health gains have been achieved by altering environments, we highlight the central role of law in shaping environmental conditions. Following a description of the conceptual framework, we present three detailed examples.

Law

Law affects the full range of institutions, organizations, and structures in society, and the resulting characteristics and actions of those organizations and structures affect the economic, social, and physical environments that the population experiences. Law shapes families, schools, churches, community organizations, businesses, and corporations. By affecting actions within such

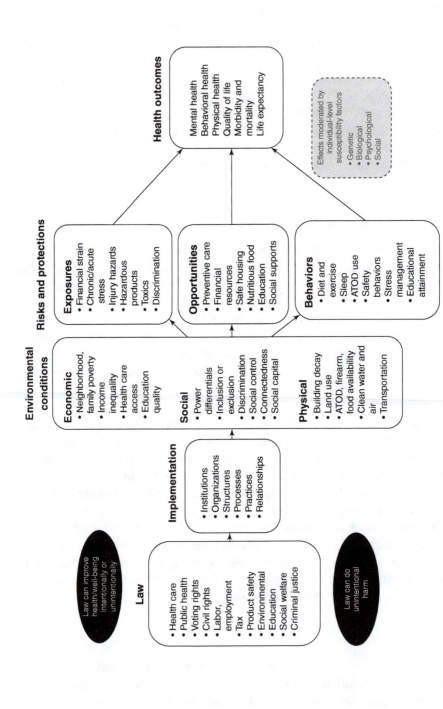

Figure 3.1. The Legal Determinants of Population Health Model.

organizations and institutions, law influences the distribution of wealth, employment, health care, education, and other resources across a population. Economic factors such as family income, relative income, degree of inequality, employment status, occupation, and education level have been independently linked with health outcomes (Adler & Newman, 2002; Solar & Irwin, 2010). Tax law and welfare regulations have direct effects on family income and resources and on the distribution of wealth within a society. One example is the Earned Income Tax Credit (EITC), first enacted in 1975, with federal and state expansions since then. The goal of the EITC is to incentivize work and raise the effective wages of low-income workers (Hotz, 2003). Multiple studies have indicated that the EITC has positive effects on maternal and child health outcomes (Arno, Sohler, Viola, & Schecter, 2009; Evans & Garthwaite, 2010; Markowitz, Komro, Livingston, Lenhart, & Wagenaar, 2017; Strully, Rehkopf, & Xuan, 2010). Social Security is another example of a policy influencing the distribution of wealth. As a result of the Social Security Act (and its amendments), monthly cash benefits are provided to the majority of retired workers in the United States and constitute the major source of income for most of the elderly. Social Security dramatically lowered the rate of poverty and reduced health disparities among the elderly (Adler & Newman, 2002; House, 2015). Another example of law influencing the distribution of resources is food assistance programs (e.g. Supplemental Nutrition Assistance Program, National School Lunch Program), which have been found to have a protective effect for low-income children's health (Jones, Jahns, Laraia, & Haughton, 2003; Komro, 2020).

Laws influence job creation, minimum wage, and collective bargaining rights. For example, in an attempt to increase jobs and reduce poverty, federal and state Enterprise Zone laws were created to target specific geographic areas where normal tax and regulatory laws are lifted (Greenbaum & Landers, 2009), although results have been disappointing (Neumark & Young, 2020). The goal of minimum wage and other labor laws is to reduce poverty and inequality at the lower end of the wage distribution (Autor, Manning, & Smith, 2010). There is growing evidence of health effects of increased minimum wage laws, including decreased smoking (Leigh, Leigh, & Du, 2019), infant mortality (Komro, Livingston, Markowitz, & Wagenaar, 2016; Rosenquist et al., 2020), and suicide (Kaufman, Salas-Hernández, Komro, & Livingston, 2020). Collective bargaining and trade union laws structure workplace relations in ways that influence wages, income inequality, and worker participation, all of which appear to affect health (Hirsch, 2008; Kahn, 2000). Occupational health and safety regulations directly affect workplace dangerous exposures, and other workplace regulations can encourage (or conversely discourage) healthy practices such as breastfeeding (Fan et al., 2020).

Federal securities laws and state corporate governance standards influence corporate conduct and affect relations between corporate executives, investors, and the public. Law attempts to curb undesirable effects of markets by reducing health, safety, and environmental risks; limiting market power; and preventing unfair discrimination. Laws that influence collective bargaining and the rights of, or limitations on, unions have an effect on power dynamics between employers and employees. Antidiscrimination and diversity policies promote the rights and freedoms of disadvantaged groups (Kalev, Dobbin, & Kelly, 2006; Moreau, 2010). Criminal law sets standards of conduct necessary to protect individuals and the community and defines formal social control structures and practices to minimize violence and injury.

Family law in the United States includes a complex mixture of state and federal laws (Estin, 2010), defining what constitutes a family, family responsibilities, and protections for children. Bogenschneider and Corbett (2010) argue for a much-expanded view of family policy and advocate for a whole field of inquiry examining social policy effects on family functioning. They define four main functions of families: family creation, economic support, childrearing, and caregiving, all of which contribute to the health and well-being of its members.

The family is only one example of a social structure affected by law. Laws define and shape a wide range of social and institutional structures and functions in society. Such laws affect population health by directly influencing broad social conditions within a society, including power dynamics, social stratification, inclusion or exclusion of specific subpopulations, and connectedness and social capital in the population, which in turn affect health outcomes (Sampson, Morenoff, & Gannon-Rowley, 2002; Solar & Irwin, 2010).

Laws and regulations provide guidelines and rules that directly alter physical conditions, thereby influencing exposures to risks or protections. Laws prohibit or regulate dangerous products. For example, many states and local governments prohibit or limit consumer fireworks due to the risk of injury and death. Laws are often successfully used to reduce the amount of hazard in products or the environment, such as regulations on the design and manufacture of products (for example, car air bags, safety locks on firearms, alcohol concentration, number of pills per prescription).

Laws and regulations protect food supplies and provide safe housing. For example, the US Food Safety Modernization Act of 2011 transformed the system of food safety oversight by shifting the focus from responding to foodborne illness to preventing it. Local and state governments define building codes and housing quality standards to protect the safety and health of residents.

Many laws directly change the physical environment, such as road design, alcohol outlet density regulation, building codes, and pollution control standards. Rules imbedded in law are also used to separate hazards from people, such as smoke-free rules to limit exposure to environmental tobacco smoke (Brownson, Eriksen, Davis, & Warner, 1997; Levy, Yuan, Luo, & Mays, 2018), minimum legal drinking age to reduce availability of alcohol to underage youth (Wagenaar, Finnegan, Wolfson et al., 1993), and pool fence requirements to protect children from drowning (Deal, Gomby, Zippiroli, & Behrman, 2000). Urban design and land use rules determine walkability and safety of neighborhoods and are shaped by public health professionals to create safe and walkable communities.

These examples illustrate the wide range of laws and regulations that affect the environments in which the population lives. We turn now to a brief discussion of implementation considerations, followed by a detailed look at environments, the most important intervening concept between law and population health when viewed from a public health perspective. Our most notable public health successes have used law to shape those environments, rather than using law to shape individual health behavior directly.

Implementation

As with all public health preventive interventions, how effective a law is in improving health depends on how well the law is implemented. Implementation fidelity is a key component to the effectiveness of any program, practice, or policy, and implementation science is an entire field of study in itself (Fixsen, Naoom, Blase, Friedman, & Wallace, 2005; Rabin, Brownson, Haire-Joshu, Kreuter, & Weaver, 2008), to which Brownson et al. (2012) provide a comprehensive introduction. A specific focus on policy implementation science is needed to study policy implementation processes, particularly how policy effects can be both health-promoting and equitably distributed (Brownson, Kumanyika, Kreuter, & Haire-Joshu, 2021; Emmons & Chambers, 2021). Laws shape environments through effects on institutions, organizations, personal and professional practices, relationships, and systems. Fidelity of implementation can be assessed through measures of exposure, awareness, receptivity, participation, enforcement, and compliance. Effects of any statute or regulation are necessarily mediated by many dimensions of the way it is implemented.

Environments

We distinguish three broad types of environments relevant to health: economic, social, and physical. We have previously summarized the links between these three domains of environmental conditions and child health and developmental outcomes (Komro, 2020; Komro, Flay, Biglan, & the Promise Neighborhoods Research Consortium, 2011). Here, we expand upon our previous work on how environmental conditions affect health outcomes more broadly across the lifespan.

ECONOMIC ENVIRONMENT

Low income and lack of resources put individuals and families at increased risk of exposure to a multitude of health-compromising factors. Socioeconomic status is linked to a wide range of health outcomes and all-cause mortality (Adler & Rehkopf, 2008). Higher incomes promote exposure to health protections, such as better nutrition, housing, education, and recreation (Adler & Newman, 2002). Lower-status jobs expose workers to both physical and psychosocial risks (Adler & Newman, 2002). Families face multiple challenges when they live in neighborhoods with a high poverty rate (Sampson et al., 2002). Residents of high-poverty neighborhoods are more likely to be exposed to health risk factors, less likely to be exposed to health protection factors, and more likely to have poor health outcomes (Krieger, Chen, Waterman, Rehkopf, & Subramanian, 2005; Sampson et al., 2002).

In addition to absolute poverty, relative deprivation and income inequality affect exposures to risks and health outcomes. Wilkinson and Pickett (2009) provide an overview of the relationship between economic inequality and various measures of health and well-being. Countries and US states with greater inequality in wealth have higher levels of health and social problems. They have lower life expectancy and higher rates of teenage births, obesity, mental illness, and homicides. In an analysis of the 50 US states, income inequality was associated with all indicators of child well-being (Wilkinson & Pickett, 2009). Material conditions, psychosocial factors, and behaviors help explain socioeconomic inequalities, with material conditions contributing most to differences in self-reported health, through direct and indirect effects (Moor, Spallek & Richter, 2017).

Low-income families are much less likely to have health insurance or access to dental and medical care, which results in many consequences, including being unlikely to have a regular source of health care; unhealthy parents, which adds to financial distress; less prenatal care, resulting in unhealthy infants and increased infant mortality; less medical and dental care for children; and poorer health outcomes among children (National Research Council & Institute of Medicine, 2002).

Household income is also linked with the quality of schools that children attend and, through earnings of offspring, contributes to the growth of income inequality in the United States. (Chetty & Friedman, 2011). Numerous studies have found a link between educational attainment and health outcomes (Egerter, Braveman, Sadegh-Nobari, Grossman-Kahn, & Dekker, 2009). Educational attainment affects health outcomes through health knowledge, literacy, and behaviors; better employment opportunities and higher income; and social and psychological factors (Egerter et al., 2009).

SOCIAL ENVIRONMENT

Social cohesion and social capital are defined as the extent of connectedness and solidarity within groups, enhancing the ability to reinforce social norms and provide help and support (McNeill, Kreuter, & Subramanian, 2006). Communities with greater social cohesion and social capital have lower overall population mortality (Lochner, Kawachi, Brennan & Buka, 2003). There is consistent evidence for a positive association between social capital and self-reported health (Rodgers, Valuev, Hswen & Subramanian, 2019). Social support has been defined as a related, yet separate dimension of the social environment (associated with but distinct from social cohesion or social capital) (McNeill et al., 2006). Social support enhances access to resources, material goods, and coping responses (McNeill et al., 2006). There is strong empirical support for the association between greater social integration and lower mortality risk (Seeman & Crimmins, 2001).

Social exclusion and discrimination break social cohesion. Discrimination creates psychological trauma, limits opportunities for advancement, and increases exposures to risks (McNeill et al., 2006). Perceived discrimination is linked to multiple deleterious health outcomes (Williams & Mohammed, 2009). Discriminatory policies and practices limit the power, status, and wealth of particular subgroups, contributing to patterns of social isolation and concentrated poverty (Wilson, 2009). As a result, residents in high-poverty neighborhoods tend to experience lower levels of physical and mental health, educational attainment, and employment than residents of other neighborhoods (Lamberty, Pachter, & Crnic, 2000; Pachter & Coll, 2009).

Physical Environment

Many aspects of the physical environment affect exposures to risks and health outcomes. Neighborhoods with greater physical disorder and decay (that is, abandoned buildings, trash, and crumbling structures) have higher levels of social and health problems, including crime, higher levels of fear, lack of social cohesion, and more physical illness (Sampson et al., 2002). Evidence suggests that improving neighborhood physical conditions can increase social cohesion and mental health outcomes (Williams, Costa, Odunlami, & Mohammed, 2008). Changing community- and street-scale urban design, and land use laws such as zoning, can achieve significant increases in physical activity and social interaction (Heath, Brownson, Kruger et al., 2006).

Availability of health-compromising products poses a significant risk for health outcomes. Tobacco availability and promotion are associated with all stages of smoking among children and adolescents, from experimentation through addiction (US Department of Health and Human Services, 2004). Ease of access and low cost of alcohol influence patterns of alcohol use and alcohol-related problems (Popova, Giesbrecht, Bekmuradov, & Patra, 2009; Wagenaar & Perry, 1994). Firearm availability, affected by numerous laws and regulations, similarly affects health. A 10-year time-series analysis of data from the 50 states indicated a significant association between firearm availability and the rates of unintentional firearm deaths, suicides, and homicides among 5- to 14-year-olds (Miller, Azrael, & Hemenway, 2002).

Residents of low-income and minority neighborhoods have limited access to supermarkets and healthy foods, and greater access to fast-food restaurants and energy-dense foods (Powell, Chaloupka, & Bao, 2007). Increasing fruit and vegetable availability in low-access neighborhoods appears to improve dietary choices (Glanz & Yarock, 2004). Research suggests that neighborhood residents with better access to supermarkets and limited access to convenience stores tend to have healthier diets and lower levels of obesity (Larson, Story, & Nelson, 2009). Residents of majority–minority and high-poverty neighborhoods face a greater risk of exposure to a range of physical toxins and carcinogens (Crowder & Downey, 2010). Living near toxic exposures is related to an increased risk for adverse health outcomes (Braun, Kahn, Froelich, Auinger, & Lamphear, 2006; Brender, Maantay, & Chakraborty, 2011).

Risks, Protections, and Health Outcomes

Economic, social, and physical environmental conditions affect exposures to health risk and protection factors, as well as affect health behaviors. Income and resources affect multiple risks and protections including affordability of nutritious food; safe housing and neighborhood quality; stress; preventive health care, screening, and treatment; and educational attainment. Social conditions affect exposure to social support, positive or negative role models, norms, and stress. The physical environment affects exposure to high-fat and high-sugar (that is, low-nutrient-density) food, physical toxins, and injury hazards. Environments not only have direct effects shaping health-relevant behaviors but also have indirect effects operating through material conditions that affect exposures to risks and protections, and those effects are moderated by other individual-level susceptibility factors (for example, genetic, biological, psychological, social). Finally, some physical and social toxic exposures have particularly large and long-lasting deleterious effects if the exposure occurs at particularly vulnerable times in the life span, such as during pregnancy or early child development.

The leading causes of morbidity and mortality are heavily influenced by exposures to risks and protections and health behaviors. Major types of exposures include physical and biological contaminants such as chemicals, gases, metals, radiation of various types, smoke, and infectious bacteria, protozoa, and viruses (related to cancers, other chronic disease, and infectious disease); access to specific foods and demands or opportunities for exercise (related to obesity and its consequences); access to alcohol, tobacco, and other drugs for human consumption (related to many acute and chronic health problems); amounts and concentrations of kinetic, thermal, and other types of energy (concentrated energy is the fundamental cause of injuries of all types); and social supports and role models. Major categories of health behaviors include alcohol, tobacco, and other drug use; physical activity; eating behaviors; sexual behaviors such as partner selection and use of condoms and contraceptives; and safety behaviors such as driving under the influence of alcohol or drugs and safety belt use.

Laws affect environments in many ways, and the resulting changes in environmental conditions and ultimate population health outcomes are complex and involve a large number of causal paths. Understanding these complex mechanisms requires drawing on knowledge and theory across many disciplines, including biological sciences, medical and clinical sciences, environmental sciences, epidemiology, psychology, sociology, anthropology, economics engineering, urban planning, architecture, education, and social work. Nevertheless, all social and physical environmental influences on health outcomes operate broadly via two causal pathways—affecting exposures to risks and protections and affecting health-related behaviors.

Studying Causal Mechanisms

We now use smoke-free laws, antidiscrimination laws, and the Earned Income Tax Credit to illustrate ways laws might affect environments, the distribution of risky and protective exposures, and health-related behaviors. In each case we draw on the overall model in Figure 3.1 to hypothesize specific causal chains that could be empirically evaluated to better understand how law influences population health.

Smoke-Free Laws

Smoke-free laws provide a straightforward example of law promoting better public health outcomes by engineering the physical and social environment. Smoke-free policies restrict smoking in venues such as workplaces, public transportation, and restaurants. There is a growing movement in the United States and other countries to extend smoke-free restrictions to outdoor public spaces such as college campuses, hospital grounds, and parks and beaches, thus creating expansive areas of involuntary tobacco abstinence.

Smoke-free laws operate primarily by influencing social and physical environments. Laws that restrict smoking influence the physical environment via the simple expedient of making it harder to find places where smoking is allowed. They also promote and support a social norm against exposing others to smoke in public spaces. The force of social norms not to smoke, and to obey the rules, appears to contribute to widespread compliance even without enforcement (Kagan & Skolnick, 1993). After implementing campus-wide smoke-free requirements, for example, hospital administrators reported more support, less difficulty, and lower costs than anticipated, as well as few negative effects and numerous positive effects on employee performance and retention (Sheffer, Stitzer, & Wheeler, 2009).

These laws are designed to reduce environmental tobacco smoke in public areas where smokers congregate (Klepeis, Ott, & Switzer, 2007). Even brief exposure to smoke can have immediate physiological effects, such as constricting blood vessels and causing platelets to clump together to form clots, which can trigger a heart attack or stroke in particularly susceptible individuals (US Department of Health and Human Services, 2006). These clinical findings are corroborated by a growing body of population-based studies documenting that hospital admission rates for cardiovascular events decline significantly in municipalities after public smoking bans are implemented (Pell et al., 2008), and these declines appear to be most pronounced among younger individuals and nonsmokers (Meyers, Neuberger, & He, 2009). Smoke-free laws lead to lower secondhand smoke exposure (Lin, Liu, & Chang, 2020), reduced smoking (Azagba, Shan, & Latham, 2020; Lin et al., 2020; Titus et al., 2019) and better health outcomes, including a lower risk of cardiovascular disease among middle-aged adults (Mayne et al., 2018).

The general idea is simple, but research is needed to elucidate more precisely the means through which these effects are won by legal intervention. Implementation is a key mediating factor for achieving success in reducing exposure to secondhand smoke (Rashiden, Ahmad Tajuddin, Yee, Zhen, & Bin Amir Nordin, 2020). Barriers to implementing smoke-free policies include lack of administrative and staff support to guide planners through the policy implementation process at their institution; lack of employee, student, or patient support and involvement; and lack of resources and tools to instruct planners how to initiate a smoke-free movement (for example, a step-by-step guide, media templates, and model local ordinances) (Harbison & Whitman, 2008; Whitman & Harbison, 2010). Increasing compliance with an outdoor smoking ban may require multiple enforcement strategies such as moving cigarette receptacles away from building entranceways, adding signage about the smoking ban, and specifying the smoke-free zone with prominent ground markings (Harris, Stearns, Kovach, & Harrar, 2009).

The major goal of smoke-free policies is to reduce exposure to secondhand smoke and its deleterious consequences. Therefore, a logical hypothesized causal pathway for the effect of smoke-free laws on population health is

> Smoke-free policies → implementation fidelity → reduced tobacco smoking → reduced exposure to smoke in public places → decreased cardiovascular risk factors or events

In addition to reducing tobacco smoke in public spaces, outdoor smoke-free policies may have other beneficial effects on the physical environment, such as reduced unintentional fires, the vast majority of which are caused by cigarettes being abandoned or carelessly disposed (Hall, 2010; Xiong, Bruck & Ball, 2017). Aside from the fire hazard, cigarette butt waste—the single most common form of litter, constituting up to 40% by weight of all litter (Chapman, 2006)—has become a growing environmental concern (Healton, Cummings, O'Connor, & Novotny, 2011). Cigarette filters are made of non-biodegradable cellulose acetate designed to capture the toxic chemicals found in cigarettes (Novotny, Lum, Smith, Wang, & Barnes, 2009), and disposed cigarette filters may leach these toxins into the environment, including groundwater supplies, causing harmful effects (Moerman & Potts, 2011; Slaughter, Gersberg, Watanabe et al., 2011). Outdoor smoking bans might reduce exposure to such environmental hazards. We are not aware of any studies to date that have examined the health effects of outdoor smoke-free policies mediated through water-borne exposures to toxins. A hypothesized causal pathway is

> Outdoor smoke-free policy → implementation fidelity → decreased cigarette butt waste → decreased exposure to toxins in water → reduced health risk

Beyond modifying the physical environment, smoke-free policies may also affect positively the social and economic environments. For example, smoking bans at workplaces may increase employee attendance and productivity (Parrott, Godfrey, & Raw, 2000); bans at hospitals may improve patient outcomes and hospital profits (Whitman & Harbison, 2010); bans at restaurants or bars may have positive effects on sales and employment (Scollo, Lal, Hyland, & Glantz, 2003); bans on beaches may increase tourism revenue (Ariza & Leatherman, 2012); and bans in any municipality may reduce cleanup and maintenance costs associated with litter abatement (Schneider,

Peterson, Kiss, Ebeid, & Doyle, 2011). These economic effects could be examined on outcomes beyond smoke exposure, such as

> Outdoor smoke-free policies → implementation fidelity → increased community resources → increased health protection factors and decreased health risk factors → enhanced population health

Most important, smoking bans directly reduce prevalence and amount of tobacco use (Azagba et al., 2020; Fichtenberg & Glantz, 2002; Lin et al., 2020) and indirectly affect public attitudes about smoking, making the practice less socially acceptable (Albers, Siegel, Cheng, Biener, & Rigotti, 2004; Heloma & Jaakkola, 2003). In turn, lower tobacco use reduces health care costs and productivity losses attributed to smoking (Centers for Disease Control and Prevention, 2008).

Antidiscrimination Laws

Discrimination—the differential and unfair treatment of groups by individuals and social institutions (Allen, 2019; Bonilla-Silva, 1997)—represents one of the most studied social determinants of health and health inequalities. Perceived racial discrimination has received substantial empirical attention as a psychological stressor that has important consequences for mental and physical health (Allen, 2019; Pascoe & Richman, 2009; Williams & Mohammed, 2009). The stress literature indicates that discrimination affects health by causing negative emotional states such as depression and anxiety, which create biological and behavioral stress responses that undermine health (Cohen, Kessler, & Underwood-Gordon, 1995). Consistent with this theorized stress mechanism, recent systematic reviews find robust associations between perceived racial discrimination and a broad array of adverse health consequences (Pascoe & Richman, 2009; Williams & Mohammed, 2009). The most persistent findings from these reviews are strong associations between perceived discrimination and negative mental health outcomes including depression and anxiety, psychological distress, and general well-being (for example, self-esteem, life satisfaction, quality of life). Weaker but consistent associations exist for physical health outcomes including hypertension, cardiovascular disease, low birth weight and prematurity, numerous diseases, physical conditions, and general indicators of illness. Furthermore, evidence from longitudinal studies suggests that discrimination precedes poor health status (Gee & Walsemann, 2009).

Intuitively, antidiscrimination laws are expected to reduce social and institutional exposure to discrimination and therefore lessen the resulting health consequences of discriminatory practices. However, despite the consistency of findings that link perceived discrimination with poor health, few published studies examine the effects of antidiscrimination laws on perceptions of discrimination and related health outcomes. And there are challenges in assessing implementation fidelity and compliance with antidiscrimination laws. Many lessons about implementing antidiscrimination policies can be gleaned from experiences with the Americans with Disabilities Act of 1990 (ADA), a wide-ranging civil rights law that prohibits, under certain circumstances, discrimination based on a physical or mental impairment. Obstacles to ADA implementation include accommodations that entail substantial cost (for example, wheelchair accessibility in a public transit system), lingering questions about who is covered, challenges and prejudices regarding mental disability, and insufficient capacity to monitor implementation and compliance (Percy, 2001). Assessing implementation fidelity of such a wide-ranging antidiscrimination law requires an examination of many processes along the implementation pipeline such as ensuring that ADA language covers the full set of organizational and individual practices that can lead to discrimination based on handicap, confirming that administrative regulations are in place and enforced, measuring adherence to implementation guidelines, monitoring compliance by governing units and business enterprises, registering complaints, and tracking settlements that have been negotiated or imposed (Moss, Burris, Ullman, Johnsen, & Swanson, 2001; Swanson, Burris, Moss, Ullman, & Ranney, 2006).

Several studies have examined the effects of antidiscrimination laws on health outcomes. In an analysis of women's health policies, Wisdom et al. (2008) found that state-level antidiscrimination laws were associated with population health status indicators for women. For example, state laws prohibiting insurance discrimination against domestic violence victims were associated with lower rates of hypertension and diabetes, while sexual orientation discrimination laws were associated with lower rates of smoking. The study authors conclude that state efforts to safeguard female residents from discrimination may not only protect civil rights but also protect public health by reducing stress for women. Similarly, King, Dawson, Kravitz, and Gulick (2012) found that diversity training policies at workplaces ameliorate minorities' experiences of discrimination as well as improve their job satisfaction, both of which could potentially reduce stress and improve health. Workplace antidiscrimination policies may also affect income and resources by mitigating financial costs of litigation (Goldman, Gutek, Stein, & Lewis, 2006), job turnover (Nunez-Smith, Pilgrim, Wynia et al., 2009), and social isolation of women and minority workers (Kalev et al., 2006). Therefore, a testable mediation model is

Antidiscrimination policies → implementation fidelity → reduced discrimination → reduced stress → improved health outcomes

In addition to reducing perceptions of discrimination and associated psychological stressors, antidiscrimination laws alter economic and physical conditions, reducing subtle nonperceived institutional forms of discrimination that foster differential access to societal goods, services, and opportunities (Allen, 2019). For example, antidiscrimination law can target racial residential segregation—the physical separation of races by imposed residence in certain areas (Williams & Collins, 2001). Racial segregation, which remains exceedingly high for African Americans in the United States, is a well-established contributor to racial differences in socioeconomic status, by limiting access to education and employment opportunities (Acevedo-Garcia, Osypuk, McArdle,

& Williams, 2008; Allen, 2019; Williams & Collins, 2001). A housing experiment addressing racial segregation showed that single-parent, minority women who took advantage of rent-subsidy vouchers (to help relocate their families to more affluent neighborhoods) were less likely to become obese or develop diabetes than were women who remained in poor neighborhoods (Ludwig, Sanbonmatsu, Gennetian et al., 2011). A hypothesized mediation model is

> Antidiscrimination policies → implementation fidelity → enhanced living and working conditions → reduced exposure to risks, increased exposure to protections → improved health outcomes

Antidiscrimination laws have been applied to many forms of discrimination, including unfair treatment attributed to age, disability, gender, gender identity, race/ethnicity, religion, and sexual orientation. Important directions for future research include (1) taking an intersectionality perspective to better understand the effects of antidiscrimination laws across multiple identities (e.g., Black men, American Indian women) (Allen, 2019); (2) further research on diversity policies within the workplace, because studies report that adults perceive more discrimination at work than any other place (Allen, 2019); and (3) understanding optimal implementation processes for achieving equality of opportunity and social inclusion (Gropas, 2021).

Earned Income Tax Credit

The federal Earned Income Tax Credit is the largest US cash-transfer program for low- and moderate-income workers. There is growing evidence that federal and state EITCs positively affect families' economic circumstances; increase participation in the labor force, particularly by single mothers; reduce poverty, including child poverty; improve educational outcomes among children; and improve health outcomes among mothers and children (Gassman-Pines & Hill, 2013; Sherman, DeBot, & Huang, 2016; Spencer & Komro, 2017). Inasmuch as it has been credited with lifting more children out of poverty than any other government program (National Academies of Sciences, Engineering, and Medicine [NASEM], 2019), it offers an example of how law in the form of the federal and state tax codes can be used in a public health model to influence health outcomes.

The EITC works primarily through altering the fiscal situation of families. The EITC is designed and implemented to promote work and lift families out of poverty. As such, most of the literature is focused on evaluating the law's effects on labor force participation and poverty levels. Evidence linking income support policies to health outcomes is growing (Arno et al., 2009), highlighting the need for research that explores this relationship and its mechanisms. A primary focus of the EITC is income support to families with young children, hypothesized to provide material resources at a critical period of child development. Those increased resources are expected to improve many dimensions of the immediate environment for such families (for example, more nutritious food, improved childcare, lower stress) with long-term positive outcomes expected as a result (Arno et al., 2009; NASEM, 2019). One hypothesized causal chain for the effects of the EITC on health outcomes is

> EITC → implementation fidelity → decreased family poverty → increased material resources → improved child development and child health → adult and lifelong health and quality of life

Alternatively, Arno et al. (2009) examined the effect of EITC on health insurance coverage for children, as a hypothesized mediator of an effect on child health outcomes. They found that single mothers with low or moderate incomes who were ineligible for the EITC program were 1.4 times more likely to lack health insurance for all of their children than single mothers who were eligible to receive the credit. They also examined EITC direct effects on infant mortality and found a statistically significant inverse association between EITC penetration and infant mortality. A causal interpretation of these results would be enhanced if they were to combine the two studies, directly examining the mediating influence of health insurance coverage on prenatal care and infant mortality, depicted as

> EITC penetration → implementation fidelity → increased health insurance coverage → increased prenatal care → decreased infant mortality

Strully et al. (2010) published an exemplary study examining the health effects of the EITC on birth weight mediated through maternal smoking during pregnancy. Low birth weight was chosen as an important outcome variable since it is predictive of various negative outcomes across the life course (for example, infant mortality, poor child health, and lifelong low educational attainment and earnings). Results of their analyses supported the mediational hypothesis. First, they found that those participants who received EITC experienced an increase in maternal employment and income, which was then associated with an increase in birth weight. They then performed a mediation analysis and found that the association between EITC and increased birth weight was partially explained by a reduction in maternal smoking during pregnancy. The mediation model tested was

> EITC → implementation fidelity → increased maternal employment or income → reduced maternal smoking during pregnancy → increased birth weight

Markowitz et al. (2017) investigated the effects of state-level EITCs on maternal health behaviors and birth outcomes stratified by generosity of the tax credits. Generosity of EITCs was defined by the amount of the tax credit and whether or not it was refundable, meaning that if one's tax liability falls to zero, the government will send a refund check for the credit amount. Nonrefundable credits provide no further income beyond a zero-tax liability. They found that the largest birth weight improvements occurred at the lowest birth weights, and that prevalence of low-birth-weight births declined as EITC generosity increased. Moreover, the largest increases in birth weight and reductions in low-birth-weight births were in states with refundable EITCs. The results indicated that few of the maternal health behaviors were affected by state EITC generosity, and the size of the EITC effects did not differ by race or ethnicity (Komro, Markowitz, Livingston, & Wagenaar, 2019). The pathway tested was

EITC → policy dimensions of generosity → maternal health behaviors → increased birth weight

Evans and Garthwaite (2010) examined direct health effects of the EITC on mothers' health outcomes. Using national data sets (that is, Behavioral Risk Factors Surveillance System and the National Health Examination and Nutrition Survey), they compared low-educated mothers with two or more children, who are eligible for the maximum EITC benefits, to mothers with only one child. They found evidence of positive health effects among those mothers eligible for maximum benefits, including fewer days with poor mental health, greater percentage reporting excellent or very good health, and lower levels of biomarkers that indicate inflammation, which is associated with stress and is a risk for cardiovascular disease. However, they did not examine mediational hypotheses. On the basis of our conceptual framework and the work by Evans and Garthwaite, we present two potential causal pathways, one examining effects on access to health care and one on social conditions:

EITC → implementation fidelity → increased social inclusion, connectedness → decreased stress → maternal health

and

EITC → implementation fidelity → increased access to health care → preventive services → maternal health

Potential health effects of the EITC may also operate via economic effects on high-poverty neighborhoods. It was estimated that federal and state EITC refunds put $9.3 million per square mile into New York City communities (Arno et al., 2009). Spencer (2007) examined the effect of the EITC on the economies of poor neighborhoods in Los Angeles. Results indicate a positive effect on poor neighborhoods, with increased EITC income associated with retail job gains. More distal effects on health indicators in the neighborhoods were not examined. A hypothesized causal chain for effects of the EITC on health outcomes within high-poverty neighborhoods is

EITC → implementation fidelity → decreased neighborhood poverty → job and business generation → increased neighborhood protective exposures → improved neighborhood health

The Earned Income Tax Credit, antidiscrimination laws, and smoke-free laws each have many possible health effects deserving further study, and we have depicted only a few possible causal paths. These are just three examples from hundreds of laws that deserve careful theorizing and empirical testing of the many possible dimensions of economic, social, and physical environments affected by a law, and how those environmental changes are reflected in aggregate levels of population health and well-being.

Conclusion

The field of public health is fundamentally interdisciplinary, integrating knowledge and theory from many sciences and disciplines to develop effective ways to create the conditions that maximize the health and well-being of the entire population. Law is a critically important force in shaping the social, economic, and physical environments in which people live, and historically, most major public health accomplishments were achieved with the help of good law. Because law shapes so many dimensions of society, and because so many dimensions of the economic, social, and physical environment affect one's odds of optimal health, opportunities for research on how law affects health abound. But research also needs to move beyond common "black box" studies that simply assess whether a given law is related to a given health outcome, as important as they are initially on new or understudied topics. Understanding the many ways law affects population health would be enhanced by increased focus on more-complex mediation studies testing specific theory-based, and potentially widely generalizable, mechanisms of effect.

Summary

Public health approaches dating back to the late eighteenth century were primarily focused on environmental conditions that increase risk of morbidity and mortality. As public health and medical breakthroughs of the early twentieth century advanced the control of infectious diseases and expanded life expectancy, public health shifted its attention from infectious to chronic disease. For several decades public health primarily focused on individual-level risk factors and intervention approaches. Now, once again, infectious diseases are of paramount concern with policy playing an important role in the control of COVID-19. The movement to reemphasize the importance of fundamental determinants of health and disease, with attention to the distribution of resources, exposures, and environmental conditions, is urgently needed to enable all people to experience optimal health and well-being.

The public health perspective highlights many mechanisms through which laws affect economic, social, and physical conditions that, in turn, affect population distributions of risky or protective exposures and risky or protective behaviors. Exposures and behaviors, in turn, affect population health outcomes. Smoke-free laws, antidiscrimination laws, and the Earned Income Tax Credit (EITC) illustrate causal pathways from law to population health outcomes.

Further Reading

CDC. Health in All Policies. Retrieved from https://www.cdc.gov/policy/hiap/index.html.

Dawes, D. E. (2020). *The political determinants of health*. Baltimore, MD: Johns Hopkins University Press.

MacKinnon, D. P. (2008). *Introduction to statistical mediation analysis*. New York, NY: Taylor & Francis Group.

Rose, G. (1985). Sick individuals and sick populations. *International Journal of Epidemiology, 14*(1), 32–38.

Solar, O., & Irwin, A. (2010). *A conceptual framework for action on the social determinants of health.* Social Determinants of Health Discussion Paper 2 (Policy and Practice). Retrieved from http://www.who.int/sdhconference/resources/ConceptualframeworkforactiononSDH_eng.pdf.

Chapter 4

Law and Society Approaches

Robin Stryker

Learning Objectives

- Identify and discuss key concepts in the law and society approach.
- Explain the way law influences public health through meaning-making, organizational politics, and "fundamental causes." Give concrete examples.
- Identify two ways in which the law and society approach dramatically expands the research agenda for law and public health research.

"Law and society" is the name given to scholarship using a wide variety of social science perspectives and methods to study law and legal institutions (Friedman, 2005). Many such approaches, including law and economics, law and psychology, and criminology, are tied loosely together through the interdisciplinary Law and Society Association (LSA). Sociologists of law founded the LSA in 1964, and sociological preoccupations with law and inequality, the politics of law, and the workings of legal culture and institutions and their effects remain central to the law and society tradition (Edelman & Stryker, 2005; Friedman, 2005; Scheingold, 2004; Silbey, 2002; Stryker, 2007). This chapter shows how theory and methods yielding insight into these core issues likewise improve our understanding of how law can diminish or improve public health. The chapter first explores key concepts and mechanisms of legal effect emphasized by law and society researchers, highlighting methodological strategies appropriate for leveraging these concepts in public health research. Second, it develops the potentially far-reaching implications of the law and society approach for policy interventions dealing with "fundamental causes" of variation in health outcomes (Burris, Kawachi, & Sarat, 2002; Link & Phelan, 1995; Lutfey & Freese, 2005).

Legal Epidemiology: Theory and Methods, Second Edition. Edited by Alexander C. Wagenaar, Rosalie Liccardo Pacula, and Scott Burris.

Concepts, Methods, and Mechanisms

Law and society researchers recognize that, as assumed by economists and criminologists emphasizing deterrence, law affects social action by shaping the instrumental costs and benefits of alternative behaviors. The unique contribution of the law and society approach, however, is to suggest mechanisms of legal effect emphasizing *meaning-making*. Key law and society concepts including legal consciousness, law as legality, organizational legalization, organizational politics, and the difference between law "on the books" and "law in action" all implicate meaning-making (Edelman & Stryker, 2005; Stryker, 2007). Meaning-making may involve either an overt politics of contested meanings or the exercise of covert power, and it is an avenue for establishing both power and resistance (Edelman & Stryker, 2005; Ewick & Silbey, 1998).

Legal Consciousness and Legality

From its beginnings, law and society research distinguished between law's meanings and practices as understood, experienced, and enacted by lawyers, judges, and other actors within legal institutions (legal culture) and those meanings and practices as understood and experienced by ordinary citizens (popular legal culture) (Friedman, 1989). Research on legal consciousness derives from interest in the latter. Scholars such as Tom Tyler (1990) investigated through survey research how attitudes about procedural and distributive justice, and support for and sense of internalized obligation to obey legal authorities, shaped obedience to law (see Chapter 6). But scholars of legal consciousness, including Austin Sarat (1990), Sally Merry (1990), and Patricia Ewick and Susan Silbey (1998), went in a somewhat different direction. They used the term *legal consciousness* to highlight how ordinary people, in interaction with each other as well as with formal legal authorities, constructed, experienced, and enacted legal meanings. Using qualitative data gathering and analytic techniques including observation, in-depth interviewing, and detailed narrative and interpretive accounts, they showed that citizen understandings of law were complex and often contradictory.

For example, Sarat (1990) conducted field research in a local welfare office and found that "the welfare poor understood that law and legal services are deeply implicated in the welfare system and are highly politicized" (p. 374). At the same time that the welfare poor experienced fear and uncertainty in the face of the welfare bureaucracy, many of them also expressed hope that (at least partly because of law) their needs would be met. Welfare bureaucrats might be seen as embodying mindless technical rule-following or as agents of need-based, substantive justice.

On the basis of in-depth, face-to-face interviews with more than a hundred people in four New Jersey counties, Ewick and Silbey (1998) found three types of everyday legal consciousness that together worked to produce what these researchers labeled "law as legality." Where "*before the law*" legal conscious-ness was marked by awe at law as a "serious and hallowed space ... removed from ordinary affairs by its objectivity," "*with the law*" legal consciousness saw the legal arena as a game and law as a resource to be mobilized strategically (pp. 47–48). "*Against the law*" legal consciousness was marked by a "sense of being caught within the law or being up against the law" and trying to "forge moments of respite from the power of law" (p. 48). The same individuals attributed multiple—and often contradictory—meanings to law in their every-day lives. The various meanings and their interrelationships formed a cultural repertoire available to be drawn on variably within and across persons and situations. The very concept of *legality* blurred the boundary between mean-ings attributed to law by formal legal actors and those by actors outside the formal legal system, and between formal law and the "law like" meanings that worked in and through other institutions, including the economy, education, religion, health and medicine, and the family. Ewick and Silbey argued that the very plurality and contradictory character of legal consciousness helped explain the power of law and the durability of legal institutions.

Building on Ewick and Silbey's explication of legality, Kathleen Hull (2003) found that many same-sex couples denied a formal legal right to marry held commitment ceremonies combining religious ritual and broader cultural enact-ments of the wedding ceremony as an alternative source of legality. The point of the commitment ceremony was to assert that they were "normal," just like heterosexuals, and to transform their social status and identities from that of single individuals to that of members of a married couple. In this case, even though the formal law did *not* recognize or endorse the identity and status trans-formation, enactment of the commitment ritual and the meanings attached to it by the community of participants ensured that "social roles and statuses ... rela-tionships ... obligations, prerogatives, and responsibilities ... [and] identities and behaviors" nonetheless bore an "imprint of law" (Ewick & Silbey, 1998, p. 20).

Given that commitment rituals enhance social support for the primary rela-tionship recognized and symbolized therein and that social support typically is positively related to health (for example, Lakey, 2010; Uchino, 2009), such ritu-als may well have unintended positive consequences for the physical and men-tal well-being of people who celebrate them. Indeed, we might go further and hypothesize that as formal law recognizes and validates same-sex marriage, the health of gay men and lesbians improves, whether or not they chose to get mar-ried (Burris, 1998a). Perceptions and experiences of marginalization and dis-crimination are associated with greater stress and feelings of insecurity (Schnittker & McLeod, 2005). By "caus[ing] wear and tear on the cardiovascu-lar, endocrine, immunologic and metabolic systems," experiencing chronic stress increases the long-term risk of maladies including hypertension, obesity, diabetes, depression, asthma, and infections (Burris et al., 2002, p. 513). By reducing perceptions and experiences of marginalization, then, the removal of federal legislation defining marriage as between a man and a woman, the further diffusion of state laws validating same-sex marriage, and a Supreme

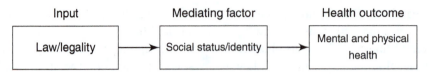

Figure 4.1. How Formal Law and Legality Influence Health.

Court decision affirming the right of gays and lesbians to marry just like anyone else may be expected to improve aggregate health outcomes among gays and lesbians, as indeed seems to be happening (Tuller, 2017).

Figure 4.1 provides a causal diagram capturing this particular hypothesized process, and any similar process through which formal law or enactment of legality makes meaning that affects social status or identity, which in turn affects mental and physical health. For the sake of simplicity, this diagram does not include the more proximate risk and protective factors, including social support and chronic stress, that may mediate between status and identity transformation and individual and group-level health outcomes.

To the extent that either formal law or broader concepts of legality do transform social status or identity or create new social categories or other types of cultural meanings, law and society scholars refer to law's "constitutive" power or effects—that is, law's power to make, and make sense of, the social world (Edelman & Stryker, 2005; Scheingold, 2004). Research on disability by David Engel and Frank Munger (2003) illustrates the promise of concepts such as legality, legal consciousness, and the constitutive power of law for research on law and public health. Where much research on the efficacy of the Americans with Disabilities Act of 1990 investigated quantitatively the statute's impact on employment outcomes of the disabled, Engel and Munger focused instead on the impact of the ADA as a vehicle for individual identity transformation. Using a narrative, life history approach, they did in-depth interviews with 60 people with diverse learning and physical disabilities. They found that the rights granted by the ADA "had a powerful effect on many of the interviewees by fostering their self-image as capable and potentially successful employees" (Stein, 2004, p. 1156, discussing Engel & Munger, 2003). However, for the ADA to enhance self-image and well-being, the disabled had to understand the rights it bestowed and that their previous exclusion from employment had been a rights violation.

Engel and Munger were not researching law and health outcomes per se. But their study, like Hull's similar study of law and same-sex couples, encourages broader investigation of potential public health consequences of law-promoted status and identity change. At the same time, it shows that the meanings individuals draw from any particular health-related law in everyday life will be contingent upon their prior life roles, experiences, and understandings. So, for example, the ADA and other disabilities-related law can be expected to shape images of disabilities and of the disabled somewhat differently for the disabled themselves, their family members, employers, and health care providers (see Engel & Munger, 1996; Stein, 2004).

Organizational Legalization

Using different methods, including surveys of organizations and various statistical modeling techniques, law and society research on law and organizations also emphasizes meaning-making as a key mechanism of legal effect. The concept of organizational legalization drew from seminal work on industrial justice by Philip Selznick et al. (1969) and focused initially on the due process grievance procedures that American firms adopted in response to post-World War II legislation and judicial rulings governing the workplace and social welfare (Dobbin & Sutton, 1998; Sutton, Dobbin, Meyer, & Scott, 1994). Organizational legalization signals that organizations *not* part of the formal legal system—for example, schools, workplaces, doctors' offices, hospitals and clinics, insurance companies, health maintenance organizations, pharmacies, day care centers, churches, and synagogues and mosques—may operate in a formal-rational way. That is, they enact and implement internally sets of "law-like" organizational rules, structures, and procedures that define and effect the rights and responsibilities of actors within the organization to each other and to the organization itself (Edelman & Stryker, 2005). Examining processes and effects of organizational legalization in response to state regulatory laws including labor, pension, employment, occupational safety, environmental, tax, insurance, information technology, health privacy and security, and family leave law has become a cottage industry (for example, Dobbin, 2009; Dobbin & Sutton, 1998; Edelman 2016; Edelman, Krieger, Eliason, Albiston, & Mellema, 2011; Kalev, Dobbin, & Kelly, 2006; Suchman, 2010).

Some of this research is qualitative, including field research and in-depth interviews attempting to assess directly the attribution and transformation of legal meaning by organizational actors, including affirmative action officers, human resource personnel, and medical professionals (Edelman, Erlanger, & Lande, 1993; Suchman, 2010). One research project observed privacy and security policy planning meetings and training sessions, toured numerous hospital clinics and wards with the hospital privacy officer, and interviewed hospital decision makers and selected front-line doctors and nurses to glean how the 1996 Health Insurance Portability and Accountability Act (HIPAA)'s security and privacy provisions were understood and were reshaping hospital practices (Suchman, 2010). This field study of a single 500-bed teaching hospital was accompanied by a survey of 320 hospitals using a multilevel stratified random sampling design that captured variations in governing state and federal law. Suchman (2010) assumed that HIPAA would affect both costs and quality of health care, and that these in turn would affect health. However, it would be impossible to say what direction these health effects would take or how large they would be without first understanding how organizational actors, meanings, and practices shaped on-the-ground implementation of HIPAA.

Figure 4.2 diagrams the causal logic of this argument, in which upstream change in regulatory law affects organization-level meaning attribution. This in turn affects organization-level policies and practices, which affect interaction among medical professionals and between medical professionals and patients.

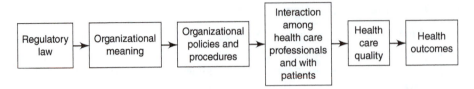

Figure 4.2. How Upstream Change in Regulatory Law Ultimately Affects Health.

These interactions affect the quality of health care provided and ultimately the health of individual patients. Suchman's field research and in-depth interviews provide empirical evidence on the first causal link only. In the full multilevel process theorized, law's effect on organizational policies and practices is mediated by (that is, works through) organization-level meaning attribution. Interaction patterns within the organization then mediate between organization-level policies and practices and health care quality.

While Suchman examined meaning-making empirically, much research on organizational legalization examines some relationship between formal legal change and organizational outcomes, while *hypothesizing* but not directly *testing* a mediating meaning-attribution process suggested by other literature. So, for example, Edelman (1992) collected survey data on organizations and then used event history analysis to model the diffusion of affirmative action policies and offices through organizational fields, as a consequence of enactment of Title VII (the employment title) of the Civil Rights Act of 1964 and of Executive Order 11246 requiring government contractors to undertake affirmative action. By 2010, Suchman had used his field research at one hospital to help him design appropriate organization-level survey questions for quantitative research that would assess systematically how a more representative sample of hospitals responded to HIPAA. To the extent that compliance with HIPAA is construed to impede efficient communication among the often-decentralized collection of doctors with different specializations, treatment clinics, and diagnostic laboratories, one can imagine that the continuity and quality of care could be affected unintentionally and adversely, increasing patient risks of mortality or sustained morbidity.

With respect to Title VII, Edelman (1992) argued that managers and human resource professionals would assimilate new federal legislation and executive orders into their prior understanding of what constituted good business practice. From the managerial perspective, a "legalized" workplace, emphasizing formalized rules and due process grievance procedures, would ensure smooth operation of the business and employee productivity. Thus, managers and human resource professionals constructed strategies of compliance that involved adding affirmative action rules and offices to other aspects of formalization within their organizations.

Much other research on organization-level meaning attribution also emphasizes this type of process, typically dubbed "managerialization" (Edelman, 1992). However, other research shows that it is not just personnel managers and human resource professionals, but also other kinds of professionals, including scientific-technical staff, who use positions in organizations as well as in their professional networks and associations to promote interpretations of regulatory law that are consistent with their professional norms, values, and identities, and also with their professional interests in expanding their authority, influence, and status (Dobbin, 2009; Kelly, Moen, & Tranby, 2011; Stryker, Docka-Filipek, & Wald, 2011). One would expect health care professionals in diverse organizational settings to be no different. And while Edelman (1992) presumed that elite meaning-making reflected covert power, others have shown how meaning-making also results from interest-based strategic action and from overt organizational and professional conflicts over the meaning of law within organizations and organizational fields, including health care (Dobbin, 2009; Kellogg, 2011; Pedriana & Stryker, 2004; Scott, Ruef, Mendel, & Caronna, 2000; Stryker, 2000).

From Organizational Legalization to Organizational Politics

To be of maximal utility for research linking law and public health, research on the legalization of organizational fields *external* to the formal legal system must be brought together with understanding of how *internal* organizational politics may affect meaning attribution within single organizations. Similarly, one must consider how variation *between* organizations in internal organizational politics and consequent meaning attribution may reverberate back to influence organizational structures, policies, and practices across the broader organizational field (Kellogg, 2011; Scott et al., 2000; Stryker, 1994, 2000).

Different professions train their members according to their own sets of professional norms and practices. Examining how the introduction of scientific technical expertise into the legal system influenced formal legal decisions and the legitimacy of law, Stryker (1994, 2000) showed that legal and scientific meanings, norms, and practices often competed to provide alternative solutions to legal issues. Parties engaged in adversarial litigation could mobilize each set of meanings, norms, and practices as resources to influence judges to rule in their favor. She termed this situation one of "competing institutional logics of law and science." More recently, she has shown how political processes of mobilization, counter-mobilization, and conflict among the competing institutional logics of law and science helped shape judicial doctrine interpreting Title VII of the 1964 Civil Rights Act (Stryker et al., 2011).

Carol Heimer (1999) showed that a similar kind of competing institutional logics analysis is fruitfully applied to health law research. She used comparative ethnographic research to study medical decision-making in the neonatal intensive care units (NICUs) of two teaching hospitals in Illinois in the late 1980s and early 1990s. She showed that formal law "gain[ed] influence by working through internal organizational processes," and that decision-making in NICUs was influenced by three separate sets of meanings, norms, and practices—those pertaining to the often-competing institutions of law, medicine, and family (p. 17).

As Heimer's study shows, the quantity of law that could potentially affect medical treatment and infant health outcomes in the NICU is fairly mindboggling. The civil law of torts operates through insurance companies, accreditation bodies, rules about standards of care, quality assurance monitoring, incident reports, hospital risk managers, hospital legal counsel, and medical malpractice litigation. Regulatory law governing medical practice operates through "consent procedures in hospitals and coordination with state officials when consent is not given by families, rules about DNR (do not resuscitate) orders, inspections, record keeping, [and] review committees [with] much overlap with mechanisms and agents of civil law" (Heimer, 1999, p. 47). Baby Doe regulations, outlawing discrimination against infants who are handicapped, and child abuse regulations that prohibit being neglectful of infants who are handicapped exemplify the category of "fiscal law—regulations about expenditure of state and federal monies" and influence infant health outcomes in the NICU through such means as withdrawal of funds, ethics committees, infant care review committees, and hotlines (Heimer, 1999, p. 47). Meanwhile, such criminal laws as those against murder and manslaughter, child abuse, and child neglect also impinge on the NICU to help protect infant patients from harm; one way they do so, for example, is through custody hearings for abusive parents.

However, Heimer found wide variability of legal penetration into the day-to-day practice of medicine in NICUs. What legitimated NICUs in the eyes of government regulators and funders was often not the same as what legitimated them to the parents of infants and professional bodies such as the American Academy of Pediatrics. Government regulatory agents were on site in NICUs very infrequently, whereas medical professionals were on site all the time. Parents mobilizing law to affect their child's treatment were, in the famous language of Marc Galanter (1974), typically "one shot players" against the "repeat player" medical professionals who had been in similar decision-making situations many times before.

Unsurprisingly, Heimer (1999) found that, although "[f]amilies, the state and hospital staff members all claim[ed] the right to make decisions about infants in NICUs, and each trie[d] to influence both individual decisions and decision making procedures ... laws end[ed] up mainly being used for the purposes of the repeat players in hospital settings—physicians rather than parents or agents of the state" (pp. 61–62). Those laws that hospital staff found less useful had much less effect. The ways that law could penetrate the NICU varied depending on the type of law and the skills possessed by those interested in using it in the medical setting, but the impact of law diminished "where legal and other institutions work[ed] at cross purposes, as when families or physicians resisted judicial intrusion" (Heimer, 1999, p. 59).

Themes of law, power, and resistance as they pertain to public health likewise are emphasized in Katherine Kellogg's (2011) field research on the impact of regulatory change restricting work hours by hospital residents. From the outside, regulating residents' working hours seems like a no-brainer. Indeed, patients' rights and residents' rights groups pushed for limiting resident work hours because residents were "overworked, sleep deprived and unduly stressed. The result [was] damage to their well-being, to medical education, to patient care, and to the entire profession" (Kellogg, 2011, p. 2, quoting commentary in the *New England Journal of Medicine*). New York passed the Bell Regulation, limiting work hours for residents to 80/week, with no reduction in pay, rather than the 100–120 hr/week typically worked. Though the Bell Regulation failed to go national, the American Council for Graduate Medical Education (ACGME) did enact a similar nation-wide regulation on hours worked.

Despite the new regulation's worthy goal of improving health outcomes for patients and residents, Kellogg found such substantial resistance to reform by defenders of the status quo within the surgical units of three teaching hospitals that two of the hospitals successfully resisted changing residents' work hours. She reported that "changing the daily work practices targeted by this regulation proved difficult because it required challenging long-standing beliefs, roles, and authority relations" (Kellogg, 2011, p. 8). Those residents with the highest status in the surgical world maintained high commitment to the "Iron Man" identity forged through weekends spent on continuous call from Friday morning until Monday night. They pushed to maintain the traditional practices buttressing their status and identity in the surgical world, and many truly believed the traditional practices were best for medical training and for patients. Reformers inside surgical units in hospitals tended to come from among those who were just starting out as interns and had not yet grasped the rules of the surgical world, female residents who were excluded from adopting the Iron Man label, residents who did not intend to make a career path of general surgery, and male residents who were especially patient-centered or who wanted to take on more responsibilities outside the hospital.

Administrators in all three hospitals planned similar compliance programs, and for a few months, change processes were similar across all three hospitals. However, over the two-and-a-half-year duration of the study, "members acted quite differently in each hospital and outcomes diverged radically" (Kellogg, 2011, p. 8). In two of the three hospitals, reformers were able to build coalitions across work conditions to promote the reduction in resident work hours, but in one of the hospitals, reformers did not achieve this key step to successful change. In only one of the two hospitals that mobilized an initial broad-based internal constituency for change could that constituency be sustained through repeated attempts to divide and undermine it by defenders of the status quo.

In short, explaining which of the three hospitals embraced the change mandated by the work hours regulation, and explaining how and why implementing the change failed in two of the hospitals, required Kellogg to examine how external legal pressures reverberated into an internal politics of contested meaning in the everyday life of the hospitals. Kellogg (2011) devotes much of her book to charting the relevant actors, resources, strategies, and tactics involved in promoting or resisting work hours change in the three hospitals and to showing what factors accounted for differences in hospital change processes and outcomes. Kellogg's own interest is in change in health care delivery, rather than in the causal link between health care delivery and health outcomes for

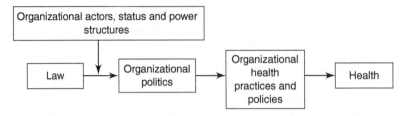

Figure 4.3. Process by Which New Health-Related Law Influences Health Through Organizational Politics.

residents and patients. However, her research exemplifies mechanisms of legal effect that operate through an everyday politics of contested meanings. These mechanisms are likely to influence on-the-ground policies and practices in many different organizational settings for health care delivery.

Figure 4.3 diagrams the more general process through which enactment of new health-related formal law sets off an internal organizational politics of contested meaning in health care organizations. As Kellogg's research shows, such internal organizational politics are not likely to be resolved uniformly. The paths and resolutions of internal organizational politics are likely to vary systematically depending upon exogenous variability in types and distributions of actors inside organizations and their resources, including the organization-level status and power structure prior to the advent of the new law. Different organization-level political resolutions in turn are likely to have different effects on organization-level health practices, and these in turn will affect the health of persons treated in each health care organization.

As in Figure 4.2, the horizontal arrows in Figure 4.3 signal that law has its effects on health *through* organization-level practices (that is, these practices mediate law's impact on health). However, unlike in Figure 4.2, law has its effects on organization-level health practices through internal organizational politics, and law's impact on organizational politics is itself *moderated* by variability in extant within-organization actors, status, and power structures that preexisted the law. In other words, just as each additional year of education may produce *different* returns in income depending upon sex or race, law may produce a *different* set of within-organization political processes and outcomes depending on the between-organization variability in actors, status, and power structures inside organizations.

To retain focus on the causal meaning of moderate versus mediate, Figure 4.3 does not depict an added complexity often characterizing legal effects through meaning attribution: that a politics of contested meanings may take place simultaneously in single organizations and at the level of the organizational field. The two are interrelated. Field-level activity influences individual organizations. But interaction internal to key individual organizations, including those that are "first movers" in constructing compliance with law, feeds back to influence the entire field (Stryker, 1994, 2000). Aggregate health outcomes for some population of individuals receiving health care across a population of health care organizations (say all surgical hospitals, for example) will depend heavily on which of a set of multiple organization-level policies and practices resulting from organizational meanings attributed through organizational politics come to dominate the organizational field.

Law on the Books and Law in Action

Whether highlighting the concept of legal consciousness, legality, organizational legalization, or organizational politics, we have seen that one way law operates in action is through meaning-making outside the formal legal system. Like Kellogg's (2011) study, many studies of law in action illuminate sizeable gaps between statutes, directives, regulations, executive orders and judicial opinions, and how compliance with them is constructed (or not) by regulated organizations. But law in action research also focuses on gaps that emerge within the formal legal system itself. Legislative law must be implemented and enforced through meaning-making by other formal legal actors including administrative agencies, courts, police, prosecutors, and prisons. Such further meaning-making will be consequential for the public health impact of all health-related legislation.

Shep Melnick's (1983) qualitative analysis of air pollution control standard setting and enforcement in US appellate and trial courts illustrates the import of formal legal meaning-making for public health. He showed that the adversarial, narrow, and reactive processes through which US pollution control takes place paradoxically led courts to extend the scope of Environmental Protection Agency (EPA) programs but diminish EPA resources to achieve pollution control. Appellate judges upheld stringent general antipollution standards set by the EPA, but the standards still had to be enforced in any particular situation through lawsuits heard in the first instance in federal district court. In such individual enforcement actions, trial judges typically engaged in equity-balancing, considering both the standards' potential health benefits and their potential economic costs to local businesses being sued. Over time, the US judiciary collectively made it clear that while general antipollution standard-setting itself allowed little role for such equity balancing, equity balancing could play a role in judicial decisions about how those general standards should apply in any particular case. Judicial interpretation of antipollution law, then, has been complex, and public health gains potentially achieved through strict standard setting may have been partially undermined through a case-by-case, equity-balancing enforcement of those standards.

Similarly, writing about water pollution control, Peter Yeager (1990) combined interpretive analysis of evolving legal doctrine with quantitative modeling of pollution charges, violations, and sanctions to show how the culture and politics of enforcement limited federal water pollution control law from substantially improving public health. Because enforcers attributed moral ambivalence rather than unqualified harm to the conduct they regulated, they adopted a more technical, less aggressive orientation to compliance rather than a possible more punitive approach. Yeager argues that in so doing, enforcers may have lessened the positive public health impact of federal clean water legislation.

Yeager also found that large corporations that were the largest polluters had the most financial and technical resources to combat the EPA in administrative enforcement. Larger companies had more access to administrative hearings than did smaller companies, and these hearings often changed pollution control requirements in favor of regulated companies. Bigger polluters thus ended up with fewer legal violations than smaller polluters. The EPA sometimes avoided going after the largest polluters because the agency knew it could win more easily in court against resource-poor smaller companies. In Yeager's estimation, the overt politics of contested meaning that played itself out through administrative and judicial enforcement, and also the more covert power of administrative enforcers to decide on targets for enforcement, ended up reproducing the very public health problems that motivated federal antipollution legislation in the first place.

Figure 4.4 combines the insights afforded by the different strands of research on law in action—the one focusing on formal legal actors and the other focusing on actors in organizations outside formal law—to depict a causal process linking law to public health through multiple and mutually influencing pathways of meaning construction.

As shown in Figure 4.4, health-related legislation is likely to set off parallel meaning construction among organizations both in the formal legal arena and outside of it. Relevant organizations outside formal law include health care providers, employing organizations, insurers, schools, churches, and families. Indeed, substantial law and society research shows that meaning-making by organizations outside the formal legal system is influenced not only by legislation but also by variation over time in interpretation and enforcement by administrative agencies and courts (Dobbin, 2009; Pedriana & Abraham, 2006; Pedriana & Stryker, 2004). At the same time, if meaning-making with respect to health-related legislation resembles meaning-making with respect to Title VII, agencies and courts interpreting and enforcing the legislation likewise will be influenced by how the organizations they are regulating construct compliance (see Edelman et al. (2011) and Edelman (2016), on judicial deference to the policies, structures, and practices put in place by business organizations constructing compliance with Title VII).

Consistent with this added complexity, Figure 4.4 illustrates that the impact of legislation on public health works through the combination of formal legal meaning-making and the making of broader, culturally infused legal meanings

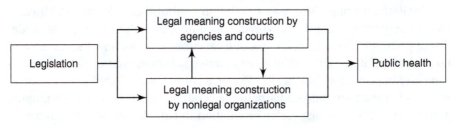

Figure 4.4. How Law Is Linked to Health Through Multiple Pathways of Meaning-Making.

by regulated organizations. The two-way vertical causal arrows in Figure 4.4 are meant to signal that the "combined" meaning attribution process that intervenes and mediates between law and public health involves a two-way street between formal legal actors and regulated actors external to the legal system.

Law, Inequality, and Health

Within the literature on the social determinants of health, one important line of research focuses on describing and explaining health disparities based on socioeconomic status (SES) (Lutfey & Freese, 2005). Findings of health gradients by income, education, and occupational prestige are commonplace, as is the knowledge that inadequate economic resources tend to translate into less and less good health care; poorer health-related education and information networks; poorer diet and lifestyle; and greater exposure to environmental toxins, crime, and violence (Burris et al., 2002; Graham, 2004; House, Kessler, & Herzog, 1990; Link & Phelan, 1995; Schnittker & McLeod, 2005).

In 1995, Bruce Link and Jo Phelan proposed that socioeconomic status be considered a "fundamental cause" of variability in individual health outcomes. By this they did *not* mean that the virtually ubiquitous positive association between SES and health (higher SES is associated with better health) invariably worked through the same mediating causal pathway. They meant instead, as Lutfey and Freese (2005) wrote, that

> some *meta-mechanism(s)* is [or are] responsible for how specific and varied mechanisms are continuously generated over historical time in such a way that the direction of the enduring association is observed.... If an explanatory variable is a fundamental cause of an outcome, then the association cannot be successfully reduced to [any one] set of more proximate, intervening causes because the association *persists* even while the relative influence of various proximate mechanisms *changes* (Lutfey & Freese, 2005, pp. 1327–1328, emphasis in original).

Karen Lutfey and Jeremy Freese investigated and built on the notion of SES as a fundamental cause of health with respect to one narrowly defined health domain: treatment of diabetes. The starting points of their research were the oft-replicated findings showing that incidence of and complications and mortality from diabetes are inversely associated with SES in the United States and other developed countries. The researchers hypothesized that in-depth qualitative, comparative research could illuminate multiple potential mediating mechanisms through which these statistical associations could work. They conducted a comparative ethnography of diabetes treatment in two endocrinology clinics: one of which treated a mostly white, middle- and upper-class population; the other of which served a mostly minority, working-class, and under-insured population. They did indeed identify a multiplicity of interconnected mediating mechanisms that would tend to reproduce poorer health outcomes among lower-SES, relative to higher-SES, diabetics. Some of these mechanisms operated at the clinic level, at which Lutfey and Freese found systematic differences in continuity of care, in-clinic educational resources, and the division of labor among doctors. These differences worked to advantage patients treated at the clinic disproportionately serving those of high SES. Other mechanisms included "differences in external constraints on potential [treatment] regimens [and] those manifesting as [between patient] differences in patient motivation ... and [apparent] patient cognitive capabilities" (Lutfey & Freese, 2005, p. 1338).

Each of these factors in turn could matter for health outcomes for multiple reasons. For example, the high continuity of care characterizing the clinic disproportionately serving a high-SES population allowed the doctors in that clinic to have better information about the patient prior to the medical interview and to get better information during the medical interview process. Because these doctors knew that they would be able to follow up personally on individual cases, they felt free to recommend more aggressive treatment regimens that provided greater control over patients' glucose levels and so had a better chance of improving patients' longer-term health outcomes than did less-aggressive treatments. Meanwhile, in the low-continuity-of-care clinic disproportionately serving a low-SES population, doctors had trouble acquiring basic information about patients, learning about patients' habits, and identifying connections between patients' habits and diabetes management. Treatment under a low-continuity-of-care regime was predicated on the assumption that all subsequent doctors who saw the patient would have the same problems. This favored a more conservative treatment regimen that provided weaker control over glucose levels, and in turn increased the risk of long-term complications (Lutfey & Freese, 2005).

The point here is not to provide a detailed accounting of all the pathways mediating between SES and health outcomes as identified in the research of Lutfey and Freese. Rather, it is to highlight just how many alternative mechanisms might contribute to the association between SES and health, and to point out that, as any one such mechanism is eliminated, another might emerge in its place, reproducing the positive association between SES and health.

This does *not* mean that addressing fundamental causes of health disparities is futile. Instead it suggests that when possible, one might want to tackle the fundamental cause itself, rather than tackling only the mediating mechanisms. If variability in the fundamental cause—in this case SES—is reduced, health disparities likewise will be reduced and probably through multiple specific pathways. One also could consider putting in place potential intervening or mediating factors that would operate as countervailing or compensatory mechanisms, reducing the more typical effect of the fundamental cause (see Lutfey & Freese, 2005).

Law provides a vehicle for both kinds of interventions. With respect to tackling directly the fundamental cause itself, if, for example, tax law were used to narrow individual-level variability in income and wealth, there would be less such variability available to act as a fundamental cause of health disparities. Instead, however, in the United States tax law has been moving in the opposite direction. Since 1981, federal tax law has increased, rather than decreased, economic inequality, and tax law may likewise have contributed to reproducing substantial wealth inequality between blacks and whites (Burris et al., 2002).

Meanwhile, where law establishes universal health insurance, this would operate in countervailing or compensatory fashion to undermine at least one of the pathways through which individual-level disparities in SES translate into individual-level health disparities. Thus, *other things equal*, the historical lack of universal health insurance in the United States (Quadagno, 2005) should make for greater health disparities associated with SES in the United States than in countries providing universal health insurance.

In *The Spirit Level*, Richard Wilkinson and Kate Pickett (2009) encourage thinking about law and fundamental causes of health—indeed about law and the social determinants of health more generally—at the aggregate level as well as in terms of individual-level health disparities. The *Spirit Level* is reminiscent of Emile Durkheim's *Suicide* ([1897] 1951) in mining different types and levels of data to converge repeatedly on the same argument. For Wilkinson and Pickett, as for Durkheim, the type and character of our social environments have profound social-psychological implications, shaping each individual's mental and physical health. Like law and society researchers, Wilkinson and Picket also highlight the roles of status, identity, and meaning-making as mediating mechanisms, in this case between economic inequality and health, rather than between law and health.

Wilkinson and Pickett argue that aggregate levels of economic inequality are associated with aggregate levels of public health through inequality's effects on social inclusion or exclusion, social status, and friendship. Increased inequality removes opportunities and inclinations for protective social interactions involving reciprocity, mutuality, sharing, social obligation, trust, recognition, and understanding of the other and others' needs. Conversely, increased inequality exacerbates status-driven comparison processes; competition and hostility; and an incapacity to perceive obligations, to trust, to take the role of the other, to involve oneself in the community, and to perceive things in terms of the community good. Increased inequality aggravates individual insecurities, the emotions of pride and shame, low self-esteem, and low sense of efficacy or high sense of grandiosity and self-aggrandizement. In short, Wilkinson and Pickett hypothesize that aggregate economic inequality relates to aggregate public health through meaning attribution embedded in situational opportunities and constraints and the nature of social interaction. These processes include socialization, behavioral experiences and attributions, individual and collective identity processes, status processes, and comparison processes.

Though the argument and evidence in *The Spirit Level* focus explicitly on economic inequality, the basic argument, by logical implication, also should apply to other social determinants of health, including race. This is so because the theorized pathways of *mediation* through meaning attribution, whether through self and identity processes, status and comparison processes, or other meaning attribution processes, flow from the "social fact" of aggregate inequality

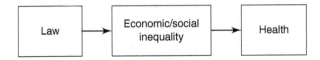

Figure 4.5. Law Affects Health Through Inequality.

levels, whether social or economic. There is, in fact, substantial research to show that health disparities are based on race, as well as on socioeconomic status (Burris et al., 2002; Schnittker & McLeod, 2005; Williams & Collins, 1995). Much, though not all, such research shows that race differences in health persist after controlling for socioeconomic status (Schnittker & McLeod, 2005).

The Spirit Level has been criticized for methodological shortcomings and has been something of a lightning rod for contending ideologies (Snowdon, 2010). Whatever one's judgment about such controversies, however, the book's underlying social scientific argument is powerful. It also is consistent with the law and society tradition's focus on meaning-making as a central mechanism by which law affects individual and aggregate health outcomes. And it is consistent with a law and society approach to the question of how law, inequality, and public health interrelate.

Above all, and paralleling the implications of SES as a fundamental cause of individual-level health disparities, Wilkinson and Pickett's theoretical argument suggests that *any* law that exacerbates or mitigates economic or social inequality is likely to enhance or conversely shrink dispersion in individual health outcomes within the population while also affecting mean aggregate health. Figure 4.5 illustrates this causal argument.

Laws that explicitly are health related and laws that apparently have nothing to do with health (for example, tax law) will have consequences for health, through their consequences for inequality. Law will have such consequences whether or not these are intended and whether or not these are recognized by lawmakers or the general public, as long as the law in question affects economic or social inequality. For simplicity, Figure 4.5 omits the many and varied mediating pathways by which inequality is known to affect health-relevant environments and behaviors and health outcomes. Guided by Figure 4.5, it only makes sense that public health effects be factored into debates over both the tax and spending sides of fiscal policy, as well as over environmental law, occupational safety and health law, disabilities law, health privacy and security law, and any law pertaining to health care, health insurance, and other health benefits.

Conclusion

The law and society tradition lays fertile ground for research on law and public health, and especially for research focused on mechanisms of legal effect emphasizing meaning-making. This chapter has shown that law affects health through meaning-making at the levels of both the individual and the organization. Likewise, it has shown that meaning-making promoted by law can operate covertly or through an overt politics of contesting meanings. It also has shown that law promotes meaning-making within the formal legal system and outside of it. The two meaning-making processes mediating between law and public health (that is, the one within the formal legal system and the other outside of it) are interrelated systematically. Each influences the other in a recursive causal fashion. Each of the various concepts emphasized within the law and society tradition, including legal consciousness, organizational legalization, and organizational politics, are associated with particular types of meaning-making at the individual level, the organizational level, or both. All of these core law and society concepts are derived from the traditional law and society concern with how law works "in action." As shown in Figures 4.1–4.5, all meaning-making processes elaborated in this chapter generate theoretical hypotheses and guide associated empirical research that links legal inputs to health outcomes.

This chapter also shows that a diversity of qualitative and quantitative methods is useful for research on law and public health framed within the law and society tradition. This is all to the good because it allows all the research design and analytic methods traditionally used in the social and behavioral sciences of health to make appropriate contributions to theory building and theory testing in the field of law and public health. Ideally, research teams are formed in which qualitative and quantitative researchers work in tandem to elucidate the various paths of meaning-making mediating between law and public health. As this chapter has shown, numerous law and society scholars whose work has been foundational use qualitative methods for grounded theorizing about legal meaning-making. But other law and society scholars have used various statistical modeling techniques to test hypotheses consistent with particular pathways of meaning-making. And, as illustrated by research on the social psychology of identity formation and its consequences, including consequences for health, it *is* possible to develop and test identity and other meaning-making processes quantitatively (for example, Stryker & Serpe, 1982; Thoits, 1986). Consistent with the proposed causal processes outlined in this chapter, various types of multilevel and dynamic modeling also can be useful.

In addition to its core emphasis on meaning-making, the law and society tradition stands out among diverse approaches to law and public health by broadening the concept of law so that it includes both formal law and law as legality. The latter concept especially calls for an appreciation of the ways beyond the most obvious that law can be "imprinted" on everyday life, whether at the level of individuals or of organizations, through cultural meanings and practices far beyond the formal legal system itself. That law truly may be "all over"—as in Austin Sarat's famous phrase (1990)—in the production of public health is a boon to research linking law and health. It is so in two far-reaching ways. First, armed with the law and society tradition's insight that the law-like rulemaking by organizations outside the formal legal system is, in fact, a form of law as legality, research on law and public health can expand its focus to the health implications of virtually all organization-level rulemaking, whether such rulemaking occurs in direct response to change in that organization's formal legal environment or not.

An example of this type of fruitful organization-based research is that of Phyllis Moen and Erin Kelly (Kelly et al., 2011; Moen, Kelly, Huang, & Tranby, 2011). The researchers took advantage of a natural experiment undertaken at the Twin Cities metropolitan headquarters of Best Buy, a Fortune 500 retail company, to study the impact of an organization-level policy initiative intended to create a new norm of flexibility about where and when employees worked (Kelly et al., 2011). Treating those participating early in the initiative as the intervention or treatment group, and those who continued prior work practices for a longer time period as the comparison group, the researchers collected pre- and post-intervention survey data and combined their survey research with qualitative observational study and interviews. Selection problems inherent in the design were lessened because employees themselves did *not* select in or out of partici-pating in the policy initiative earlier versus later. Instead, unit supervisors com-mitted to the initiative earlier versus later depending on factors that should have been unrelated to employee health outcomes (Kelly et al., 2011; Moen et al., 2011).

While Moen and Kelly did not frame their research within the law and society tradition, their findings nonetheless are consistent with that tradition's emphasis on meaning-making as a central pathway by which law affects health. Employees participating in the policy initiative experienced reduced work–family conflict and enhanced sense of control over their schedules (Kelly et al., 2011, p. 265). Hypothesizing that variation in work–family conflict and schedule con-trol reflected broader notions of variations in job strain and stress; the research-ers also found that employees participating in the policy initiative slept more, exercised more, saw a doctor more when they were ill, and refrained more from coming to work when ill than did employees who did not participate in the initiative. The policy effects were mediated in part by the meaning-making inherent in perceiving negative spillovers between work and home and in per-ceiving schedule control (Moen et al., 2011).

The second way that the law and society tradition dramatically expands research on law and public health stems from the insight that any law affecting economic and social inequality is also likely to affect public health. Here, the mechanism of legal effect is through inequality as a mediating "fundamental cause" of health disparities. Inequality itself then influences health through a multiplicity of resource and meaning-making mechanisms such as those signaled by Link and Phelan (1995), Lutfey and Freese (2005), and Wilkinson and Pickett (2009). In short, law and public health researchers are encouraged to consider how many laws apparently unrelated to health may nonetheless have substantial public health effects. Indeed, those who are concerned about public health might want to promote considerations of health impact, akin to analogous considera-tions of environmental impact, across a wide swath of public policy making.

Summary

"Law and society" is the term for scholarship using a variety of social science methods to study law and legal institutions. The unique contribution of this approach is its focus on meaning-making as a mechanism of legal effect.

A foundational assumption is the need to focus on law in action rather than solely on law on the books. The latter ("law on the books") refers to the institutionalized doctrine of legal codes and judicial opinions; the former ("law in action") shows how law operates in practice. Key law and society concepts, including legal consciousness, law as legality, organizational legalization, and organizational politics, elaborate how law operates in action through meaning-making. Meaning-making may involve an overt politics of contested meanings or the exercise of covert power and is an avenue both for establishing power and for resisting authority. Meaning-making happens both within the formal legal system, for example, through administrative and court enforcement, and outside formal law, for example, through construction of compliance by regulated organizations. Each of these meaning-making processes influences the other.

The concept of legal consciousness highlights how ordinary people construct legal meanings. The same individuals attribute multiple—and often contradictory—meanings to law in their everyday lives. The various meanings and their interrelationships form a cultural repertoire available to be drawn on variably in different situations. To the extent that either formal law or broader concepts of legality transform social status or identity or create new social categories or other types of cultural meanings, law and society scholars refer to law's "constitutive" effects—that is, law's power to make, and make sense of, the social world. Intriguingly, recent research holds open the possibility that, even to the extent persons respond to current marginalization with the hope that fair and just law might improve things in future, rather than with legal cynicism, they may experience better mental health (Upenieks, Sendroiu, Levi, & Hagan, 2021).

Law and society research on law and organizations also emphasizes meaning-making. Organizations that are not part of the formal legal system may enact and implement internally sets of law-like organizational rules, structures, and procedures that define and effect the rights and responsibilities of actors within the organization. From the managerial perspective, a "legalized" workplace, emphasizing formalized rules and due process grievance procedures, ensures smooth operation of the business.

To be of maximal utility for research linking law and public health, research on the legalization of organizational fields external to the formal legal system must be brought together with understanding how *internal* organizational politics may affect meaning attribution within single organizations. Similarly, one must consider how variation between organizations in internal organizational politics and consequent meaning attribution may reverberate back to influence organizational structures, policies, and practices across the broader organizational field.

Law and society research can further inquiry into how law operates as or upon social determinants of health. The "fundamental cause" framework of social epidemiology is consistent with the law and society tradition's focus on meaning-making as a central mechanism by which law affects individual and aggregate health outcomes. And it is consistent with a law and society approach to the question of how law, inequality, and public health interrelate. Any law that affects economic or social inequality also is likely to affect mean aggregate public health as well as dispersion in health outcomes within the population.

Further Reading

Burris, S., Kawachi, I., & Sarat, A. (2002). Integrating law and social epidemiology. *Journal of Law, Medicine & Ethics, 30*, 510–521.

Kellogg, K. C. (2011). *Challenging operations: Medical reform and resistance in surgery.* Chicago, IL: University of Chicago Press.

Sarat, A. (1990). "… The law is all over": Power, resistance and the legal consciousness of the welfare poor. *Yale Journal of Law & the Humanities, 2*, 343–379.

Valverde, M., Clarke, K. M., Darian-Smith, E., & Kotiswaran, P. (2021). *The Routledge handbook of law and society.* Milton Park, UK: Taylor & Francis Group.

Chapter 5

Criminological Theories

Wesley G. Jennings   Tom Mieczkowski

Learning Objectives

- Identify how deterrence and labeling theory inform public health law research.
- Illustrate conceptual mechanisms through which deterrence and labeling affect public health outcomes.
- Assess how deterrence and labeling theory can be applied to criminal and noncriminal events from a public health perspective.

Criminology is the scientific study of the nature, extent, causes, and control of criminal behavior. Criminal law and public health overlap in a number of important ways. Crime causes both physical and psychological harm to victims. Violent crimes—murder, rape, assault—cause millions of deaths and injuries every year, particularly in the United States (Burris, 2006; Grinshteyn & Hemenway, 2019). Criminal laws and their enforcement can cause unintended harm, as exemplified by deleterious effects of drug control measures on HIV risks for injection drug users (Allen et al., 2019; Burris, Blankenship, Donoghoe et al., 2004; Davis, Burris, Kraut-Becher, Lynch, & Metzger, 2005). Criminal law is also an important regulatory tool used to discourage unsafe behavior, such as driving while intoxicated.

Criminology as a field of research also has important connections to public health science. Epidemiology and criminology overlap both in methods and substantive scope in the effort to investigate the nature, causes, extent, and control of harmful behavior. Some criminologists have gone so far as to propose a framework of "epidemiological criminology" to link the fields (Akers & Lanier, 2009; Anderson, Donnelly, Delcher, & Wang, 2021). For students and practitioners of legal epidemiology, criminology offers theoretical models and research tools for understanding how all regulatory rules—criminal, administrative, and civil—influence behavior. This chapter focuses on two key theories—deterrence and labeling—that can be used in public health law research to improve rigor and explanatory power. The chapter begins with a detailed description of these two key theoretical approaches. This is followed by a presentation of causal diagrams based on deterrence and labeling perspectives, as well as a diagram that integrates both. The discussion includes examples of ways to empirically examine these concepts. We close by pointing to broader applications.

Theory in Criminology

Theory in criminology builds on key propositions emerging over the past few centuries—ideas that also informed other social science disciplines. And theoretical developments in closely related fields such as sociology and psychology shaped the development of criminological theory (Akers, Sellers, & Jennings, 2020).

Theoretical Roots of Deterrence

The possibility of an empirical criminology was created by the emergence of two intellectual forces—naturalism and rationalism—both of which are associated with the historic period of the seventeenth century commonly referred to as "The Enlightenment." Both of these strands are essential in understanding the foundation of the explicit and implicit theoretical dynamics of deterrence within contemporary criminology.

Prior to The Enlightenment, any set of ideas that might be called a "proto-criminology" would exclusively be identified with mystical views of the nature of causation in the physical world and supernatural causation of human behavior. In the case of overt, specific, and recognizable deviant and criminal behaviors, the sources of these were regarded as Satanic—either primarily mediated through spirit forces, such as possession by devils or demons, or secondarily induced by an actor or set of actors. These actors were mediators of supernatural forces and brought these forces into the persona by some form of act—for example, through sorcery, witchcraft, or the like.

Furthermore, there existed for more than a millennium an official Christian doctrine regarding innate and universal human characteristics that were criminogenic. Mystical Christian views imbued humankind with an "inclination towards evil" in an anticipation of the Hobbesian view, which suggested that evil, criminal, or deviant behavior itself ought not to be viewed as aberrant but was rather the natural expression of human nature as formed by the Deity. Thus, conformity to societal norms expressing "good" behavior was something that needed to be compelled—largely by a combination of self-discipline and internalization of norms, coupled with threats of supernatural punishment—in effect, a deterrence theory.

The Enlightenment began replacing these views in a gradual fashion, selectively negating many of the underlying assumptions of medieval supernaturalism. Perhaps with the exception of Beccaria (1764), it exhibited a slow pace of displacement rather than revolutionary transformation. Among the foundations of this change were arguments that causation of events was the result of a logical order to the world—once the underlying logical mechanism was known to the perceiver, the dynamics of events generally were not random and were comprehensible within a naturalistic paradigm. From this circumstance two critical ideas became established in comprehending the meaning of crime. First, human conduct obeyed a logic of cause and effect. Second, this sequence of causation was embodied within a natural, as opposed to supernatural, view of the world. The correct and consistent perception of this logic is the basis of rationality and consequently predictability in nature. Implicitly (but not explicitly) supernatural factors are dismissed or saved as some ultimate or ontological principle.

When the rationality of this view was extended to human behavior, two behavioral elements were established as explanations of human criminality. The first was that responsibility rested within the criminal actor—that such people were not acting under the influence of a force alien to them (such as possession by a spirit) and that there was logic to the choices they made. This logic was identified by Bentham (1789) as a "hedonistic calculus," an element built into the very nature of human beings. The choice to act out criminally was a product of the rational summing of the coexisting elements of pleasure and pain, the anticipated rewards of the criminality combined with the potential risk of apprehension.

Influenced by this conceptualization of "human nature," criminological ideas (still reflected in current deterrence theory) used this logic of motivation as the basis of human action in a completely naturalistic paradigm. Indeed, the history of all criminology can be seen as a movement from supernatural and mystical explanations toward naturalistic and secular conceptions of human conduct. This was neither sudden nor abrupt—indeed, it is still linked in the form of conceptions of the morality of law in contrast to purely behavioral law. However, causation outside of a naturalistic paradigm is no longer a part of the actual legal sphere.

LEGAL DETERRENCE

Two fundamental ideas are linked together in the concept that undergirds legal deterrence. These are the hedonism of Hobbes and the utilitarianism of Bentham.

These two ideas created and allowed for a purely naturalistic setting in which the behavior of humans can be reduced to two governing principles— one active, and one passive, one micro-oriented, one macro-oriented. The Benthamite principle of utilitarianism focuses on the logic of the individual actor and uses this as the foundation of criminal behavior. Any subsequently observed large-scale social effects emerged from these individual properties.

Characterizations of the large order consistent with this view are best expressed by Hobbes, who saw the emergence of civil society as itself an extension of the principle of rationality—a rational agreement in the form of a contract designed to shape, and especially to deter, violent and destructive human conduct.

Utility

Benthamite utility is a mechanism that explains individual conduct as a rational choice that is the net outcome of an assessment of pain and pleasure. Its role in modern criminology is incorporated in behavioral psychological mechanics as applied to criminal conduct and the imagination and prospective thinking of the criminal actor. Manipulating this utility (via a punishment-or-pleasure schedule or structure) is the underlying basis of deterrence. It is complicated by a variety of nuances around Bentham's ground-state mechanism of a hedonistic calculus. Among these are a series of elaborations that include differentials in perception of what is pleasurable and what is painful, how the temporal ordering of experiences of pleasure and pain influence behavior (such as lag), and the complexity of phenomena that contain simultaneous elements of both pleasure and pain.

Conflict

The Hobbesian belief in the fundamentally anarchic and self-serving orientation of the human psyche can be coupled with the Benthamite hedonistic calculus. It is the fusion of these two views that completes the intellectual foundation of deterrence. Utility shapes the individual behavioral dynamic and Hobbesian control shapes the social policy component.

The Hobbesian view of the "natural state" of human life is grim. Hobbes's most noted observation comes from his work *Leviathan* and its most famed paraphrase, the "war of all against all," which would be the defining characteristic of social life without constraints. The motive of survival and the pursuit therefore of self-interest and self-advancement determine the dynamic of human conduct. In criminology, this most often is colloquially expressed by the statement that it is not criminal behavior that begs an explanation, but rather noncriminal behavior that is enigmatic. Indeed, Hobbesian views are comfortable with this quip. Conformity to the law is extracted through the threat of punishment. Absent that, one would fully expect an anarchic "war of all against all" as the natural product of human nature. The law serves as a protective buffer or insulator against the natural enmity that one human most likely will feel toward others. It is only through a filter of self-utility that relationships exist in the state of nature. Other forms of human conduct are compelled by the law and rely on Bentham's calculus to extract conformity. The law shifts the assessment of pleasure and pain from a variety of interactions sufficiently into the "pain" category and thus extracts obedience and conformity in ways that would be absent in natural settings.

In law, using deterrence as a social management strategy is based on the ideal of a functional consequence arising out of the act of punishment. It is therefore distinguished from retribution—which sees the pain of punishment as an end in and of itself—and incapacitation in that deterrence is anticipatory and forward looking while incapacitation is reactive. Deterrence arises out of the pain of punishment inflicted by law and is generally considered to have two objectives, the so-called specific deterrent effect and the general deterrent effect. These two objectives differ in their target and typically are assessed using different units of analysis. Specific deterrence focuses on the individual actor, while general deterrence focuses on the aggregate. An evaluation of the deterrent effect of a particular punishment (or the threat of a punishment) on an individual would measure the reduction in offending by that person. A general deterrent effect would be observed as a drop in the crime rate over the aggregate of individuals who are under the domain of that particular law.

Since deterrence is "forward looking" and seeks to prevent criminal behavior, it intrinsically involves the notion of risk. A person can only be deterred from a crime by a complex consideration of the relative risks and rewards of a particular crime. Thus, deterrence is always imperfect, since it involves prediction of an outcome that cannot be known with certainty. In addition, it is clearly the perception of risk that is critical in forming intent to commit a crime or desist from criminal behavior. If one assumes that the perceptive mechanisms are functioning appropriately (that there are shared social perceptions of risks and rewards), then the evaluation of risk is based on a calculation involving several elements or variables. These are variations on the context variables identified by Bentham as the basis for the assessment of pleasure or pain. Within criminology the most important of these are certainty (the degree to which the person believes the authorities will detect and respond to the act) and celerity or propinquity (that the time between the act and the response will be short, therefore little time will be had to enjoy the reward of the behavior or avoid punishment). The severity of punishments were to be meted out in relation to the pleasures or social harms associated with the crime—the measure of punishment being defined by the amount of pain necessary to negate the pleasure gain from the criminal act. The principle of equity is also at play in that the punishment is determined by the nature of the act and not the nature of the actor. The social status of the person does not play a role in determining the nature of the punishment, but solely the nature of the crime itself.

These fundamental properties of deterrence are largely identified with the classical school in criminology (Bentham and Beccaria), and in Beccaria's work "On Crimes and Punishments" were summarized as the cornerstone of an equitable and effective criminal justice system. Tied to a belief in the fundamental rationality of humankind, this model would in almost all cases expect that a rational offender will be deterred from criminality because it would always engender a higher cost than gain. This deterrent effect would operate directly on the individual (specific) as well by example on the society as a whole (general). Only the irrational, viewed effectively as "insane," would be exempt from this governor of behavior. Careful calibration of crimes and pleasures would deter all others.

Theoretical Roots of Labeling

Labeling, as the term is used in criminology, is a theoretical paradigm that is a complex amalgamation of philosophical, sociological, and psychological dimensions primarily concerned with the organization and influences of perception on action (Lemert, 1951, 1967). It considers how meaning is attached to perception, and how a series of perceptions and their associated meaning is organized into a coherent set of abstract forms and expectations that then constitute or influence the basis of human social and psychological activity. Labeling is primarily concerned with the negative consequences that come from classifying—via language—human actors as "criminals," "deviants," or similar pejoratives and how these labels then shape the person's future behavior. It incorporates elements of symbolic interactionism—how social exchange itself forms realities and identities in the spirit of Mead's (1934) *Mind, Self, & Society*—and power theory.

Power theory is incorporated into labeling because the creation and meaningful application of specific labels have varying consequences to the extent that institutions of power are the creators of the labels. In effect, not all labelers can create equivalent consequences for the labeled. The reification of a criminal identity, for example, has greater consequences to the extent an institution of power, such as the criminal justice system, is the creator of a label, as compared to a neighbor or casual acquaintance. Thus, labeling's criminological ideas come from phenomenology, and much of its language is found particularly in interactionist perspectives within sociology. It also has applications in various conflict and power theories.

Labeling as it applies to criminology is best thought of as a perspective that is infused into a variety of criminological theories. In its most radical form, it can be seen as essentially a postmodernist perspective that largely rejects what has often been called the "received view" that an empirical and objective reality can be ascertained and described without regard to the orientation of the perceiver. Postmodern and associated labeling theories generally do recognize that some components of the physical world are imposed or "objective" (and cannot be modified by perception). However, the meaning attached to these empirical experiences is not contained within the experiences themselves, but rather in the interpretation of those experiences. While objective conditions may be recognized as existing, notably in the physical world, the meaning of these objective conditions arises from their perception, context, and other interpretative dynamics. Since a great deal of human life occurs within social and psychological contexts, the phenomenological aspects of labeling cannot be dismissed as sophistry, which some critics have done.

It is also important to mention that labeling is distinct from, yet similar to, the rational choice perspective. Essentially, labeling theory adds a layer of complexity to the rational choice perspective by focusing on how individuals respond to and internalize identities that are applied to them by others. This response often can be counterproductive, or, in other words, law and social control have the potential to backfire due to labeling effects, which is unique from what Hobbesian thinkers would theorize. More specifically, labeling in criminology typically combines both power perspectives and phenomenological perspectives, and can be seen as, in some sense, a tautological dynamic system. In some ways, both of these perspectives can be integrated, but at times the different emphasis (alternately on power or on phenomenon) can create very distinct and opposed ideas of the nature of crime.

Labeling, and the related stigmatization, can have deleterious effects on certain segments of the population such as drug users as it may negatively influence their willingness to seek or attend drug treatment or mental health services or gain access to health care. Furthermore, this stigma can adversely affect the perceptions of community members toward harm reduction strategies, including needle exchanges or safe drug consumption areas, because community members may perceive these approaches as promoting drug use rather than prioritizing treatment or prevention (Joyce, Sklenar, & Weatherby, 2019). In addition, the racial bias and disparities in drug-related criminal justice involvement continues to plague socially disadvantaged and minority communities (Rosenberg, Groves, & Blankenship, 2017). Without addressing these injustices surrounding systemic problems related to poverty and a lack of employment opportunities for these communities, labeling and stigmatization will continue to disproportionately affect these communities.

POWER PERSPECTIVE

The power perspective, as it involves criminological labeling, adds the dimension of consequence. If one accepts that perceptions themselves lack intrinsic meanings (and meaning comes from the integration of these perspectives into a coherent "narrative" of the world), the power perspective notes that not all constructed narratives carry the same consequences. Some come to have more power than others and are thus deterministic of what constitutes reality. Power theory added to labeling focuses on how any activity is organized and then infused with meaning that has a consequence for all members of a society.

Thus, it can be said that no act is intrinsically criminal. Criminal acts come to be labeled as such because of the context in which they occur, and the meaning is associated with the activity and its context. Those who control this process of contextualization are the determiners of what is criminal. Meaning is constructed and then imbued into activity, but not all meanings have the same weight, consequences, or validity. For example, homicide—an objective act—may be criminal (in a robbery attempt) or may be honored (in warfare). This is a relativist theory of moral or criminal conduct that is malleable and for which the concept of absolute evil is greatly reduced, if not entirely absent.

PHENOMENOLOGICAL APPROACH

Philosophically, labeling arises out of phenomenology. Phenomenology as a philosophy is concerned with the nature of consciousness, how the experience of the conscious is organized, and how meaning is derived from or arises from the experiences of perception and sensation. Phenomenology is itself not an entirely unified philosophical perspective. The basic ideas on phenomenology as applied to social experience are associated with a nominalist view of the social world. This influence, the shaping of reality of perception and organizing acts of perception into a coherent system, leads to constructionist ideas of social reality.

The phenomenological approach to labeling that is also relatively well established is in social constructionist ideas of crime on the aggregate level. The aggregate level of social construction focuses on the reification of social institutions and the concepts of order and meaning that are gleaned through socialization. For criminological purposes, for example, the concept of a "criminal justice system" is a reified social institution—in effect, a separate reality. It is passed on generationally; it consists of physical structures and an aggregation of individuals, it is spoken of as an objectified entity, and so on.

This dynamic can be extended to both individuals and aggregations; in criminology this has been vigorously applied to subcultural groups. This is especially of interest in criminology since much of criminality is analyzed in reference to the power of organized criminality and the developmental influences that crime-prone organizations have on developing criminal definitions within the individual. Indeed, one of the most practical implications of labeling theory is the degree to which identity can coalesce around criminal group life. Ultimately, the labeling perspective in criminology can be summarized as a theoretical framework for explaining crime and criminal law and the notion of the label "criminals" itself as a direct result of social construction. Furthermore, those individuals who create these labels can be in positions of power, and those that are labeled can respond to this negative labeling process by developing and internationalizing deviant identities.

Theory for Legal Epidemiology

Recognizing that there is a considerable amount of geographical variability and complexity in how laws and legal practices affect populations, it is not possible to develop a "one size fits all" schematic design. Nevertheless, it is possible to categorize and depict two causal diagrams (one diagram from a deterrence theory framework and one diagram from a labeling theory framework) when there is some degree of communality in the process of how laws and legal practices affect population-based public health outcomes. These two theoretically distinct yet complementary causal diagrams are shown in Figures 5.1 and 5.2, in which the independent variables on the left side of the causal diagrams can generally be considered as laws, actions of legal agents, or both, and the dependent variables on the right side can be any of a number of population-based public health outcomes. However, relationships between laws and legal practices and population-based public health outcomes are not necessarily this direct or parsimonious. Rather, a series of key mediators plays a role in how this relationship occurs. Following a description of these two

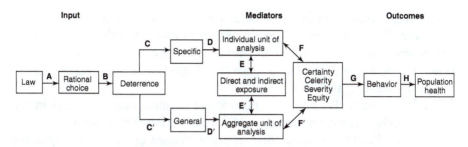

Figure 5.1. Deterrence Theory.

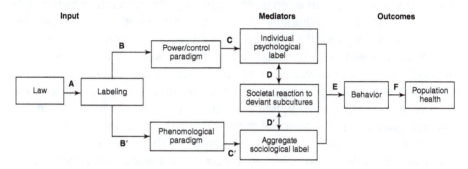

Figure 5.2. Labeling Theory.

causal diagrams, a theoretically integrated causal diagram meshing deterrence and labeling theories is also presented.

Deterrence Theory Causal Diagram

The first path of the deterrence-based causal diagram (path A in Figure 5.1) assumes that individuals make rational choices about behavior. The rational criminal actor is assumed to be guided by a utilitarian assessment of pain and pleasure, which forms the basis of legal deterrence (path B). Paths C and C' represent the two distinct forms of deterrence-based laws and legal practices: general deterrence or specific deterrence. Paths D and D' depict the operation of these two distinct forms of deterrence: general-deterrence-based laws and legal practices target an aggregate-level unit of analysis (speed limit signs aimed at all drivers), whereas specific deterrence-based laws and legal practices target specific individuals as the unit of analysis (electronic monitoring devices ordered for individual offenders).

Paths E and E' and F and F' represent the key mediators in the causal chain between deterrence-based laws and legal practices and population-based public health outcomes. Specifically, paths E and E' signify that both direct and indirect forms of exposure to deterrence-relevant processes can ultimately affect behavior, and it is possible that these two modes of deterrence (aggregate-level and individual-level) can operate simultaneously (Stafford & Warr, 1993) and be considered as a feedback loop. That is, direct personal experience of being pulled over by the police or arrested affects that person. In addition, the direct experience of particular individuals affects others when they witness the experiences of others or hear about enforcement or punishment actions through other secondary or tertiary communication channels such as the media. Finally, just as deterrence effects on individuals can shape social diffusion to the population, the degree of general deterrence can shape how individuals respond to threats of punishments.

Although paths E and E' are categorized as important mediators in the relationship between deterrence-based laws and legal practices and population-based public health outcomes, their roles are affected by the variability in the core deterrence-based theoretical components of certainty, celerity, severity, and equity. Behavior is affected along path G by the degree to which people believe that (1) legal authorities will detect and respond to the crime (certainty); (2) time between the crime and the non-pleasurable punishing response will be short (celerity); (3) punishment for harm associated with the crime outweighs the pleasure involved in the commission of the crime (severity); and (4) punishment is determined by the nature of the act, not the nature of the actor (equity). Note that the notion of equity may also be conceived as a moral principle guiding the operations of punishment rather than deterrence.

The relative strengths of effect of certainty, celerity, severity, and equity on behavior is not fully known. Neither is exactly how the four components interact to synergistically increase or diminish effects. The death penalty lacks celerity but is viewed as having the ultimate degree of severity and is presumed to influence an individual's decision to commit homicide and to deter homicides in the aggregate among members of the general population. Nevertheless, the subject of the death penalty remains controversial among researchers and policy makers, particularly concerning its relative ineffectiveness as a mechanism for realizing deterrence without preventing a deleterious side effect, brutalization. In summary, deterrence-based laws and legal practices ultimately affect population-based public health outcomes, such as violence (path H), through a series of mediating mechanisms operating at the individual and aggregate levels of analysis.

Labeling Theory Causal Diagram

The first path of the labeling-based causal diagram (path A in Figure 5.2) indicates that laws and legal practices prescribe labels for criminal actors. For example, the word *delinquent* or *criminal* is a label that distinguishes the actor from *nondelinquents* or *noncriminals*. Path B and B' represent two complementary, but distinct, labeling paradigms through which laws and legal practices can operate. In the power paradigm, the effect of the label is influenced by the consequence associated with the activity on which the label is applied. Labels emerging from laws and legal practices often differentially target groups with the least amount of power in society. For example, vagrancy is labeled as a crime because the actors are predominantly poor and transient individuals with little to no power in comparison to those who are actively involved in the law-making. In contrast, path B', from the phenomenological paradigm, focuses on the reification of social institutions. Social institutions are created because of laws and legal practices that apply labels to different forms of behavior. For instance, special gang police units form because the label "gang" has been applied to individuals who are involved in a variety of "socially unacceptable" behaviors such as graffiti and violence and do so in a group context with an organizational structure.

Labeling can affect an individual's self-concept or identity (path C). This process has been succinctly characterized by American sociologist W. I. Thomas as a "situation defined as real is real in its consequences" (Thomas & Thomas, 1928, p. 572). The label applied from the external source becomes incorporated into one's self-identity. Thus, the label becomes a self-fulfilling process. For example, an individual has been labeled a deviant because he frequently gambles; therefore, he internalizes this label and continues to gamble because he has been labeled a deviant. Labeling also operates in the aggregate (path C'). For instance, a juvenile spending a great deal of time hanging out with her peers in an unsupervised capacity has been socially constructed as deviant in the sense that unstructured socializing is assumed to be a direct correlate for criminal behavior. Therefore, this behavior that has been socially constructed as deviant behavior has an effect on group behavior in the aggregate.

Although effects of labeling have been described separately for the individual and aggregate levels, it is important to acknowledge a possible feedback loop between social reaction to deviant subcultures (path D') and individual psychological labels (path D). For example, socially constructed labels can also possess power—sometimes great power. The expression of this is described in criminology as "societal reaction"—the label attached to persons, events, or institutions evokes specific responses from a general audience of observers. These observers then proceed to organize their beliefs and behaviors toward the labeled object in accordance with accepted and reified social constructs. Situations and persons, for example, may be perceived as threatening or comforting depending on a series of visible signs that are present to an observer. This is the process of labeling as a reactive state. Taken together, these mediating sociological and psychological mechanisms attenuate the relationship between the labeling that directly results from laws and legal practices (on the left side of Figure 5.2) and health-relevant behavior and, ultimately, population health.

Integrating Deterrence and Labeling Theory

While deterrence- and labeling-based theories of legal effects can be considered separately, and are at times diametrically opposed to one another, there is room for conceptual integration. First, in a theoretically integrated model, the left side of the causal diagram remains unchanged from the deterrence model. Specifically, path A (Figure 5.3) represents the link between laws and legal practices and deterrence (path B) via rational choice assumptions. The next phase of the causal diagram presenting the key mediators disaggregates deterrence into its individual-level form aimed at achieving specific deterrence

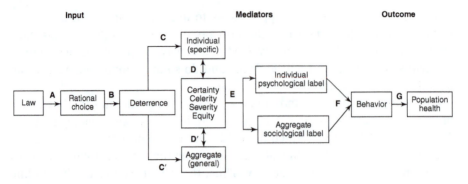

Figure 5.3. An Integrated Model from Criminology.

(path C) and its aggregate-level form, in which the intention is general deterrence (path C′).

Acknowledging the possible varying levels of influence and application of the recursive components of deterrence theory exhibited in paths D and D′ (certainty, celerity, severity, and equity), the next key mediating mechanism is drawn from the labeling perspective. Similar to the deterrence perspective, these mechanisms can operate at the individual psychological level or the aggregate sociological level (path E). Therefore, this integrated causal diagram is conditioned on the primacy of deterrence in laws and legal practices, yet this causal chain also permits the meditational effects of both deterrence and labeling concepts in ultimately affecting behavior (path F) and population public health outcomes (path G).

These effects are not necessarily operating in a purely linear fashion. The synergistic relationship between deterrence and labeling could be conceptually considered in relation to what regulatory researchers call the enforcement pyramid (Ayres & Braithwaite, 1995; Braithwaite, 2020). At the base are well-intentioned actors who are attempting to obey the law because they accept that as the right thing to do. Above them is a smaller group of "rational actors" who will obey because they calculate that the benefits of disobedience are lower than the costs of lawbreaking. At the top of the pyramid are a small group of bad actors who, for reasons of their own, are determined not to obey the law. These distinct types of actors require different regulatory strategies, and the key to regulatory efficiency is to apply the correct strategy or mix of strategies.

Actors disposed to obey the law require the least regulatory energy. The main thing is to make sure they know the correct course of action. Labeling, which tells them which activities are proscribed, may be enough in most cases to secure compliance. Rational actors, deterrence tells us, may need to be reminded that detection and punishment are available. When actors in the lower levels of the pyramid do break the rules, regulators initially can use relatively lighter sanctions—warnings, shaming, civil penalties—on the assumption that labeling or deterrence will be sufficient to get these actors back on the right track. If these base-of-the-pyramid strategies are not effective, then regulators can move up the pyramid to enforce more punitive strategies (license revocations, fines, and so on) with the ultimate and most severe deterrence strategy being at the peak of the pyramid (imprisonment or incapacitation). However, a synergistic process allows regulators to move up and down the pyramid with a number of enforcement options of varying degrees of punitiveness that theoretically would lead to favorable public health outcomes while avoiding deleterious effects of labeling and shaming.

Measuring Deterrence and Labeling

Incorporating concepts from criminology when evaluating public health effects of law requires their measurement. In this section, we review a few examples of how deterrence and labeling concepts have been measured for research.

Deterrence

There is little argument that drinking and driving and its related motor vehicle crashes and fatalities still remain a significant public health concern (Wagenaar, Maldonado-Molina, Erikson et al., 2007; Hadland et al., 2017). Therefore, it comes as no surprise that the application of legal sanctions for drinking and driving is widespread, and sanctions have been imposed for multiple purposes including deterrence, punishment, retribution, and incapacitation (Ross, 1982). As they relate to deterrence specifically, examples of legal sanctions for drinking and driving include fines, loss of license, jail time, and associated large-scale media campaigns publicizing the penalties and their enforcement (Freeman & Watson, 2006). Three studies in particular have examined the deterrent effects of penalties such as these at the individual level (specific deterrence) (Freeman & Watson, 2006; Piquero & Pogarsky, 2003) and aggregate level (general deterrence) (Wagenaar et al., 2007) that have broader relevance for legal epidemiology (see also Paternoster & Piquero, 1995; Piquero & Paternoster, 1998).

Using the following hypothetical vignette scenario among a large sample of college students, Piquero and Pogarsky investigated the deterrent effects of varying penalties and other components of deterrence (such as certainty and severity):

> Suppose you drove by yourself one evening to meet some friends in a local bar. By the end of the evening, you've had enough drinks so that you're pretty sure your blood alcohol level is above the legal limit. Suppose that you live about 10 miles away and you have to be at work early the next morning. You can either drive home or find some other way home, but if you leave your car at the bar, you will have to return early the next morning to pick it up (Piquero & Pogarsky, 2003, pp. 162–163).

Regarding the certainty of punishment, the respondents answered the following question after being presented with the hypothetical scenario: "If you drove home under the circumstances described above, what is the chance (on a scale from 0 to 100) you would be pulled over by the police?" The severity of the punishment was assessed with the following question: "If you are convicted for drunk driving, you will not go to jail or receive a fine. However, your driver's license will be suspended for … [either one or twelve months]." Furthermore, Piquero and Pogarsky included measures of vicarious or indirect punishment experiences, which are also influential deterrence concepts (Stafford & Warr, 1993), by asking the respondents to report the percentage of people they knew who had ever been charged with drunk driving and the percentage of people they think had driven while intoxicated on at least several occasions. Finally, the likelihood of committing the crime was measured by asking the respondents to estimate on a scale of 1–100 the likelihood they would drive home under the circumstances provided in the scenario above.

Freeman and Watson (2006) provide a replication and extension of Piquero and Pogarsky's work, in which they recruited 166 recidivist drunk drivers who were all participants in a court-appointed probation order for a drinking and driving offense. These researchers collected a variety of deterrence-relevant information measuring perceptions of legal sanctions, experiences with direct and indirect punishment, and perceptions of the severity and celerity of punishment. Items in Freeman and Watson's deterrence questionnaire include

- My penalties for drunk driving have been severe.
- I drink and drive regularly without being caught.
- My friends often drink and drive without being caught.
- Out of the next hundred people who drink and drive in Brisbane, how many do you think will be caught?
- The time between getting caught for drunk driving and going to court was very short.
- My friends have been caught and punished for drunk driving.
- The penalties I received for drunk driving have caused a considerable impact on my life.
- When I drink and drive I am worried that I might get caught.
- The chances of me being caught for drunk driving are high.
- It took a long time after I was caught by the police before I lost my license.

In contrast to the studies reviewed on individual-level deterrence, Wagenaar et al. (2007) provided an empirical examination of the general deterrent effects of statutory changes in DUI fine and jail penalties (that is, severity) on alcohol-related crashes in the aggregate across states. Results indicated that mandatory fines appeared to have a general deterrent effect, while mandatory jail sentences generally did not. These studies illustrate evaluations of deterrence-theory-based laws at either the individual level (specific deterrence) or the aggregate level (general deterrence).

There are a number of examples of how deterrence applies in areas other than drinking and driving. For example, speed limit signs are posted to deter drivers from exceeding a safe traveling speed. Speed limits operate as a specific deterrent process for drivers who have previously received a speeding ticket themselves and as a general deterrent for drivers who have heard of others being caught and punished for exceeding the posted speed limit. The certainty, severity, and celerity of punishment and related fines, license suspensions, and so on all have an influence on the degree to which public health benefits of posting speed limit signs is realized.

Electronic monitoring devices for convicted offenders also have an inherent deterrent element. These devices make it difficult or impossible for monitored individuals to leave their homes or workplaces in order to offend. Assuming that these devices are properly operating and being monitored, any departure from the permitted area would result in an immediate alarm to the authorities (certainty). Following this alarm, the probation or parole officer normally would swiftly respond to the alarm (celerity), document violation of the offender's probation or parole, and return the offender to jail (severity).

Researchers have also begun to study relative weights of certainty, severity, and celerity in affecting deterrence. A number of examples of reliable and valid measurement tools and scales can be found in the following sources (Durlauf & Nagin, 2011; Nagin, 2010; Nagin & Pogarsky, 2001; Roche, Wilson, & Pickett, 2020). Furthermore, systematic reviews and meta-analyses provide helpful resources on how to measure elements of deterrence (Andrews, Zinger, Hoge et al., 1990; Braga, Weisburd, & Turchan, 2018; Cullen, Pratt, Miceli, & Moon, 2002; Cullen, Wright, & Applegate, 1996; Howe & Brandau, 1988; Howe & Loftus, 1996; Klepper & Nagin, 1989; Nagin, 1998; Nagin & Pogarsky, 2001; Pratt & Cullen, 2005; Pratt, Cullen, Blevins, Daigle, & Madensen, 2006; Pusch & Holtfreter, 2021; Williams & Hawkins, 1986).

Labeling

There can be little argument that sex offender registration and community notification provide one of the most identifiable and current examples of labeling in criminology. Although sex offender registration is not necessarily a new idea (Logan, 2009), the universal requirement for convicted sex offenders to register with law enforcement, have their identifying information posted on publicly accessible, Internet-based registries, and (at least in some jurisdictions) have community organizations and residents notified of their identities and residential locations (Terry & Ackerman, 2009) has presented a real-world experiment on the effects of such laws on population-based public health outcomes such as sexual violence.

A growing number of studies have begun to question the effectiveness of universal application of sex offender registration and community notification policies due to their misperception regarding sex offender specialization and recidivism (Bouffard & Askew, 2019; Zimring, Jennings, Piquero, & Hays, 2009; Zimring, Piquero, & Jennings, 2007). Furthermore, research has identified a number of collateral consequences for sex offenders as a direct result of having been labeled a "sex offender" and experiencing the associated negative and stigmatizing effects of this label. For example, Tewksbury (2005) collected information from a mailed survey administered to offenders listed on the Kentucky Sex Offender Registry and asked them about their experiences since becoming a registrant. There was a wide range of negative experiences reported, with the most common experiences including loss of job (43%); denial of promotion at work (23%); loss or denial of place to live (45%); treated rudely in a public place (39%); asked to leave a business (11%); lost a friend who found out about registration (55%); harassed in person (47%); assaulted (16%); received harassing or threatening telephone calls (28%); received harassing or threatening mail (25%).

Considering the prevalence of such negative experiences, reintegration and avoidance of long-term stigmatization among labeled and registered sex offenders might be difficult at best (Braithwaite, 1989). Furthermore, such negative experiences likely lead to a reduction in protective factors and a corresponding increase in risk factors for re-offending. Reducing re-offending probably requires creating conducive conditions for successful societal reintegration (Fox, 2017; McAlinden, 2006).

Laws on sex offender registration and community notification illustrate how a theoretically integrated model may be tested. The research question is whether these laws reduce rates of sexual violence (a population-based public health outcome) by providing a specific deterrent effect (preventing sexual violence recidivism among sex offenders) and a general deterrent effect (deterring would-be first-time sex offenders) while avoiding unduly stigmatizing labeling effects and preventing registrants' successful reintegration into society. Recent empirical evidence on sex offender registration and community notification laws suggests that deleterious consequences of the labeling effects of these laws may be exceeding the beneficial deterrence consequences (Call, 2018; Hamilton, 2020; Sandler, Freeman, & Socia, 2008; Schramm & Milloy, 1995; Tewksbury, 2005; Tewksbury & Jennings, 2010; Vasquez, Maddan, & Walker, 2008; Zgoba, Veysey, & Dalessandro, 2010).

Legal Epidemiology Research Challenges

Theory, as the term is used in all social sciences including criminology, should be viewed with modesty and constraint, because, unlike in many physical sciences, theoretical ideas of causation of crime and the quantitative and qualitative relationships between important concepts and constructs are not fully defined or measured. Operationalizing and measuring constructs related to human conduct are typically more ambiguous and more difficult than measuring constructs related to the physical world. Theory in criminology and the social sciences, as a consequence, is underdeveloped, suggesting cause–effect relationships without necessarily providing an ability to precisely predict prospectively.

There are inherent tensions between crime control and public health objectives that can present problems for legal epidemiology. Consider the tug-of-war between harm-reduction strategies and political incentives to appear tough on crime. "Get tough" measures such as drug crackdowns are often serious impediments to achieving beneficial crime control and public health objectives. Ultimately, scientists, practitioners, and lawmakers should make a more concerted effort in developing partnerships to design research programs addressing shared crime and public health issues, as well as implement effective laws and policies that strike a balance between crime control and public health objectives.

Conclusion

This chapter described how theories and methods from the field of criminology, particularly deterrence and labeling theories, help explain how law influences behavior. Following a discussion of the effects of criminal and non-criminal laws and a review of theoretical frameworks for deterrence and labeling theories, we presented three causal diagrams that graphically depicted ways law can affect population health outcomes via the complex mediating mechanisms emerging from deterrence and labeling theories. Examples of ways to measure and empirically examine these concepts were also provided. Finally, we discussed the theoretical and methodological challenges that exist as well as offering a series of recommendations and directions for future research for those interested in examining public health effects of laws in light of prominent theories in criminology.

Relevant public health law and the research on its effects can both inform and be informed by criminology. This mutually beneficial relationship centers on how each discipline informs the theoretical thinking and empirical knowledge base upon which each relies to deepen their contributions to public life. For example, each discipline shares a concern for health in prospective thinking about policy. The very concept of deterrence in criminology is a prospective and preventive approach completely consistent with the public health concern with prevention. Ideally, policies directed at criminal behavior as well as unhealthy behaviors are most effective when they prevent negative effects rather than having to deal with corrective ex post facto actions. Furthermore, criminological ideas regarding labeling have important implications for generalized patterns of behavior that can be elements in prevention policies. This is well illustrated by the labeling efforts directed at tobacco use as a public health concern. Labeling unhealthy and antisocial behaviors as unhealthy and undesirable are common mechanisms for both disciplines.

It is clear that the nexus between criminology and legal epidemiology extends beyond these abstract domains. Persons drawn into the criminal justice system bring with them serious public health issues. For instance, this population exhibits greater degrees of morbidity than the general population and often is involved in higher rates of unhealthy behavior compared to the general public. They are also less likely to have any form of health insurance outside the general public assistance offered to the indigent. In sum, they offer special challenges to public health policy while simultaneously being potentially less tractable to the usual health delivery services available to citizens. In addition, offenders' motivation for a healthy lifestyle, perceptions of self-interest, and patterns of thought may be radically different from the typical population-wide patterns that public health practitioners often assume. As a result, there are many ways in which criminological theory, data, and research help advance public health law and improve population health outcomes. Finally, a long history of mistreatment, prejudice, and social bias exacerbates criminal justice system involvement and associated public health consequences among racial and ethnic subpopulations. Elevating recognition of the role of such biases is central to effectively using criminological theories not only to advance public health but also to right systemic injustice.

Summary

Criminology is the scientific study of the nature, extent, causes, and control of criminal behavior. Two theories—deterrence and labeling—are widely used by criminologists to explain the influence of criminal law on behavior. Public health law researchers investigating effects of regulations and sanctions on health behavior can draw on these theories and the research methods and tools criminologists have devised to test them.

- Deterrence posits that the choice to act out criminally is a product of the rational assessment of the anticipated rewards of criminality versus the potential costs imposed by law. Manipulating this calculation (through punishment and the perceived likelihood of detection) is the underlying basis of deterrence.

- Labeling theory explains crime and criminal law as products of a social process of meaning-making. Certain behaviors, not necessarily intrinsically harmful, are labeled as "crimes" and those who commit them as "deviants." Labeling theory explains how these labels emerge and how people's identities and behaviors are influenced by them.

- The two theories can be integrated to explain how ideas about crime, fears of punishment, and expectations of detection work in relation to each other to shape individual and aggregate behavior in response to law.

Further Reading

Braithwaite, J. (1989). *Crime, shame, and reintegration*. Cambridge, UK: Cambridge University Press.

Nagin, D. S., Cullen, F. T., & Jonson, C. L. (Eds.) (2018). *Deterrence, choice, and crime, volume 23: Contemporary perspectives*. Milton, UK: Routledge.

Stafford, M., & Warr, M. (1993). A reconceptualization of general and specific deterrence. *Journal of Research in Crime and Delinquency, 30*(2), 123–135.

Wagenaar, A. C., Maldonado-Molina, M. M., Erickson, D. J., et al. (2007). General deterrence effects of U.S. statutory DUI fine and jail penalties: Long-term follow-up in 32 states. *Accident Analysis and Prevention, 39*(5), 982–994.

Yao, J., Xiao, T., & Hou, S. (2021). Risk perceptions and DUI decisions of drivers in different legal environments: New evidence on differential deterrence from a Chinese sample. *Accident Analysis & Prevention, 157*, 106188.

Chapter 6

Procedural Justice Theory

Tom R. Tyler   Avital Mentovich

Learning Objectives

- Define and describe the components of procedural justice.
- Illustrate the significance of legitimacy and self-regulatory behavior in developing, implementing, and enforcing public health law.
- Design a legal epidemiology study that incorporates procedural justice in examining compliance to a public health law.

Law is a prominent intervention tool through which citizens, acting through their democratically elected government, can seek to achieve public health goals (Burris, Wagenaar, Swanson et al., 2010). To take a straightforward example, governments create regulations banning smoking in public places, and provide penalties, typically a fine, for those who disobey those rules. The government similarly promotes public health by regulating the quality of drugs that are sold in America, again creating rules and enforcing them through a system of fines and, in extreme cases, criminal penalties. These regulations are an effort by government to improve public health by putting the force of law behind stopping unhealthy behaviors.

The COVID-19 pandemic highlighted the many ways that governments seek to manage people, with requirements ranging from wearing a mask and social distancing to self-reporting symptoms. Research in the United States and Europe documents the important role that perceived obligation to obey the law and legal authorities can play in motivating compliance with COVID-19-related rules (Folmer et al., 2021; Kooistra et al., 2021; Reinders et al., 2020; Van Rooij et al., 2021). It also makes clear that there are other forces that can be important, particularly when trust in law is low, including strong community norms (Ho, 2021) and trust in science (Bicchieri et al., 2021).

Legal Epidemiology: Theory and Methods, Second Edition. Edited by Alexander C. Wagenaar, Rosalie Liccardo Pacula, and Scott Burris.

It might be initially imagined that the way these laws influence behavior is straightforward. If a law or regulation is passed and backed up by threats of fines, arrest, or incarceration, behavior will change. If wearing safety belts is mandated, people will wear belts to avoid getting a ticket. The threat of a sanction certainly can work but obtaining a high level of compliance with the law is complex and can be difficult; the ability of law to shape public behavior is the result of many interacting factors that vary depending on local conditions, the behavior, and the target population. Studies suggest that the limits of mandated compliance are typically linked to capacity. When the government cannot effectively monitor and sanction people, coercion does not work. This is particularly true when the government is trying to manage behavior that is widespread within the population, such as everyday mask wearing or social distancing.

From a social psychological perspective, the effectiveness of the legal system depends at least in part on the willingness of citizens to voluntarily consent to the operation of legal authorities and to actively cooperate with them. Social psychologists posit that behavior is determined by two main forces. The first is the pressure of the situation or the environment, and the second includes the motives and perceptions that the person brings to the situation. In Lewin's famous equation, behavior is understood to be a function of the person and the environment: $B = f(P, E)$. An expanded conception of the *person* term includes the set of social and moral values that shape the individual's thoughts and feelings about what is ethical or normatively appropriate to do. The *environment* includes the way legal officers and institutions behave in their creation and enforcement of rules.

Where compliance with the law is concerned, two values constituting what sociologist Max Weber called "legitimacy" are of particular importance to defining P: the individual's sense of obligation to obey authorities, and his or her sense of trust and confidence in legal authorities (Weber, 1968). These feelings of legitimacy, and the willingness to comply with law, are influenced by the legal environment. There are a variety of reasons that people might view an authority as legitimate. Research has made a compelling case for the positive effect of perceptions of procedural justice on an individual's sense of a rule's legitimacy and his or her compliance with it. This chapter will examine the complexity of compliance and propose an approach to studying health-related behavior that has been effective in other settings. This approach is known in the literatures on law, regulation, and social psychology as "procedural justice."

Complying with the Law

The problems involved in obtaining compliance with the law in everyday life involve a wide variety of regulations, ranging from traffic laws (Tyler, 2006a) to drug laws (MacCoun, 1993). While most people comply with the law most of the time, legal authorities are confronted with sufficient noncompliance to be challenging to regulatory resources. In situations such as the use of illicit or addictive substances, levels of noncompliance are high enough to suggest a substantial failure of current regulatory strategy (MacCoun, 1993). People do indeed comply with the law in the presence of a legal authority, but the same people often revert to their prior behavior once that authority is absent (McCluskey, 2003).

If citizens fail to sufficiently obey legal restrictions, further intervention by legal authorities eventually will be required to obtain the desired level of compliance. Continued monitoring and enforcement are sometimes feasible. For example, smoking bans in workplaces or restaurants are enforceable because these are inherently social settings and behavior is monitored. Similarly, smoking or mask wearing on airplanes can easily be monitored by smoke detectors or enforced by flight attendants. In other cases, ranging from speeding to substance abuse, consistent oversight and enforcement have been more difficult. The problem may be in developing strategies of monitoring or enforcement—hidden behaviors may be difficult to detect, for example, or we may know how to monitor the behavior—speeding for instance—but lack the resources to maintain enforcement at a sufficiently high level to achieve deterrence. These difficulties have been strikingly revealed in the COVID-19 era by the challenge of enforcing rules about mask wearing, social distancing, and vaccination.

There are two principal models for compliance or rule adherence. The first is deterrence theory, also referred to as a sanction-based or command-and-control model. The assumption underlying this theory is that we shape behavior by varying the risks associated with breaking rules, the gains associated with adherence, or both (see Chapter 5). The legal system attempts to project credible risks for wrongdoing. As any driver knows who has stopped talking on a cell phone as a patrol car came into view, rule adherence can be influenced by whether people perceive that rule breaking will be detected and punished.

It is sometimes possible to motivate compliance by creating a risk of punishment for non-adherence (a fine for smoking) or incentives for adherence (payment for exercising at the gym). Studies demonstrate, however, that regulating behavior through threat serves to undermine people's commitment to norms, rules, and authorities (Frey, 1997, 1998; Frey & Oberholzer-Gee, 1997). This is an important deleterious side-effect of a deterrence-based regulatory approach. While it would be optimal from a regulatory perspective if the use of threats did not influence people's values, research suggests that the strength of people's internal motivations for rule following can be lowered when compliance is framed in terms of the possible risk of sanctioning for rule breaking (Schmelz, 2021).

From a motivational perspective, instrumental approaches such as deterrence are not self-sustaining and require the maintenance of institutions and authorities that can keep the probability of detection for behavior that threatens public health at a sufficiently high level to constantly motivate the public through external means (that is, the threat of punishment or provision of incentives). Over time it becomes more and more important to have such external constraints in place, as whatever intrinsic motivation people originally had is gradually "crowded out" by external concerns. In other words, the very behavior of surveillance creates the conditions requiring future surveillance.

There are two distinct points to be made about instrumental approaches. The first is that motivating compliance via the use of incentives and sanctions is a suppression strategy. It requires the continual presence of credible self-interest risks to maintain desired behavior. Sanction-based approaches do not build legitimacy or promote norms. Second, sanction-based strategies can undermine whatever internal norms and values are already motivating people. To the degree that incentives and sanctions crowd out the field, the role of norms and values lessens over time.

Self-regulation offers an alternative to the deterrence model. In a self-regulatory model people are seen as motivated to follow rules because their own values suggest to them that doing so is the appropriate action to take. Voluntary healthy behavior that is motivated by a person's own attitudes and values is superior from a regulatory perspective to behavior that has to be coerced. When values are the motivator of behavior, rule adherence does not need to be sustained either by enacting a credible system of monitoring and sanctioning or by developing a way to incentivize desired behaviors. A variety of "nudges" designed into environments can enhance the prevalence of healthy behaviors consistent with commonly held values (Thaler & Sunstein, 2009). When healthy behavior is motivated by nudges, as when it is shaped by values, a key issue is the ability to create sustained change.

The general legal question is how to motivate everyday adherence to legal rules, or self-regulation. The key issue is how to create and maintain values that motivate people to take personal responsibility for behaviors that promote the public's health (Tyler, 2006a, 2006b). A good deal of research in the legal arena indicates that self-regulatory motivations are activated when people believe that legal authorities are legitimate and they therefore have an obligation to conform to the law (Tyler, 2007, 2008). Consequently, people who identify with legal authorities and imbue the legal system with legitimacy will voluntarily abide by laws and defer to authorities (Darley, Tyler, & Bilz, 2003; Jost & Major, 2001; Tyler, 2006a; Tyler & Blader, 2000).

Legitimacy

The issue of legitimacy is widely studied in the arena of law, and it is clear both that the legitimacy of legal authorities (for example health officials, police officers) and of the law itself shapes law-related behavior (Tyler, 2006b). Modern discussions of legitimacy are usually traced to the writings of Weber (1968) on authority and the social dynamics of authority (for example, Zelditch, 2001). Weber, like Machiavelli and others before him, argue that successful leaders and institutions do not rely solely or even primarily on brute force to execute their will. Rather, they strive to win the consent of the governed so that their commands will be voluntarily obeyed (Tyler, 2006a). Legitimacy, according to this general view, is a quality that is possessed by an authority, a law, or an institution that leads others to feel obligated to accept its directives. When people ascribe legitimacy to the system that governs them, they become willing subjects whose behavior is strongly influenced by official (and unofficial) doctrine. They also internalize a set of moral values that is consonant with the aims of the system (Jost & Major, 2001). Although the concept of legitimacy has not featured prominently in recent discussions of social regulation with respect to law-abiding behavior, there is a strong intellectual tradition that emphasizes the significance of developing and maintaining positive social values toward cultural, political, and legal authorities (Easton, 1965, 1975; Krislov, Boyum, Clark, Shaefer, & White, 1966; Melton, 1986; Parsons, 1967; Tapp & Levine, 1977).

A values-based perspective on human motivation therefore suggests the importance of developing and sustaining a civic culture in which people abide by the law because they feel that legal authorities are legitimate and ought to be obeyed. For this model to work, society must create and maintain public values that are conducive to following behavioral norms. Political scientists refer to this set of values as a "reservoir of support" for government and society (Dahl, 1956). Studies indicate that values shape rule following (Sunshine & Tyler, 2003a, 2003b; Tyler, 2006a, 2006b; Tyler & Fagan, 2008), and that the influence of values is stronger than the effect of risk estimates (Sunshine & Tyler, 2003a).

Some laws merely facilitate social coordination—for example, making sure that everyone drives on the same side of the road. In these instances, the particular form of appropriate behavior is not the key issue. Rather, the important thing is that people agree upon what is appropriate and behave accordingly. While the law enforces such rules, enforcement is not a major societal issue because people have little or no motivation to undermine or disobey such rules. There is very little to be gained by driving on the wrong side of the road. Similarly, some laws are directed at acts that are deemed inherently wrongful, such as murder or the adulteration of food. Most people don't intend to break these rules, and have no objection to deterring the few who do through surveillance and harsh punishment.

Legitimacy becomes more contested when the function of the law is to restrict behavior that is not seen as inherently wrongful and may even offer benefits to the actor. Legal intervention in matters like this is most likely to seem legitimate in situations in which behavior harms others directly. For example, the case for restricting smoking via law became more compelling when smoking was recognized to have second-hand effects. This recognition of harm to non-smokers legitimated the introduction of smoking bans in public places in ways that the harm of smoking to smokers was never able to do. The public reasoning is that people have the right to choose to harm their own health but they are not entitled to choose to harm others.

Many public health measures address harm to people other than the actor, but just as many are partially or primarily paternalistic—aimed at encouraging people to avoid harming themselves by making healthier choices. Paternalistic public health restrictions present an interesting case for legitimacy-oriented approaches to compliance. They regulate everyday personal activities, promoting desirable health-related behavior (exercise, healthy diet, safe sex) or discouraging undesirable behavior (overeating, smoking, and drinking in excess).

Sometimes the behavior—smoking, drunk driving, unsafe sex—threatens harm to others, but often the person most immediately at risk of harm is the actor him or herself. In some cases, for example COVID-19, the harm to oneself and to others is intermingled and there are several reasons to follow rules.

There is vigorous philosophical debate as to whether it is proper for government to interfere with individual choices that do not pose a risk to others (Epstein, 2003; Thaler & Sunstein, 2009). A committed anti-paternalist may regard any such law as illegitimate, regardless of its good intentions or the severity of the risk to the actors. But even those who are prepared to accept some paternalism as a matter of principle (or who don't even think about the issue) may not share the health policy maker's sense of the risks of a specific behavior or the advantages of giving it up. Smoking, drinking, and eating are all things that people enjoy doing. Convincing them to change gratifying behaviors voluntarily is no easy task. Indeed, forcing them to change their own behavior against their desires risks undermining the legitimacy of legal authority.

Interventions that merely provide information have limited effects. Despite the fact that people are the primary beneficiaries of their own better health, studies make clear that people often fail to engage in practices that ensure that health (Brewer, 2017). This is true in terms of everyday life, in which people drink too much, use unhealthy drugs, have sex without protection, become obese, and smoke. Even with the benefit of simple guidance, such as the food pyramid developed by the United States Department of Agriculture, people do not conform to eating regimes intended to prevent or minimize health problems that are prevalent across the population.

The threat of punishment seems to work poorly for cases where the behaviors are ubiquitous and difficult for authorities to observe and monitor. Both practically and politically, many important health-related behaviors, such as overeating of unhealthy foods, are going to be hard to directly address through laws that punish those who engage in the behavior. People like high-fat foods, for example, and the food industry deploys huge resources to retain that support and forestall regulation. Even if there were widespread popular support for punishing those with unhealthy lifestyles, it would be hard to devise or enforce any suitable regulations on consumers. Problems of surveillance are likely to be particularly important, given that activities such as being a couch potato, snacking, and having sex tend to happen in the privacy of the home. Regulating food producers and distributors rather than individual consumers is likely perceived as a more legitimate and is probably a more effective use of threats of punishment. On the other hand, it is important to recognize that deterrence-based approaches can have substantial benefits by significantly shaping behavior when the right conditions exist.

These factors predict that public health efforts to regulate unhealthy behaviors are likely to look similar in the future to how they have looked in the past. Activities that are seen as innately bad and dangerous to others will be prohibited. Paternalistic public health regulations that seek to motivate an individual to forego a short-term benefit in return for a long-term one will continue to rely more on "soft" regulatory techniques. These include warning and informational labels or signs, official guidelines, and attempts to make healthy behavior a default option. In a few cases, involving products that have been perceived to have a risk-utility profile akin to cigarettes—trans fats, to take a recent example—bans may be enacted. Similarly, "sin taxes" may on occasion be extended to new products, like sugar-sweetened beverages, to increase the incentive to avoid them. Getting support for these measures, and getting the desired level of compliance and behavioral change, will depend to a great degree upon the extent to which people either trust scientists who point out the risks and urge safe behavior, or take the view that they ought to obey the law because it is the law—in other words, on government legitimacy.

Gaining public support for lifestyle changes is likely to be especially challenging when authorities are arguing for some behavior change that is good for a person. Liberal paternalism tries to convince a person that their own self-interest is better served by some type of lifestyle change. In contrast the authorities can also try to motivate a person to change in ways that accord with their own views about how that person should live. Both types of changes can be attempted through appeals to values, by offering incentives or threatening sanctions or by modifications in people's everyday environment that shape their choices. Whatever approaches are used, accepting change is likely to be harder when it is not possible to suggest that the change benefits the changer. Arguing that a person should lose weight so they will live longer is different than asking someone to promise to donate their organs when they die because that will help someone else.

It is trust in the motivations and character of both legal and non-legal authorities (the US Food and Drug Administration, the Centers for Disease Control and Prevention, the Surgeon General) and others in the public health system of regulation that matters most when everyday people as well as organizations responsible for healthy behaviors (for example schools, corporations) are trying to decide whether to accept the decisions and guidance of such authorities. People should not need to feel obligation to obey decisions that are in their own interest, but mistrust of the motivations of public health authorities may lead to suspicion about their recommendations and may undermine the willingness to follow their directives and advice. Therefore, people can be motivated to engage in healthy behaviors and not to engage in unhealthy behaviors by their feelings of responsibility and obligation to government authorities.

The extension of a values-based model to public health and public health law suggests that public health laws and behavioral guidelines are most likely to gain compliance if they are perceived as legitimate. It is therefore important for public health authorities and institutions to consider the factors that shape their legitimacy—and important for health researchers to study them. Further, the role of law can be a facilitative one. If desirable practices for creating and sustaining legitimacy are identified, the legal system can create and implement structures for mandating those practices. Murphy et al. (2021) provide an excellent example of research on legitimacy. Among a sample of Australians, compliance with COVID-19 restrictions was found to be most strongly motivated by normative concerns linked to the duty to support legal authorities; legitimacy mattered more than either self-interest or health concerns in shaping the public's behavior.

Procedural Justice

If public health authorities know that they can benefit from being viewed as legitimate, they need evidence-based guidance as to how they can facilitate such public views. Studies suggest that legitimacy can be built through procedural fairness. Authorities can gain a great deal in terms of legitimacy when they follow clear norms of procedural justice, including impartiality, transparency, and respect for human dignity (Tyler, 2003). Thus, implementing fair procedures as well as providing favorable or fair outcomes can provide a solid basis for establishing system legitimacy with public health authorities. Questions about the extent to which procedural justice is enacted by health authorities, and the effects procedural justice has on health behaviors, constitute an important agenda for legal epidemiology. This section discusses some theoretical and methodological aspects of this agenda.

Elements of Procedural Justice

Procedural justice is the study of people's subjective evaluations of the justice of procedures—whether they are fair or unfair, ethical or unethical, and otherwise in accord with people's standards of fair processes for social interaction and decision making. Subjective procedural justice judgments have been the focus of a great deal of research attention by psychologists because they have been found to be a key influence on a wide variety of important group attitudes and behavior (Lind & Tyler, 1988). In particular, they shape legitimacy (Tyler, 2000).

Procedural justice has been especially important in studies of decision acceptance and rule following, which are core areas of legal regulation. A central point for legal authorities is that people are responsive to evaluations of the fairness of procedures, even when authorities do not provide the outcomes people hoped for. Tyler and Huo (2002) for example, studied people's experiences with the police and courts. In the case of the police, they found that the primary way that people had personal experiences with the police was by calling them for help, or going to court about a problem. However, when people called the police for help, approximately 30% of the time they reported a negative outcome (that is, a problem not solved). From a legitimacy perspective, police inability to help was not a central concern; rather, people evaluated the police by the justice of their procedures for managing the request for help. The same result emerges in situations in which legal authorities are responding to a public request for assistance. People are found to regard the police/judges as legitimate if they believe that the police/judges exercise their authority through fair and impartial means, not by their satisfaction with the outcome (Sunshine & Tyler, 2003a; Tyler, 2006a). Indeed, the evidence suggests that procedural justice judgments are more central to judgments of legitimacy than are such factors as the perceived effectiveness of the police in combating crime, and procedural justice is more important for courts than issues of cost or time to resolution. With all these types of contact, decision favorability was not key. To the extent that people perceive law enforcement officials as legitimate, they are significantly more willing to comply with the law in general (Sunshine & Tyler, 2003a; Tyler, 2006a).

When people indicate that authorities are or are not procedurally fair, what do they mean? Recent discussions identify two key dimensions of procedural fairness judgments: fairness of decision making (voice, neutrality) and fairness of interpersonal treatment (trust, respect) (Blader & Tyler, 2003a, 2003b). Studies suggest that people are influenced by both aspects of procedural justice.

Procedures are mechanisms for making decisions. When thinking about those mechanisms, people evaluate fairness along several dimensions. First, do they have opportunities for input before decisions are made? Second, are decisions made following understandable and transparent rules? Are decisions themselves explained? Third, are decision-making bodies acting neutrally, basing their decisions upon objective information and appropriate criteria, rather than acting out of personal prejudices and biases? Fourth, are the rules applied consistently across people and over time?

Quality of interpersonal treatment is found to be equally important. It involves the manner in which people are treated during a decision-making process. First, are people's rights respected? Second, is their right as a person to be treated politely and with dignity acknowledged, and does such treatment occur? Third, do authorities consider people's input when making decisions, and are decision makers responsive to people's needs and concerns? Finally, do authorities account for their actions by giving honest explanations about what they have decided and why they made their decisions? Do they make clear how they have considered people's arguments and why they can or cannot do as people want? Judgments about the character and motivation of the decision maker—issues of trust in their intentions—is an aspect of interpersonal treatment.

If people only viewed those authorities who make decisions with which they agree as legitimate, it would be difficult for authorities to maintain their legitimacy, insofar as the authorities are required at times to make unpopular decisions and deliver unfavorable outcomes. With state and local health authorities, for example, the effective practice of reducing chronic and fatal illnesses resulting from smoking or second-hand exposure to smoke has involved prohibiting the sale of tobacco products to minors. Mandating people to take actions that require effort, willpower, and potentially enduring pain, or at least lack of benefit, requires that those individuals have a basis for viewing the authority involved as someone who ought to be deferred to and accepted.

Tyler, Mentovich, and Satyavada (2011) examined the role of procedural justice in promoting deference to doctor's recommendations by interviewing patients about their own doctors. They found that the procedural justice of the doctor was a strong predictor of both believing that the doctor had a competent treatment plan and accepting his or her treatment recommendations. The quality of interpersonal treatment was found to be especially important. Further, patients who believe their doctor acted fairly were less likely to indicate that they wanted to change doctors. Mentovich, Rhee, and Tyler (2014) extended the examination of procedural justice to people's health plan choices. They asked people to compare different health care plans that varied along two dimensions: the degree to which people had a choice of doctors and the cost or average life expectancy of the plan. The study found that people choose the high choice plan even when it cost more or offered them on average less expected future life. This emphasizes the degree to which people value choice more than material costs or health gains.

Moderators of Procedural Justice

The underlying assumption behind procedural justice mechanisms is that experiencing just procedures reaffirms people's identity and feelings of status and inclusion within a society (Bradford, Murphy, & Jackson, 2014). This suggests that people need to feel that they are members of a group and that the authorities with whom they deal represent that group for procedural justice to work. An example supporting this argument is provided by an experimental study reported in Smith, Tyler, Huo, Ortiz, and Lind (1998). An experiment was conducted in which University of California, Berkeley, undergraduates were treated disrespectfully by an experimenter who was wearing either a University of California, Berkeley (in group) or a Stanford (out group) sweater. As predicted the self-esteem of participants declined, but only when the experimenter was an in-group authority. Disrespect from an out-group authority had no identify implications. Similarly, Tyler, Lind, Ohbuchi, Sugawara, and Huo (1998) compared cross-cultural to within-cultural negotiations. They found that when people were negotiating with members of their own group procedural justice mattered more than when they were negotiating with a member of a different group. This was equally true for American and Japanese participants. A consequence of this finding is the recognition that it is important to create and build a shared group identify that includes relevant authorities. When that does not happen procedural justice effects are likely to be weaker or nonexistent.

Group identity is a matter of degree. Even people who feel marginal within or alienated from a society may still care about procedural justice, although perhaps to a lesser degree. For example, Murphy, Bradford, Sargeant, and Cherney (2021) found that immigrants in Australia were less identified with law and legal authority than long-term residents. Their degree of identification influenced the degree to which procedural justice shaped cooperation with the police. In the case of COVID-19, McCarthy, Murphy, Sargeant, and Williamson (2021) found that the procedural justice of police treatment influenced compliance even among the most defiant members of Australian society.

Procedural Justice in Organizations

Research in organizational settings suggests a very promising direction for law in motivating healthy behaviors. Such research shows that the manner in which authority is exercised in organizations influences the way people within them feel about themselves, including shaping their feelings of self-esteem and self-worth (Tyler & Blader, 2000). These findings have developed within the psychological literature on procedural justice, but are of obvious relevance to health given the increasing recognition of the effect of workplace hierarchy on the health outcomes of employees (Commission on Social Determinants of Health, 2008).

Studies show that creating procedurally just organizations enhances the physical health of people within those organizations. In a laboratory study, Vermunt and Steensma (2003) examined the influence of procedural justice upon the level of stress participants experienced when involved in a difficult mental task. They used physiological measures of stress and found that fairness mitigated stress levels. Schmitt and Dorfel (1999) studied factory workers and found that procedural justice lowered psychosomatic problems (for example, sick days taken; days at work when the worker "felt sick"). In a similar study of workers in health centers in Finland, Elovainio, Kivimäki, Eccles, and Sinervo (2002) found that procedural justice lowered occupational strain. Meier, Semmer, and Hupfeld (2009) found that lower procedural justice in a sample of employees was linked to higher depressive moods among those with high but unstable self-esteem. Suurd (2009) found that procedural injustice was related to psychological strain in a sample of military personnel. Other studies link procedural justice to mental health (Eib, Bernhard-Oettel, Magnusson Hanson, & Leineweber, 2018; Ndjaboue, Brisson, & Vézina, 2012).

This connection between the procedural justice of organizations and stress among their members is strongly supported by a series of epidemiological studies. Kivimäki, Elovainio, Vahtera, Virtanen, and Stansfeld (2003) studied a sample of 1,786 female hospital employees and found that low procedural justice was linked to higher levels of psychiatric disorders. Kivimäki, Ferrie, Head, and others (2004) studied 10,308 civil servants and found that procedural justice was related to self-reported health. Similarly, Liljegren and Ekberg (2009) found that procedural justice was related to self-reported health in a sample of Swedish workers. Kivimäki, Ferrie, Brunner, and others (2005) found that in a study of 6,442 British civil servants procedural justice was related to coronary health disease. Further, it has been found that procedural justice is linked to smoking, with those who feel unfairly treated 1.4 times as likely to be heavy smokers (Kouvonen et al., 2007); to drinking, with the unfairly treated 1.2 times more likely to be heavy drinkers (Kouvonen, Kivimäki et al., 2008); and to problems with sleeping at night (Heponiemi et al., 2008).

In light of the findings above, important questions emerge for legal epidemiology researchers in relation to how organizations can best promote fair procedures, what particular effects such procedures can have, and whether law should mandate justice within organizations. In their study of mandated justice, for example, Feldman and Tyler (2010) use a combined survey and experimental design to examine whether the influence of fair procedures in a work organization is influenced by whether the decision to create fair procedures is the choice of management or the result of government-mandated rights. Their findings suggest that government-mandated fair workplace procedures have a stronger impact on employee behavior in the workplace and attitudes toward the company. New research is needed to produce evidence on whether mandated procedures have a direct impact on employee health.

Researchers can also explore the question of whether voluntary corporate efforts yield better results than mandated efforts. Research on "new governance" has revealed less of an emphasis on formal legal regulation and more on the voluntary efforts of both civic groups and market-driven business organizations to create and maintain internal procedures for enforcing, among other things, standards of ethics and social responsibility (Braithwaite, 2008; Gunningham, 2007; Lehmkuhl, 2008; Parker, 2002; Shamir, 2008). These new forms of governance highlight the importance of reconsidering the degree to which the state should intervene directly within work organizations by mandating appropriate procedures.

The literature on governance also highlights the idea that procedural justice can occur in two ways. First, people can experience fair procedures when policies are being created. Here the emphasis has been on community participation and allowing community input when policies are being created. Second, the authorities involved in implementing policies can act fairly. It is not enough, for example, to implement a smoking ban using fair procedures. Procedural justice also involves allowing affected parties to participate in discussions about whether there should be rules regulating smoking and what those rules should be.

Measuring Legitimacy and Compliance

Tyler's central work on the concept of legitimacy and compliance and how to measure them is his book titled *Why People Obey the Law* (2006a), which explored the question of why people comply with the law. The research for this book employed a large-scale survey (Tyler, 2009). The questionnaire was administered via telephone in two waves, the first with a random sample of 1,575 Chicago residents and the second with a random sample of 804 citizens who were re-interviewed 1 year later.

This research was focused empirically on peoples' experiences with and attitudes toward the police and the courts as well as peoples' compliance with the law (see Tyler, 2006a, appendix A). Many questions were designed to measure the concept of fairness, such as the following:

Overall, how fair were the procedures used by the police to handle the situation when they stopped you? Were they:

___ Very fair

___ Somewhat fair

__ Somewhat unfair, or

__ Very unfair

__ Do not know (Tyler, 2006a, p. 180).

What emerged both during and after the research for *Why People Obey the Law* is that while having a fixed set of responses is helpful, it is also important not to have yes-or-no questions but rather to use scales so that there is variation in the responses obtained. For example, instead of soliciting a "yes" or "no" answer to the question of "Were the police dishonest," it's more useful for analytical purposes to ask, "Would you say you 'agree strongly,' 'agree,' 'disagree,' or 'disagree strongly'?" Also, breaking scales up into smaller questions can help simplify the response format. For instance, the researcher could ask a question with one of two possible answers (for example, "Is the person honest or dishonest"), and then depending on that answer, ask a follow-up question with scales that measure levels of dishonesty (for example, "very dishonest," "somewhat dishonest") (Tyler, 2009). This allows respondents to make a series of simpler judgments.

Measuring compliance is also challenging and requires appropriate scaling. During the first wave of the Chicago study, it became clear that people did not want to admit to illegal behavior. For example, when asked, "Have you taken inexpensive items from stores without paying for them," all 1,575 respondents indicated "never," suggesting that shoplifting never occurs. Therefore, scaling was introduced to the questionnaire for the second wave to capture not simply whether someone did something wrong or not, but rather if they broke the law "almost never" or "practically almost never," and so on. By differentiating more at the "never" end of the scale it was possible to capture more variance in self-reported behavior.

Overall, measuring peoples' compliance behaviors through self-reporting is limited in that behavior is not directly observed, but it nonetheless remains useful if no direct evidence of behaviors is available. Evidence of compliance behaviors provided by others, including legal authorities, is one way of compensating for this limitation (Tyler, 2009). Tyler, Sherman, Strang, Barnes, and Woods (2007), for example, have used police arrest data to index compliance. Another common, useful technique is asking about one's friends or peers— "How many of your friends use heroin (or shoplift, and so on)?"—and use that indirect measure as an index of the person's own behavior or to more accurately estimate population prevalence. The idea is that when estimating what others are doing they use their own behavior as a guide. And because they are not being asked directly about themselves, self-presentation issues are less salient and responses are more accurate.

Mechanisms Through Which Law Affects Public Health

The roles of procedural justice and legitimacy as mechanisms through which law influences public health are captured in Figure 6.1. Path A captures the behavior of public health authorities toward citizens and groups in terms of the

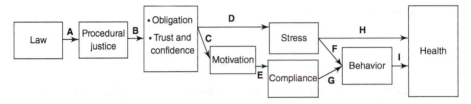

Figure 6.1. Procedural Justice Mechanisms Through Which Law Affects Public Health.

core dimensions of procedural justice (impartiality, transparency, respect, fairness). Such authorities may be individual agency personnel tasked with law enforcement or organizations that have the authority and responsibility to create and sustain healthy corporate environments for workers. Path B represents the legitimacy (obligation, trust, and confidence) of legal authorities, which flows from their procedurally just character, and with the existence of system legitimacy, people are motivated to comply with the law (path C).

The type of motivation captured here is internally driven and value-based (as opposed to instrumentally driven and based on the threat of punishment or the receipt of incentives). On the basis of this motivation, people comply with the law (path E), thereby undertaking the prescribed healthy behaviors (path G) that affect different public health outcomes (fewer deaths, fewer injuries, lower rates of communicable disease) (path I) depending on the area of intervention. We also reviewed studies pointing to the role of procedural justice, trust, and ultimately legitimacy in reducing stress (path D). Less stress can yield direct health benefits such as fewer psychiatric disorders (path H), and it can also lead to healthier behaviors including drinking less often (path F), which in turn contributes to population-level health outcomes (path I) such as lower death rates from impaired driving.

The various paths in this causal diagram point to areas of needed empirical research. While the mechanisms discussed here are theoretically grounded in a range of empirical contexts, including compliance with criminal laws and the associated outcome of public safety, attention should be placed more squarely on factors shaping compliance with public health directives. The diagram presented here provides a framework for conceptualizing research questions in this area, ones that will require the development of appropriate instruments for measuring peoples' experiences with, and attitudes toward, public health authorities.

Conclusion

This chapter has discussed changes in health behavior that are motivated by attitudes and values. This is in contrast to behavior that has to be coerced. Self-regulation is activated when people believe that legal authorities are legitimate, but such legitimacy cannot be assumed. Many public health directives are paternalistic, asking individuals to change behaviors that are personally gratifying and that may pose no direct threat to the health of others. Gaining compliance with them requires legitimacy. That legitimacy could be the legitimacy of science and/or the legitimacy of government. Therefore, failure to build legitimacy with either of these sources of authority not only undermines compliance with a particular law but risks undermining the overall legitimacy of the entire public health system of regulation and advice.

Research on compliance has shown that legal authorities can gain a great deal in terms of legitimacy when they follow clear norms of procedural justice, including impartiality, transparency, and respect for human dignity (Tyler, 2003). Questions about the role of procedural justice in shaping system legitimacy warrant greater attention in legal epidemiology, as do questions about the effects of legitimacy on health behaviors. Public health agencies can attend to procedural fairness and legitimacy not only in the actual enforcement of the law but also in the formulation of behavioral guidance (such as recommended vaccination schedules). The logic model presented here offers a framework for studying law's effect on public health through the mechanisms of procedural justice and legitimacy.

The most relevant empirical evidence on procedural justice as a mechanism for shaping health behaviors comes from studies conducted in organizational settings. A number of studies show that creating procedurally just organizations enhances the physical and mental health of people within those organizations. A key question for legal epidemiology is whether government should mandate the use of fair procedures and the creation of a climate of ethicality in an effort to produce desirable health outcomes within both public and private organizations.

In summary, the law can shape health-related behavior through providing incentives for healthy behavior and sanctions for unhealthy behavior. However, the argument we are making, drawing upon the literature on self-regulation, is that the best approach is to promote favorable attitudes and values, changing what people feel they should do with respect to their health behaviors. This involves creating trust and confidence in health authorities. How precisely this should be done in relation to various health behaviors is an important area of empirical inquiry.

Summary

The effectiveness of behavioral regulation depends in significant part on the willingness of citizens to consent to the commands of legal authorities and to actively cooperate with them. Two values constituting what sociologist Max Weber called "legitimacy" are of particular importance to compliance: the individual's sense of obligation to obey authorities, and his or her sense of trust and confidence in legal authorities. While it is sometimes possible to motivate compliance by creating a risk of punishment for non-compliance, regulating behavior through threats can undermine people's own commitment to norms, rules, and authorities. Voluntary healthy behavior that is motivated by a person's own attitudes and values is superior from a regulatory perspective to behavior that has to be coerced. When values are the driver of behavior, rule adherence does not need to be sustained either by enacting a credible system of surveillance and sanctioning or by developing a way to incentivize desired behaviors.

Legitimacy is a quality that is possessed by an authority, a law, or an institution that leads others to feel obligated to accept its directives. Self-regulatory motivations are activated when people believe that legal authorities are legitimate and they therefore have an obligation to conform to the law, and when people have trust and confidence in those authorities. People who identify with legal authorities and imbue the legal system with legitimacy will voluntarily abide by laws and defer to authorities. Legitimacy can be built through procedural fairness. Procedural justice is the study of people's subjective evaluations of the justice of procedures—whether they are fair or unfair, ethical or unethical, and otherwise in accord with people's standards of fair processes for social interaction and decision making. The two key dimensions of procedural fairness judgments are fairness of decision making (voice, neutrality) and fairness of interpersonal treatment (trust, respect). Robust tools have been developed to measure procedural justice and have been used in important health research.

Further Reading

Tyler, T. R. (2006). *Why people obey the law*. Princeton, NJ: Princeton University Press.

Tyler, T. R., Goff, P., & MacCoun, R. (2015). The impact of psychological science on policing in the United States: Procedural justice, legitimacy, and effective law enforcement. *Psychological Science in the Public Interest, 16*(3), 75–109.

Weber, M. (1968). *Economy and society*. Berkeley, CA: University of California Press.

Chapter 7

Economic Theory

Frank J. Chaloupka   Rosalie Liccardo Pacula

Learning Objectives

- Identify how economic theory intersects with public health law.
- Evaluate effects of economic incentives and disincentives on public health outcomes.
- Examine information failure, externalities, internalities, and market power as they affect a public health problem.

Economics is the study of how society allocates scarce resources. Economic players interact through the supply of and demand for various goods and services. A key assumption of modern economic theory is that individuals are seeking to maximize their own well-being subject to the constraints they face. Individual consumers aim to maximize the satisfaction ("utility," in the language of economics) they gain from consuming goods and services, subject to the prices they face in the market, time constraints, health and/or legal risks, and their own incomes and wealth. Producers aim to maximize the profits they receive from supplying goods and services to the market, subject to the costs of inputs into production, available production technologies, and demand for the products they produce. Under ideal conditions, the result of economic players acting to maximize their own well-being in freely operating markets will be an efficient allocation of scarce resources. When markets are not operating under ideal conditions, laws and regulations can change the relative costs and benefits that influence decisions consumers and producers make and, as a result, lead to an allocation of resources improved from that, which would result from unregulated markets. If the market is operating under ideal conditions, laws and regulations will result in a less optimal allocation of resources compared to that which would result from the free market.

Economics, law, and public health intersect because many markets do not operate under ideal conditions. Instead, there are a variety of "market failures" that lead to an inefficient allocation of resources in a way that creates public health consequences. Economic agents are assumed to have full information and to act rationally when making decisions. Full information about the short- and long-term costs and benefits of consuming or producing some products is often limited, and individuals make choices they later regret. The full costs of consuming or producing are often not borne by those making the consumption or production decisions (negative externalities). Conversely, consumption or production of some goods or services generates benefits that go beyond the individual consumer or producer (positive externalities). Producers benefiting from limited competition due to extensive regulation and/or licensing requirements (barriers to entry) and economies of scale will supply less of a good to the market and charge more for it than would be optimal from a societal perspective. As with full information, the rationality of agents has been shown to be limited, particularly when making decisions that are complex or involve psychological factors, like strong emotions (Kahneman, 2011; Thaler & Sunstein, 2009). When faced with these more difficult situations, agents tend to succumb to status quo bias, framing effects, misperception of risks, and heuristics to make their decision rather than objective factors or information. When such market failures exist, laws and regulations can effectively lead to changes in consumption decisions, production decisions, or both that can lead to a more optimal allocation of resources than would result from the free market.

The public health consequences that result from market failures are enormous. Drug overdose fatalities arise in part from imperfect information about the risks of substances in legal markets and the contents of substances obtained through illicit market (Alpert, Powell, & Pacula, 2018; Pacula & Powell, 2018; Powell & Pacula, 2021). Driven by overdose, unintentional injuries became the third leading cause of death since 2015, at least until the pandemic hit (Ahmad & Anderson, 2021), generating a decline in US life expectancy for the first time in six decades (Case & Deaton, 2020). Other chronic diseases, such as heart disease, cancer, respiratory disease, and diabetes remain leading causes of death and disability in the United States (Ahmad & Anderson, 2021; Heron, 2021), in part a result of lifestyle choices and health behaviors, including smoking, low physical activity, poor nutrition, high blood pressure, and excessive drinking (Mokdad et al., 2018).

Over the past few decades, health economists have made substantial contributions to our understanding of how laws, regulations, and other policies can address the market failures that continue to lead to poor health behaviors and therefore improve public health. Economists have also contributed, through behavioral economics, to a better understanding of how regulations and law might reduce the influence of psychological factors impairing decision-making and improve the context in which people make choices, nudging them to make better decisions when it comes to health behaviors. This chapter introduces the concepts used by economists in this research. It begins by providing a discussion of the economic rationale for government intervention in a variety of markets where individual behaviors lead to public health consequences. This is followed by a discussion of policy interventions that address these market failures, beginning with demand-side approaches to promoting public health through legal interventions and emphasizing the concept of the "full price" of consumption. Legal approaches to addressing the supply side of these markets are then briefly reviewed. Examples of where economic theory and research has helped inform public health law are provided throughout.

Laws, Regulations, and Economic Behavior

Homo Economicus, the informed, rational, and self-interested economic agent (i.e., individual or firm) is at the heart of much of classical economic theory (Persky, 1995). By seeking to maximize their own self-interest subject to constraints, interactions with other economic agents will lead to the efficient allocation of society's scarce resources.

Laws and regulations will alter the conditions under which the economic agent makes these decisions, as illustrated in Figure 7.1. Law can change the information environment by mandating more information of a particular kind or by restricting the flow of other information. Laws can require that the contents of particular products are listed on product packaging, while others can require that packages include standard dosing or warnings about the consequences of consumption. Mass media and other public education campaigns provide information that can alter consumers' perceptions of the relative costs and benefits they receive from consuming a given product, resulting in different consumption choices. Other policies can restrict producers from conveying information by limiting the content of or channels through which they advertise their products or how these products are labeled.

Laws and regulations can influence the choice architecture in which the consumers or producers make decisions, thereby making it easier for agents to make choices that improve their welfare (Thaler & Sunstein, 2009). In the case of public health, applications have been applied in the design of school lunch cafeterias, where healthy food options are placed at the start of a buffet line or at eye level for youth (Metcalfe, Ellison, Hamdi, Richardson, & Prescott, 2020; Skov, Lourenco, Hansen, Mikkelsen, & Schofield, 2013); star ratings on food of high nutritious quality in grocery stores (Rahkovsky, Lin, Lin & Lee, 2013); adding caloric intake on menus (Krieger et al., 2013), and nudging Medicare enrollees to enroll in higher quality health insurance plans (Howell et al., 2017). Laws and regulations supporting such programs and policies effectively seek to retain the individual's opportunity to choose but create a choice environment ("architecture") around the individual that *nudges* them toward healthier behaviors.

Laws and regulations can enhance or constrain the market power of producers or consumers. Antitrust laws aim to prevent producers from gaining significant market power or abusing the market power that they do have. At the

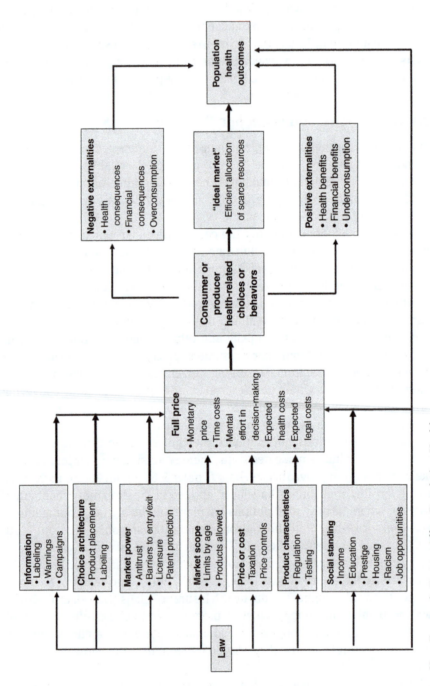

Figure 7.1. How Economic Factors Affect Population Health.

same time, collective bargaining laws allow unions to gain market power that enables them to offset the "monopsony" power that large firms have. By erecting entry barriers that reduce the number of firms in a given market, policies can increase market power for those that are operating in the market. Licensure requirements that establish density standards, for example, will limit the number of firms in a given market, reducing competition from potential entrants and generating market power for those with licenses. In many countries, governments monopolize a variety of product markets, in some places to limit exposure to a product (e.g., for alcoholic beverages), and in others to benefit from efficiencies that can occur due to economies of scale (e.g., tap water, or broadband internet access). Exclusive-territory policies provide market power within a given geographic area while limiting the ability of firms to compete outside of that area.

The scope of a particular market is something else that can be changed via law and regulation. Laws can prohibit some from participating in given markets by setting minimum age requirements for purchase or use of particular products. Likewise, labor laws may set minimum and maximum ages for workers in particular fields. Laws can also alter the characteristics of a product. Some may prohibit various ingredients, while others may mandate certain product safety features.

Laws and regulations can directly alter the prices of a product or key inputs into the production of that product or can affect the costs associated with consuming that product. Excise taxes add to the price consumers pay for products, while subsidies reduce prices. Minimum wage laws raise the labor costs faced by firms, while rent control laws limit the price received by property owners. Tax credits for education reduce the costs of schooling for students and their families. Minimum price laws or bans on quantity discounts raise consumer prices.

The theory that resources will be optimally allocated by the interactions of unfettered supply and demand depends on several key assumptions: that individuals have all of the information that they need to make fully informed choices; that they fully understand and can adequately process this information; that they behave rationally, weighing the short- and the long-run costs and benefits of their decisions; that the individual consumer bears the full costs and receives the full benefits of his or her consumption; that the individual producer likewise bears the full costs and gains the full benefits of producing; and that neither the producer nor the consumer has market power that allows them to influence prices. Of course, absent from these theories of market efficiency is the notion of social equity, or consideration of the initial endowment point ("standing") from which consumers and sellers enter the market for exchange. Greater attention is now being given to the problem of social inequity, with a growing body of RCT, natural experiments, and long-term observational data demonstrating the degree to which income, education, housing, and race influence the economic opportunities, education, and health that individuals experience later in life (Campbell, Conti, Heckman, Moon, Pinto, Pungello, &

Pan, 2014; Chatterji, Kim, & Lahiri, 2014; Chetty, Hendren, Jones, & Porter, 2020; Chetty, Hendren, & Katz, 2016; Chetty, Hendren, Kline, & Saez, 2014; Chetty, Hendren, Lin, Majerovitz, & Scuderi, 2016; Chetty et al., 2017; Cutler and Vogl, 2011; Sanbonmatsu et al., 2011). Similarly, research shows that race, prestige, and housing influence the full cost people face when obtaining or consuming particular goods, for example the legal risk of using illicit drugs (Eckel & Grossman, 2008; Geller & Fagan, 2010; Goel, Rao, & Shroff, 2016), purchase of fresh fruits and vegetables (Cantor et al., 2020; Dubowitz et al., 2015; Powell, Han, & Chaloupka, 2010; Powell, Slater, Mirtcheva, Bao, & Chaloupka, 2007), and health care received (Ayanian, Weissman, Chasan-Taber, & Epstein, 1999; Trivedi, Zaslavsky, Schneider, & Ayanian, 2006; Yearby, 2018). Perfectly competitive markets focused on efficiency alone do a poor job of addressing these various types of inequities (Sen, Sen, Foster, Amartya, & Foster, 1997), which some have argued provides justification for government intervention to redistribute wealth, income, or social opportunities (Feldstein, 2012; Folland, Goodman, & Stano, 2016). Debates continue in the economics literature as to whether income redistribution represents a superior tool to other available policies (e.g., price subsidies, free health insurance) for addressing public health needs, given disincentives such income supports can create. Rebecca Blank (2002) has argued that under certain conditions income redistribution can be an important complement to other policies aimed at addressing social inequities.

Market Failures

Economists refer to situations in which one or more of the key assumptions generating efficiency in perfect competition are violated as market failures, which result in an inefficient allocation of resources. This is where economics, law, and public health intersect. While laws and regulations are adopted for a variety of reasons, including redistribution, the existence of market failures provides an economic rationale for governments to intervene in markets to improve efficiency as well. Examples of market failures and key legal mechanisms for addressing them are described next.

Information Failures

Imperfect or asymmetric information regarding the health risks that result from consuming a variety of products is one market failure that generates considerable public health consequences. Perhaps the clearest example is cigarette smoking. Cigarette smoking in the United States rose rapidly in the first half of the twentieth century and, given the lags between onset of smoking and onset of lung cancer and other diseases caused by smoking, it wasn't until the 1950s that strong evidence linking cigarette smoking to lung cancer first appeared in the scientific literature. Consequently, individuals made decisions to smoke with far from full information about the health risks from smoking. In the decades since, the evidence linking cigarette smoking to an ever-increasing number of diseases has grown, but many individuals continue to underestimate this risk, particularly in low- and middle-income countries. Moreover, many of those who have a general appreciation of these population risks fail to adequately internalize the threat to their own health.

This information failure has been further complicated by information asymmetries among consumers and producers. The release of millions of pages of internal tobacco company documents in various lawsuits provided clear evidence that cigarette companies were aware of these risks and altered product design in a way that alleviated consumers' health concerns while failing to significantly reduce or eliminate these risks. Filtered low tar and nicotine cigarettes were marketed as less harmful but were, in fact, as deadly as the cigarettes that they replaced. Despite the increasing scientific evidence to this effect, many smokers continue to see these as less harmful than full-flavored cigarettes.

Market failures due to imperfect or asymmetric information are further complicated in many markets by the fact that initiation of use for many of these products begins in childhood or adolescence, a time when many are prone to heavily discount the short- and long-term health consequences that result from consumption. For example, past year prevalence rates of nicotine and cannabis vaping doubled between 2017 and 2019, according to data from the Monitoring the Future Survey, with nicotine vaping rates reaching 35.1% of all high school seniors (Miech, Johnston, O'Malley, Bachman, & Patrick, 2019), and past year cannabis vaping rates reaching 20.8% of high school seniors (Miech, Patrick, O'Malley, Johnston, & Bachman, 2020). Data for 2020 show a leveling off at these higher rates for nicotine but continued small increases in adolescent cannabis vaping (Miech et al., 2021). While the scientific evidence examining the long-term health effects of vaping is uncertain at this time, there is growing evidence that use of either substance during adolescence is associated with several negative health outcomes, including greater risk of addiction to each (American College of Pediatricians, 2018; U.S. Department of Health and Human Services, 2012). Moreover, cannabis use during adolescence has been found in a couple of recent studies to be associated with subsequent onset of nicotine and cigarette use (Terry-McElrath, O'Malley, & Johnston, 2020; Weinberger, Zhu, Lee, Xu, & Goodwin, 2021), raising the possibility that long-term gains achieved with reductions of youth smoking may be offset by the latest vaping trend.

Discounting of risk among young people is even further complicated by an under-appreciation of the addictiveness or habitualness of the use of harmful products. Orphanides and Zervos (1995) provide a nice theoretical framework for how "imperfect foresight" can result in many youths experimenting with addictive substances, with some becoming addicted. In their model, the risk of becoming addicted varies among individuals, as do each individual's subjective beliefs about his or her potential to become addicted. As an individual experiments with a potentially addictive substance, this subjective belief is updated through a Bayesian learning process. Those who underestimate their potential for addiction can end up addicted. Thus, rather than the "happy addict" implied by economic models that assume well-informed individuals making rational decisions with perfect foresight (Winston, 1980), individuals who become addicted to substances regret ever having started. Empirical evidence is consistent with this type of "learning and regret," with considerable majorities of adult smokers, for example, wishing that they had never started smoking (Fong, Hammond, Laux et al., 2004) and favoring higher cigarette taxes as such taxes induce them to quit (Gruber & Mullainathan, 2005). Similarly, while only 3% of those smoking daily as high school seniors thought that they would definitely be smoking in 5 years, almost two-thirds were still smoking 7–9 years later (Johnston, O'Malley, Bachman, & Schulenberg, 2011).

Externalities

Externalities occur when individual consumers or producers do not bear the full costs of their consumption or production (negative externalities) or when there are benefits from consumption or production that go beyond the price paid by the individual consumer or the income accrued to the producer (positive externalities). From a societal perspective, when externalities exist, economic agents left to their own devices will generate an inefficient allocation of resources. The inefficiencies that arise in the presence of various externalities create public health consequences.

When there are negative externalities in consumption, there are costs that result from consumption that are not borne by the individual consumer, resulting in greater-than-optimal consumption at a lower-than-optimal price. There are countless examples of negative externalities from individuals' consumption that generate sizable public health consequences. Nonsmokers, for example, experience lung cancers, cardiovascular diseases, and other adverse health effects when exposed to tobacco smoke pollution (Carreras et al., 2019). Innocent bystanders experience violence and/or death caused by excessive alcohol consumption (Cook, 2007) and drug consumption (Dobkin & Nicosia, 2009). Poor diet and low physical activity increase risks of diabetes and obesity, which cause negative externalities on others through higher medical costs paid for by public and private third-party payers (Cawley, 2015).

Negative externalities can also occur in the production of goods, specifically when there are costs to society that are not reflected in the input costs paid by producers. There are numerous examples of air pollution, water pollution, and soil pollution caused by producers of goods who emit various toxins with massive health consequences (Clay, Lewis, & Severnini, 2016; Smit & Heederik, 2017), the costs of which are not considered in their production process nor are they incorporated into the market price of the products sold by them. This leads producers to over produce these goods.

Alternatively, positive externalities in consumption imply that persons other than the individual consumer of a given good or service benefit from that consumption. Positive externalities in consumption lead to under-consumption of a product. One example of a positive externality in consumption is the reduction in the risk of infectious disease to others that results from an individual receiving a vaccination for that disease, which has led to vaccinations being heralded as 1 of the 10 great public health achievements (CDC, 2011b). Early evidence suggests that vaccines for COVID-19 have similarly reduced the spread and severity associated with it (Gupta et al., 2021; Scobie et al., 2021). Thus, the benefits to society are considerably larger than those to the individual. Positive externalities in production occur when a producer does not receive the full benefit of production, resulting in less-than-optimal output at a higher-than-optimal price. Pharmaceutical drugs that reduce the public health burden caused by numerous diseases, such as COVID-19, provide examples of positive externalities in production. A pharmaceutical company concerned that the substantial investment it needs to make in developing a new drug would not be recouped if its competitors could easily copy and market the drug once it hit the market will under-invest in research and development, leading to fewer such drugs being supplied. Investment and/or subsidies provided by the government can increase incentives for such investment.

Health behaviors that create significant public health consequences can also generate sizable financial externalities. The magnitude and persistence of opioid drug overdose deaths, for example, has led not only to 3 years of consecutive declines in US life expectancy recently (Case & Deaton 2017, 2020), but also substantial losses in terms of lost employment (Aliprantis, Fee, & Schweitzer, 2019; Kaestner & Ziedan, 2019); increases in foster care placements and reductions in child welfare (Crowley, Connell, Jones, & Donovan, 2019); and the spread of hepatitis C and other infectious diseases (Powell et al., 2019; Liang & Ward, 2018). All these consequences impose costs on social welfare and social insurance systems.

While many in the public health community focus on the overall economic costs that result from various health behaviors, economists generally distinguish between internal costs (those borne by individual consumers) and external costs (those borne by others). This distinction has important implications for policy. For example, smokers' higher health insurance premiums, greater out-of-pocket costs, and lower wages, at least for the most part, do not constitute a market failure but rather reflect the increased health risks they incur by smoking, their greater use of health care, and the lost productivity that results from the increased absences resulting from diseases caused by smoking. Financial externalities are limited to the lost productivity and costs of treating the consequences of exposure to tobacco smoke pollution among nonsmokers and the costs of treating smoking-attributable diseases in smokers that are paid for through public health insurance programs. Some economists have gone further to look at net external costs, offsetting the increased costs at a point in time with the reductions in social security payments and Medicare spending that result from smokers dying younger than nonsmokers (for example, Manning, 1991).

Internalities

More recent economic models have incorporated the experimental evidence from behavioral economics that imply that much of what have traditionally been considered internal costs are more appropriately treated as "within-person externalities" (Bhargava & Loewenstein, 2015; Herrnstein, Loewenstein, Prelec, & Vaughan, 1993) caused by an individual's failure to fully consider the effect of current behavior on future outcomes, thereby imposing external costs on oneself (for example, Gruber & Köszegi, 2008). These "internalities" result from at least two factors: the time inconsistency inherent in individual's preferences, and systematic biases that occur when people make psychologically difficult choices.

Traditional economic models assume that individuals exponentially discount the future costs and benefits of their consumption decisions, implying that their decisions will be consistent over time. Behavioral economic experiments, however, demonstrate that preferences are not consistent over time and that individuals are conflicted between their desire for short-run gratification and their recognition of long-term consequences. These more recent models allow for hyperbolic discounting of future costs and benefits, producing a more accurate depiction of how individuals actually behave, and capturing the conflict between short-run gratification and long-run regret reflected in many health behaviors. In these models, the long-run consequences to the individual that result from unhealthy choices in the short run can be viewed as external to that individual's future self. This new approach has significant implications for public health policies in that it implies greater scope for government intervention than implied by traditional models. For example, Gruber and Köszegi (2008) show that on the basis of this approach, optimal cigarette taxes could be 20 or more times higher than they would be using traditional economic models.

Ongoing developments in behavioral economics have also acknowledged people's cognitive limitations when faced with complex or psychologically burdensome choices. Founded on the principles of prospect theory developed by Kahneman and Tversky (1979), these models assume economic agents behave in a manner more consistent with *bounded rationality*, in that they tend to unconsciously fall back on heuristics, framing, loss aversion, and reference points to make cognitively difficult decisions. Richard Thaler and Cass Sunstein (2009) provided numerous examples of how very small changes in the choice architecture facing individuals in these situations can nudge them to make healthier choices, such as placing leafy green vegetables at the start of the buffet line in school lunch cafeterias and replacing sweets at the checkout counter with fresh fruit. A number of recent efforts have been undertaken to integrate these sorts of nudges into broader policymaking (Matjasko, Cawley, Baker-Goering, & Yokum, 2016). In the case of public health, applications have been applied in the use of star ratings on food of high nutritious quality in grocery stores (Cawley et al., 2015; Rahkovsky et al., 2013); adding caloric intake on menus (Krieger et al., 2013), and improving the quality of health insurance plans in Medicare (Howell et al., 2017). The evidence on the effectiveness of some of these nudges on broad population behaviors is limited (Ledderer, Kjær, Madsen, Busch, & Fage-Butler, 2020; Metcalfe et al., 2020; Skov et al., 2013), in part due to lack of consideration to the mechanisms leading to the poor health behaviors in particular instances as well as cultural sensitivities to nudging (Ledderer et al., 2020). However, the idea of using public health law to influence choice architecture to nudge healthier choices remains a popular notion in that such interventions overcome the problems caused by bounded rationality, reducing the influence of emotions, impulsiveness, environment, decision fatigue, and other circumstance that cause individuals to make unhealthy choices, while maintaining the individual's choice.

Market Power

Economists consider perfectly competitive markets to be optimal in that these lead to the most efficient allocation of resources—one in which the marginal benefits from consuming are equated to the marginal costs of producing. When producers are faced with more limited competition, they are said to have market power. This market power allows them to charge higher prices than would result in a more competitive market, while less is produced and consumed.

While ideal in theory, perfectly competitive markets rarely exist in the real world; some degree of market power is inevitable, and the extent of this market power can have public health implications. For example, in the pharmaceutical industry, some have argued that the branding of prescription drugs and the extensive direct-to-consumer marketing of these drugs results in a market failure by creating perceptions among consumers that comparable, less costly generic drugs are not a good substitute for the branded drug (for example, Institute of Medicine Committee on the Assessment of the US Drug Safety System, Baciu, Stratton, & Burke, 2007).

Policy Interventions to Address Market Failures

When considering laws and other policies that would reduce the public health consequences of market failures such as those just described, economists distinguish between "first best" and "second best" interventions (Jha, Musgrove, Chaloupka, & Yurekli, 2000). First-best interventions are those that narrowly target the market failure at issue and do not have broader effects. For example, mandating nutrition labeling on packaged foods and beverages is a way of providing consumers with information to make better, informed choices on the basis of a product's caloric, fat, and nutrient content.

However, a one-to-one correspondence between market failures and interventions does not always exist, or sometimes the first-best intervention that does exist fails to reach key populations. In these cases, second-best interventions, which typically take a blunter approach and have broader effects, may be more effective. Policies such as taxes and subsidies that alter prices of healthier and less healthy options are perhaps the best examples of a highly effective, second-best intervention.

Laws, regulations, and other policies targeting market failures that generate significant public health consequences address failures that occur on both the demand side and the supply side of the market. This section provides an overview of key policy domains and provides examples in which economic research has played an important role in policy development and implementation.

Demand-Side Policies

When it comes to public health laws that target the demand side of the market, economists emphasize the concept of *full price* as the mechanism through which these policies influence health-related behaviors and their consequences. Full price includes not just the monetary cost of a product but also the other costs associated with obtaining and using that product. Particularly important among these other costs are time costs and the potential health and legal consequences of consumption.

EXCISE TAXES

In *An Inquiry into the Nature and Causes of the Wealth of Nations*, the father of modern economics Adam Smith (1776) wrote, "Sugar, rum, and tobacco are commodities which are nowhere necessaries of life, which are become objects of almost universal consumption, and which are therefore extremely proper subjects of taxation." Smith was focused on the revenue-generating potential of taxes, but in recent years it has become clear that taxes are also a highly effective policy for improving public health. Pigou (1962) was the first to suggest that levying taxes on products that generated negative externalities in consumption would improve economic efficiency. However, conventional wisdom long held that consumption of harmful, addictive substances such as tobacco, alcohol, and other drugs would be unresponsive to the changes in prices resulting from taxes and other factors. Extensive economic research conducted over the past few decades, however, clearly demonstrates that higher taxes and prices lead to significant improvements in public health by reducing the use of harmful products—even addictive substances. Given the huge public health burden it causes, much of the economic research has focused on cigarette smoking and other tobacco use, showing that higher tobacco product taxes and prices lead adult tobacco users to quit, keep former users from restarting, prevent initiation and uptake among young people, and lead to reductions in consumption by those who continue to consume (International Agency for Research on Cancer [IARC] & World Health Organization, 2011). Effects of higher taxes and prices on overall cigarette smoking in the United States over the past several decades is illustrated in Figure 7.2.

Several studies go further in showing that higher tobacco taxes, because of declines in tobacco use that result from them, lead to reductions in the public health and economic consequences of tobacco use (IARC & World Health Organization, 2011). The extensive evidence base demonstrating the effectiveness of tobacco taxes in reducing tobacco use has contributed to nearly every state and the federal government increasing their cigarette and other tobacco taxes over the past two decades, with average state cigarette taxes rising nearly fivefold since 1990, while the federal tax has increased more than sixfold.

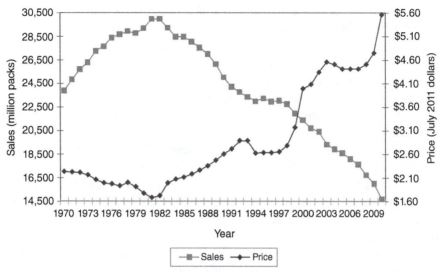

Figure 7.2.   Cigarette Prices and Cigarette Sales, United States, 1970–2010.

Source: Tax Burden on Tobacco, Bureau of Labor Statistics, and author's calculations.

Similarly, numerous studies have found that increases in alcoholic beverage prices that result from higher alcoholic beverage excise taxes reduce the prevalence, frequency, and intensity of drinking (Cook, 2007; Wagenaar, Salois, & Komro, 2009). Additional research shows that higher taxes and prices improve public health by reducing the consequences of excessive alcohol use, including motor vehicle traffic crashes and other injuries, liver cirrhosis and other alcohol attributable mortality, violence and other crime, and risky sex and sexually transmitted disease rates (Wagenaar, Tobler, & Komro, 2010; Xu & Chaloupka, 2011). Despite this evidence and in contrast to the sharp rise in tobacco taxes observed over the past two decades, average alcoholic beverage taxes have declined after accounting for inflation, contributing to increases in drinking and its consequences (Xu & Chaloupka, 2011; Xuan, Chaloupka, Blanchette, Nguyen, Heeren, Nelson, & Naimi, 2015).

The public health success with tobacco excise taxes, coupled with increased recognition of the obesity epidemic in the United States, has increased interest in using taxes as a policy tool for improving diet by reducing consumption of high-calorie, low-nutrient-density foods and beverages. Much of the debate to date has focused on sugar-sweetened beverages, given their relatively high levels of consumption, evidence that their consumption contributes to weight gain, their low or no nutritional value, and economic research demonstrating that beverage consumption responds to price (Chaloupka, Powell, & Chriqui, 2011; Dubois, Farmer, Girard, & Peterson, 2007). Currently, most states tax these beverages under their sales tax systems, with a few states levying small excise or similar taxes. However, existing taxes are small, and sugar-sweetened beverages are taxed the same as artificially or unsweetened beverages. As a result, existing economic research finds that existing taxes have little to no impact on weight outcomes; estimates from some studies, however, do indicate that more significant taxes (for example, one or two cents per ounce) would likely lead to population-level reductions in obesity (Powell & Chriqui, 2011). Studies of tobacco and alcohol demand that account for the addictive aspects of consumption conclude that the long-run impact of tax and price increases is greater than the short-run impact. In general, and consistent with economic theory, studies that have looked at the differential impact of taxes and prices on population subgroups find that young people, less-educated populations, and those on low incomes are relatively more responsive to price. With respect to cigarette smoking, for example, estimates suggest that youth smoking is two to three times more sensitive to price than is adult smoking. The finding that lower socioeconomic groups respond more to price is particularly important in the context of the more recent economic modeling that allows for time-inconsistent preferences described earlier. Specifically, it implies that low-income populations benefit the most from the self-control that results from higher taxes so that these taxes are progressive, rather than regressive as implied by conventional models (Gruber & Köszegi, 2008).

Finally, nearly all estimates of the price elasticity of overall demand for tobacco products, alcoholic beverages, and sugar-sweetened beverages indicate that demand is in the inelastic range, implying that a given price increase leads to a less-than-proportional reduction in aggregate consumption. This, combined with the fact that taxes account for only a portion of prices, implies that increases in taxes on these products will generate significant new revenues in the short-to-medium term. Some states, particularly with respect to tobacco, have earmarked a portion of tax revenues to support some of their other prevention, treatment, and control efforts, adding to the public health benefits of higher taxes.

SUBSIDIES

Increasing the consumption of products that improve public health can be accomplished by reducing prices of these products through subsidies. Given costs associated with their implementation however, subsidies to promote healthier behaviors have not been as widely used as taxes have been to discourage unhealthy consumption. Nevertheless, some governments do use subsidies to promote public health, typically targeting them to narrow segments of the population. Perhaps the best examples are the various food assistance programs run by the US Department of Agriculture aimed at preventing food insecurity and its consequences, including the Supplemental Nutrition Assistance Program (SNAP); the Special Supplemental Nutrition Program for Women, Infants, and Children (WIC); and the National School Lunch and Breakfast Programs. More recently, in efforts to promote healthier diets and curb obesity, some states and localities have begun experimenting with additional subsidies within these programs that further lower the prices of fruits, vegetables, and other healthier options. Limited economic research indicates that reductions in the prices of fruits and vegetables lead to increases in their consumption and at the same time result in healthier weight outcomes in at least some populations, suggesting that efforts to expand these subsidies may be an effective approach for reducing obesity (Powell & Chriqui, 2011).

Experimental evidence, however, raises some questions about the effectiveness of subsidies, particularly relative to taxation, to improve diet and reduce obesity. Using an experimental grocery store selling widely purchased foods and beverages, Epstein et al. (2010) found that taxing less-healthy products led to reductions in purchases of these products, overall calories purchased, and proportion of fat purchased. In contrast, subsidies on healthier products, while increasing purchases of these products, led to increased purchases of less-healthy products as well, resulting in an increase in overall calories purchased while not improving the overall nutrient composition of foods purchased, suggesting that subsidies would be ineffective in reducing obesity. While a clearly artificial setting that forced participants to spend the savings they accrued on the subsidized product on other items in the experimental store rather than on other necessities, this does suggest that subsidies will likely have a smaller overall effect than taxes, given the income effect created by the subsidy.

Tax Credits and Deductions

Income tax credits and deductions are another tax policy that can be used to reduce the price of healthy behaviors in a way that promotes public health. For example, a recent paper by von Tigerstrom et al. (2011) describes the national and provincial income tax credits introduced in Canada that are designed to promote physical activity. Credits are provided that offset the costs of enrolling in various organized physical fitness, sports, and other recreational programs, as well as for the costs of public transit. While little empirical evidence exists on effects of these credits, the authors nicely describe why such credits are unlikely to have population-level effects on activity and obesity. Among the factors they note are the lag of a year or more between the time when costs are incurred and the benefit is received, the modest size of the credit relative to the costs of the programs it covers, the likelihood that it will be largely taken advantage of by those already enrolled in programs rather than increasing participation in these programs, and the likelihood that many new program participants will simply be substituting from other forms of physical activity to activity in programs covered by the tax credit.

Other Pricing Policies

Governments have a variety of other policy options for manipulating prices in a way that promotes public health. Many states, for example, have adopted laws setting a minimum retail price for cigarettes (CDC, 2010). If the minimum price were set higher than the prices that would otherwise result from a freely operating market, cigarette smoking and its consequences could be reduced. In practice, however, these laws appear to have little effect on cigarette prices, with prices in the states that have adopted them similar to prices in states without them, after accounting for differences in state cigarette taxes. The one exception is the few states that include price promotions in their policies, keeping price-reducing promotions from lowering the price below the minimum.

Similarly, as a part of the three-tier system states adopted for alcohol distribution following the repeal of prohibition, a number of states implemented policies setting minimum prices or requiring minimum markups on alcoholic beverages at various points in the distribution chain, while others banned quantity discounts at the wholesale level. One result of these policies is higher retail prices for alcoholic beverages which, given the evidence discussed, will result in reductions in harmful drinking and its consequences (Chaloupka, 2004). These policies, however, have come under increasing attack in recent years, given the limits they place on competition, with some states repealing them and court rulings in others invalidating them, despite their benefits for population health.

Policies like these, while indirectly raising prices and reducing consumption of targeted products, are likely to have smaller effects than tax policies that directly increase prices. The revenue generated from tax increases goes to governments, some of which use these revenues to support programs that add to the public health benefits of the tax. In contrast, policies that set higher-than-free-market-level prices generate additional profits for those involved in manufacturing and distribution of those products. These additional profits can be used to support increased marketing and other efforts that increase demand, partially offsetting the reductions in consumption that result from the higher prices.

TIME COSTS

Policies that raise the full price of consumption by adding time or inconvenience can similarly reduce consumption in a way that improves public health. For example, comprehensive smoke-free policies that ban smoking in private workplaces increase the cost of smoking by requiring smokers to leave their workplace and go outdoors to smoke, adding both time and inconvenience, particularly in inclement weather. Growing evidence clearly shows that comprehensive smoke-free policies are effective in reducing both adult and youth smoking while reducing nonsmokers' exposure to tobacco smoke pollution, directly addressing one of the externalities caused by smoking (IARC & World Health Organization, 2009).

PERCEIVED HEALTH COSTS

As discussed earlier, imperfect or asymmetric information creates a market failure that can have a negative effect on public health. When clear science is available regarding real health risks, governments can address information failures by adopting policies that disseminate information on the health impact of various products or behaviors or by limiting producers' ability to spread inaccurate or unsupported information about the health benefits of their products. Some of these options are highly cost-effective, given their low cost of implementation and broad reach. Others are costly but still cost-effective, given the effects of the information on behavior. Still others have proven to be relatively cost-ineffective, given their high costs and lack of demonstrated effect.

How effective and cost-effective these information interventions are depends on the type of information provided, the channels used to provide that information, and the audience being targeted.

Mandating the provision of information on product packaging, advertising, or elsewhere is one relatively low-cost approach to addressing information failures. For example, requiring health warning labels on all cigarette packages provides information about the harms that can result from smoking. In the United States, however, these labels have had little or no impact on smoking, given that the labels are not that visible and the information provided on them is relatively well known. International experiences, however, provide more support for the potential of pack warnings to reduce smoking. The International Tobacco Control Policy Evaluation Project's (ITCPEP) (2009) review of the evidence on warning labels produced several clear conclusions, including that pictorial warning labels are more effective than text-only warnings in raising and sustaining awareness about the risks of tobacco use; larger and more comprehensive (for example, more rotating messages) warning labels increase knowledge about the harms from tobacco use; and pictorial warnings increase motivation to quit, including strengthening quit intentions and increasing the likelihood of a quit attempt. Larger, graphic warning labels of this type will soon be coming to the United States as a result of a mandate by the Food and Drug Administration (FDA).

Alternatively, governments can limit the provision of potentially misleading information that leads to reduced risk perceptions. For example, there is considerable evidence that the use of misleading descriptors on tobacco product packaging and advertising (for example, light, low tar, mild) leads some users to perceive some products as less harmful to health or less addictive than others, and to view these products as alternatives to quitting. In 2010, the FDA implemented a ban on the use of these descriptors in the United States. However, such bans may not go far enough, as tobacco companies have adapted to the ban on descriptors by using colors in their product names or packaging to suggest similar concepts, leading some tobacco control professionals to call for "plain" or "generic" packaging that would eliminate all brand-related imagery.

Governments can go further and limit or prohibit a variety of advertising and other marketing efforts that can similarly distort risk perceptions, although how far such policies can go is questionable, given First Amendment protections of free speech in the United States, which have been expanded by the courts in recent years to include commercial speech. To date, most such efforts have been voluntary, industry-initiated limits that aim to reduce children's exposure, such as the Children's Food and Beverage Advertising Initiative (CFBAI) that aims to reduce television advertising of less healthy foods and beverages during children's programming. Given the narrow focus of the CFBAI on children's programming, there has been little improvement in the nutritional quality of the products youth are seeing advertised on television, suggesting that such voluntary initiatives have little public health impact (Powell, Schermbeck, Szczypka, Chaloupka, & Braunschweig, 2011).

Alternatively, public education campaigns can be implemented to raise awareness of the harms from consumption of tobacco, alcohol, other drugs, and other products, or to raise awareness of the benefits of healthier behaviors such as physical activity. These can take many forms, from school-based education programs aimed at influencing youth behavior to large-scale, mass-media campaigns that target broader audiences and that can influence social norms. A mix of such efforts has been widely implemented for tobacco, with comparable, albeit more limited efforts targeting other health behaviors. Evidence is mixed with respect to the effectiveness of school-based programs in promoting healthier youth behavior. For example, Thomas and Perera's (2006) comprehensive review of school-based tobacco education programs found that some programs had short-term but not sustained effects and that the largest and most rigorous intervention reviewed produced no evidence of a long-term effect on smoking behavior. School-based programs that have been found to be successful in the short term tend to emphasize the role of social influences and development of specific skills to resist these influences; such programs are most effective when implemented as part of a more comprehensive strategy that includes control policies and broader education efforts. In contrast, mass-media campaigns that use a variety of communications channels (including television, radio, print, billboards, and the Internet) have repeatedly been shown to reduce tobacco use (National Cancer Institute [NCI], 2008).

EXPECTED LEGAL COSTS

Policies that raise the expected legal costs of engaging in a particular behavior will add to the full price, reducing the likelihood and frequency of engaging in that behavior if enforced (Becker & Stigler, 1974). Economic theories of crime emphasize two key factors that influence expected legal costs: the probability of being caught and convicted and the swiftness and severity of the penalty imposed (see Chapter 5) (Becker, 1968; Cook, Machin, et al., 2012). Increasing either factor raises the expected legal costs and, as a result, reduces targeted behaviors and their public health consequences. The legal costs could apply to producers and/or sellers (covered below) but are frequently applied to consumers of both legally regulated consumption goods and illicit goods.

Policies targeting drinking and driving are good examples of laws that raise anticipated legal costs in a way that promotes public health and that addresses the related negative externalities. Policies implementing sobriety checkpoints and breath testing and other efforts to detect drunk drivers raise the probability of detection, while lowered *per se* illegal blood alcohol content laws increase the probability of conviction. Policies that specify mandatory minimum fines or jail terms can raise expected penalties, while administrative license revocations increase the swiftness of the penalty. Extensive research by economists and other social scientists has demonstrated that these types of laws, particularly those that involve swift and certain penalties (Midgette, Kilmer, Nicosia, & Heaton, 2021; Wagenaar & Maldonado-Molina, 2007), have reduced the likelihood of drinking and driving and the traffic crashes that result from it, and, as a result, have improved public health.

However, there is also a growing literature that suggests that there is a downside to using legal costs as a way of raising the full price of unhealthy behavior. It is clear in the case of drug laws, for example, that these policies have disproportionately targeted people of color (Geller & Fagan, 2010; Tonry, 1994). Moreover, it is frequently argued that illicit markets allow the sale of less safe consumer products due uncertain quality (Galenianos, Pacula, & Persico, 2012). The health risks associated with criminalization are not limited to drugs. Several studies have found that the criminalization of other behaviors, in particular prostitution, can generate significant health risks in terms of the spread of sexually transmitted diseases (Cameron, Seager, & Shah, 2021; Immordino & Russo, 2015), thus imposing an even larger burden on already marginalized populations.

Supply-Side Policies

Laws, regulations, and other policies targeting the supply side of the market also have considerable potential to influence public health. These policies work to increase supply and to reduce the monetary and time costs of a given product, leading to increased consumption, while those that restrict supply work in the opposite direction, resulting in a higher full price and reduced consumption.

SUPPLY CONSTRAINTS

Policies that constrain supply can take many forms, from outright prohibition to efforts to control distribution through licensing, legal sanctions, and regulation. Some efforts are broad-based, such as the short-lived Eighteenth Amendment, which banned the manufacture, distribution, and transportation of alcoholic beverages or the current policies that make sale and distribution of a wide variety of drugs illegal. Others can be more narrowly focused, such as bans on the sale of alcohol to those under 21 years of age and the increasingly prevalent restrictions on the sale of at least some sugar-sweetened beverages in schools. The number of outlets selling a particular product can be restricted by requiring a license to operate and restricting the number of licenses available, as many jurisdictions do with alcoholic beverages. Similarly, the location of outlets can be limited through zoning laws that prohibit certain types of establishments in residential areas or near schools. In the case of alcoholic beverages, some states further constrain supply by monopolizing the wholesale and, in some cases, retail distribution of some beverages.

These types of supply constraints ultimately affect consumption of targeted products through their effects on several aspects of full price. Those that limit the number or location of outlets raise the time costs associated with consumption by reducing physical access. Those that prohibit the sale or distribution of various products can add to the expected legal costs. By reducing competition, constraints on supply result in higher prices. Numerous studies by economists, social scientists, public health researchers, and others have shown that constraints on supply, by increasing full price, reduce consumption and associated public health consequences.

However, at least some policies that constrain supply can create other health, social, and economic problems, in addition to the desired impact in reducing demand and its public health benefits. These consequences result from the profit opportunities created by supply constraints. This is most apparent in the markets for illicit drugs, in which high profits from the sale and distribution of these drugs result in considerable violence as existing suppliers try to protect their position and new players try to gain a foothold (Grogger & Wilils, 2000). However, the unintended consequences of supply constraints have also been seen recently in restrictions on prescription opioids through medical channels, which caused many legitimate medical consumers in need of pain relief to seek alternatives through illicit markets (Alpert et al., 2018; Powell, Alpert, & Pacula, 2019). Thus, the actual benefit of some supply restrictions is much debated.

SUPPLY STIMULI

Finally, there are a variety of laws that seek to increase the supply of some goods and services to improve public health. By increasing supply, time costs are reduced and increased competition can lower prices, thereby increasing use. Various supply-side policies are being employed, for example, in efforts to promote healthier eating and increased activity to reduce obesity. Communities are offering tax incentives and changing zoning policies to attract supermarkets and other stores offering a greater variety of higher-quality, lower-priced fruits, vegetables, and other healthier foods and beverages in food deserts—neighborhoods where residents have little or no access to healthier options. Similar approaches are being used to attract physical fitness clubs and other establishments offering sport and recreational opportunities. Others are requiring or investing in changes to the built environment that increase the venues in which their residents can be active, from local park and recreation facilities to increased presence of sidewalks and trails.

Other laws aim to stimulate the supply of new drugs to promote public health by treating a variety of non-infectious diseases and preventing the spread of infectious diseases. Particularly important is patent protection afforded to producers who develop new drugs in exchange for disclosing the science behind it. By granting monopoly control over the distribution of a drug for a limited period of time, patents generate profits that offset the research and development costs that led to the new discovery. At the same time, the information disclosed as part of the patent increases the likelihood of additional advances.

Measurement Issues

Much of the economic analysis of public health law focuses on how law alters the full price of health-related behaviors. Consequently, developing measures of full price is central to economic analysis of these behaviors. Some aspects of full price are relatively easy to measure, while others can be more challenging.

Monetary prices of products that are legally sold are readily available in various databases. Particularly useful are the scanner-based databases that record the monetary prices of all transactions, along with detailed information on characteristics of products and various price-reducing promotions. Prices for some products can also be derived from consumer expenditure survey data, directly obtained in surveys of individuals or collected observationally at the point of sale. For products subjected to excise taxes, the taxes themselves can be a good proxy for price in the absence of significant geographic differences in the costs of production and distribution, as in the case of cigarettes or alcoholic beverages. Prices for illegal products are more challenging to collect and are subject to considerable variation depending on the quantity and quality of the product. Nevertheless, economists have tried to develop price measures for illegal products, most notably illicit drugs, on the basis of information collected from undercover purchases and seizures, as well as from individual self-reporting (Caulkins, 2007; Dobkin & Nicosia, 2009).

The time costs of acquiring or consuming a good are another key component of full price. For legally available products, economists often use measures of outlet density as a proxy for time costs involved in acquiring the good, with greater physical density reflecting lower costs of obtaining a given product. For example, many economic analyses of drinking and its consequences control for alcohol outlet density, which can vary considerably across jurisdictions depending on differences in alcohol control policies. Others will use measures derived from questions about perceived availability collected in surveys, particularly for illegal products. The time spent consuming a good is not something that has received as much attention, and may be more difficult to measure given confounding with the social context with which a good is used (e.g. drinking alcohol at home versus drinking at a bar or pub).

Expected health costs are a more challenging component of full price to measure. Economic time-series studies of health behaviors often use indicators of health "shocks" as proxies for new information about the health consequences of a particular behavior. Many economic time-series studies of cigarette demand, for example, included indicators for things such as the release of the 1964 Surgeon General's report and televised advertising about the health consequences of smoking broadcast under the Fairness Doctrine in the late 1960s. More recent studies have tried to capture exposure to mass-media counter advertising campaigns and other public education campaigns, with exposure varying both cross-sectionally and over time. For example, exposure to campaigns that highlight the consequences of illicit drug use is assessed using Nielsen data on gross or targeted rating points measuring potential exposure to the televised advertising that is a key part of these campaigns. Still others use measures of perceived harm obtained from various surveys.

Economic theories of crime provide a nice foundation for developing measures of expected legal costs (see Chapter 5). These theories emphasize the importance of the risks of being caught and convicted, along with the swiftness and severity of the sanctions levied upon conviction. Economic analysis of the effects of drunk driving policies, for example, capture these multiple dimensions of expected legal costs with indicators for policies such as preliminary breath test laws (that increase the probability of arrest), *per se* illegal BAC laws (that raise the probability of conviction), administrative license sanctions (that impose relatively swift sanctions), and mandatory minimum penalty laws (that can increase the severity of the sanctions).

Conclusion

Economic theory provides a helpful framework for assessing effects of a number of public health laws. It highlights market failures that exist in the markets for a variety of goods and services, the use of which have considerable implications for population health. Information failures lead to overconsumption of products such as tobacco, alcohol, and sugar-sweetened beverages, resulting in many health, economic, and social consequences. Other information failures result in under-consumption of products such as fruits and vegetables, condoms, and smoking cessation services that, if consumption were increased, would improve public health. Similarly, use of many products can have harmful effects on others, while use of other products can create benefits among those that go beyond the individual consumer. Market failures create a clear economic rationale for governments to intervene through the use of laws, regulations, and other policies so as to minimize the inefficiencies that result and, by doing so, to improve public health.

Economic theory provides guidance on the types of policies likely to be effective in addressing market failures and in improving public health. The key economic mechanism through which these policies work is by affecting the full price of a behavior. Policies that increase the full price of unhealthy behaviors or reduce the full price of healthier behaviors have the potential to significantly improve public health. Particularly important are policies that directly influence prices of various goods and services, such as taxes on unhealthy products and subsidies for healthier options. Other interventions that raise time costs associated with obtaining and consuming, alter perceived health consequences and benefits of consumption, and raise the expected legal costs of consuming can also change behaviors in a way that improves public health. Laws that create incentives for increased supply of goods or services with public health benefits, thereby lowering the prices and the time costs of using them, can similarly improve the public's health.

Summary

Economics is the study of how society allocates scarce resources. Modern economic theory rests on the assumption that individuals seek to maximize their own well-being, subject to the constraints they face. Under ideal conditions, in freely operating markets, this will result in an efficient allocation of scarce resources. Economics, law, and public health intersect because many markets do not operate under ideal conditions. Instead, there are a variety of "market failures" leading to an inefficient allocation of resources—and negative public health consequences.

Market failures include imperfect information and informational asymmetries, negative and positive externalities, time inconsistencies in individual preferences (internalities), and excessive market power. Law can address market failures by changing the relative costs and benefits that influence the decisions consumers and producers make. Law can also

- Change the information environment by mandating or restricting information;

- Create or constrain the market power of producers or consumers;

- Change the scope of a market by prohibiting participation by certain purchasers, certain producers, or certain products;

- Alter the characteristics of a product, the prices of a product, key inputs into the production of that product, or the costs associated with consuming that product.

Laws targeting market failures that generate significant public health consequences address failures that occur on both the demand side and the supply side of the market. On the demand side of the market, economists emphasize the concept of full price as the mechanism through which these policies influence health-related behaviors and their consequences. Full price includes not just the monetary cost but other costs associated with obtaining and using a product. The experience of excise taxes on cigarettes and alcohol illustrates the potential for impact. Subsidies, tax credits and tax deductions, and various other mechanisms may also be used to influence consumption decisions. Policies that raise the full price of consumption by adding time, inconvenience, or expected legal costs associated with the behavior can similarly reduce consumption in a way that improves public health.

Supply-side policies use economic levers to increase the supply of healthy products and decrease the supply of unhealthy ones. Policies that constrain supply can take many forms, from prohibition to efforts to control distribution through licensing, legal sanctions, and other approaches. Supply stimuli used in public health include tax incentives and zoning changes. These types of supply constraints or stimuli ultimately affect consumption of targeted products through their impact on several aspects of full price. Measures of full price are essential to economic analysis of legal interventions in public health. The role of economic structures in creating inequities in income, education, and access to the broad range of social opportunities necessary for optimum health and well-being has recently begun to gain renewed attention and deserves to be an increasingly important focus of legal epidemiologists and economists interested in discovering effective ways to improve population health.

Further Reading

Chaloupka, F. J., Tauras, J. A., & Grossman, M. (2000). The economics of addiction. In P. Jha & F. J. Chaloupka (Eds.), *Tobacco control in developing countries* (pp. 106–130). Oxford, UK: Oxford University Press.

Cook, P. J. (2007). *Paying the tab: The costs and benefits of alcohol control*. Princeton, NJ: Princeton University Press.

Gruber, J., & Kőszegi, B. (2008). *A modern economic view of tobacco taxation*. Paris: International Union Against Tuberculosis and Lung Disease.

Jha, P., Musgrove, P., Chaloupka, F. J., & Yurekli, A. (2000). The economic rationale for intervention in the tobacco market. In P. Jha & F. J. Chaloupka (Eds.), *Tobacco control in developing countries* (pp. 153–174). Oxford, UK: Oxford University Press.

Matjasko, J. L., Cawley, J. H., Baker-Goering, M. M., & Yokum, D. V. (2016). Applying behavioral economics to public health policy: illustrative examples and promising directions. *American Journal of Preventive Medicine, 50*(5), S13–S19.

Chapter 8

The Theory of Triadic Influence

Mark B. Schure   Kazi Faria Islam   Brian R. Flay

Learning Objectives

- Identify and describe diverse behavioral mechanisms by which laws and regulations influence population health behavior.
- Illustrate, using the theory of triadic influence, how a specific public health law may influence institutional, social, and personal behavior.
- Illustrate effects of law-related social media dissemination in altering health-related behavior.
- Apply measures of social psychological and sociological constructs in evaluations of public health laws.

Social psychology has played a central role in both describing and predicting health behaviors, and those behaviors are related to a range of important health outcomes (Flay, Snyder, & Petraitis, 2009; Glass & McAtee, 2006; Jolls, Sunstein, & Thaler, 1998; Petraitis, Flay, & Miller, 1995). Public health increasingly has acknowledged the important effects of laws and regulations in improving population health (Burris, Wagenaar, Swanson et al., 2010; Wagenaar & Burris, 2013). Laws and regulations affecting sanitation infrastructure, food safety, and immunizations historically have had dramatic positive effects on reducing communicable diseases (Cutler & Miller, 2004; Gostin, Burris, & Lazzarini, 1999; Sperling, 2010; Stern & Markel, 2005). With the rise of chronic diseases as major public health issues (Anderson & Horvath, 2004), population behavior and sociocultural environmental exposures became crucial targets for prevention efforts (Brownson & Bright, 2004; DiClemente, Crosby, & Kegler, 2009).

Legal Epidemiology: Theory and Methods, Second Edition. Edited by Alexander C. Wagenaar, Rosalie Liccardo Pacula, and Scott Burris.
© 2023 John Wiley & Sons, Inc. Published 2023 by John Wiley & Sons, Inc.

The behavioral sciences have made enormous contributions in guiding public health efforts to address these modern-day issues, and social psychology is likely to play an increasingly important function in understanding the mechanisms by which legal systems influence health behaviors and outcomes.

This chapter first classifies laws and regulations according to the specific types of causal mechanisms by which they are believed to effect behavior change. We present relevant theories from the field of social psychology to illustrate how various behavioral and social mechanisms might facilitate, for good or worse, specific health-related behavioral changes. We offer the Theory of Triadic Influence (TTI) (Flay & Petraitis, 1994; Flay et al., 2009) as a comprehensive and integrative model for understanding the interconnections between many social psychological and sociological theories. Finally, we discuss measurement of relevant constructs.

Health-Behavior Laws and Regulations from a Social Psychological Perspective

From a social psychological perspective, laws and regulations that influence health behaviors can be differentiated by the distinctive mechanisms involved in changing specific behaviors. While the specific targets of laws and regulations may differ, the behavioral mechanisms are often similar.

Prevention and Safety Laws

Prevention and safety laws are some of the most common "interventional" public health laws. For example, immunization laws are aimed at preventing the spread of communicable diseases. Driver safety regulations aim to reduce death and disability among motorists and pedestrians. Safety regulations are also an important component of occupational health, intended to reduce harmful exposures and injuries in work settings. From a social psychological perspective, the most likely mechanism of action of safety laws is that they provide people with the information they need to understand the benefits (reduced chances of injury or death) of complying with a particular law and the costs (penalties or possibility of litigation or tort) if they choose to not comply. A recent example of such safety laws by governments is mandatory mask wearing to reduce transmission of the SARS CoV-2 virus.

Environmental Exposure Regulations

Historically, environmental exposure regulation has been one of the legal foundations for preventing public health problems. For example, sanitation laws ensured a standard for clean water and proper disposal of waste products. Such feats were accomplished by substantial funding for proper urban infrastructure (Perdue, Gostin, & Stone, 2003). In modern times, the revelation that lead, which was formerly used in many household and industrial objects, was harmful to health drove authorities to set regulations to ensure that lead would no longer be utilized in the manufacturing of most products (Lewis, 1985). Laws that prohibit smoking in public buildings have reduced toxic exposures and altered specific behaviors of those affected (Frazer et al., 2016).

Intuitively, most environmental regulations would seem to influence social and individual behavior through the same informational and motivational mechanisms described above for prevention and safety laws. For example, motivations to comply with regulatory standards are conditioned on the desire to avoid penalties or litigation. As information and awareness of environmental toxins increases, causal pathways are also likely to occur through changing social norms, thereby affecting the behavioral patterns of whole populations. For example, notable shifts in adults' attitudes and practices regarding childhood exposure to tobacco smoke have occurred with increased awareness of the harmful effects of secondhand smoke (Frazer et al., 2016; McMillen, Winickoff, Klein, & Weitzman, 2003).

Access and Availability Laws

Laws and regulations affect access to and the availability of health-enhancing and health-inhibiting products and resources in multiple ways. For example, Wagenaar and Perry (1994) demonstrated how legal availability laws (age limits), economic availability laws (alcohol tax), and physical availability regulations (zoning for liquor businesses) altogether affected youth's access to and consumption of alcohol. Laws influence access to health care (e.g., health insurance parity laws), food choices (e.g., school and workplace vending rules), and exercise opportunities (e.g., land use laws). Laws against possession of tobacco, alcohol, or other drugs also come with penalties intended to deter the behavior itself.

From a social psychological perspective, access, availability, and possession laws have their effects through two mechanisms. First, they change people's perceptions of the availability of, and expectancies about, the *personal* costs and benefits of using a product or service. Second, they influence people's motivation to comply or cooperate and one's expectancies about the *social* costs and benefits of adopting the behavior or not. Although personal versus social costs and benefits are considered as two separate causal pathways in social psychological theories (Fishbein & Ajzen, 1975), they are considered as one pathway by other social scientists such as economists, as components of subjective-expected utility theories (Bauman & Fisher, 1985; Savage, 1954; Starmer, 2000; Stigler, 1950). According to Tyler (1999), perception processes also involve evaluations that reflect pride and respect within the organizational or cultural system, and those evaluations become strong influences on motivation to cooperate.

"Soft" Laws (Information and Labeling)

"Soft" regulatory strategies rely on choice architecture, education, and the provision of information without legal penalty to the ultimate targets of individual behavior change (although they are typically mandatory and penalty-based with respect to the parties providing the product or service). These laws are used in many areas, including food nutrition and calorie labeling, alcohol and tobacco warning labeling, and other product contents labeling. Laws and regulations are often linked to or require the dissemination of messages encouraging individuals to adopt a healthier behavior or to comply with a particular law. From a social psychological perspective, the causal pathway from regulation to behaviors passes through attitudes and norms. The ideas of "libertarian paternalism" (Jolls et al., 1998; Rebonato, 2014) and soft regulatory strategies "nudging" people to make the "right" decisions (Thaler & Sunstein, 2009) are interesting perspectives on this.

Social Psychological Causal Mechanisms

We focus on the "changes in behavior" mediator in the Burris et al. (2010) model of public health law research (see Figure 1.1). Some effects of laws and legal practices on behavior are mediated by changes in the physical and social environment. We also describe theory-based mediators (of which there are many) for the effects of laws and environmental changes on behavior. To this point, we have suggested only two primary causal pathways by which laws related to prevention and safety, environmental exposure, access and availability, and possession may have their effects. First, information about required behaviors and the costs of noncompliance informs attitudes toward a behavior, and second, compliance requires consideration of social norms (even those with a legal basis) and the motivation to comply or cooperate with them. We now introduce two more. To the extent that laws change the behavior of specific individuals, we may also observe a secondary effect on the behavior of others that arises from people learning by observing others (Akers, 1977; Bandura, 1977b). A final causal pathway involves self-efficacy, which is the confidence one has of being able to successfully engage in any specific behavior (Bandura, 1977a).

Evaluative Theories

Consideration of the costs and benefits of a behavior is common to multiple social psychological theories, including expectancy-value, subjective utility, and decision-making theories. Expectancy-value theories posit that people's choices are influenced by their beliefs and values regarding a specific behavior or activity (Feather, 1982; Wigfield, 1994; Wigfield & Eccles, 2000). For example, applied to alcohol consumption behavior, the positive expectations of feeling good and enhanced social interactions act as behavioral motivators, and the negative expectations of acting inappropriately or "nursing" a hangover the next day act as behavioral restraints (Jones, Corbin, & Fromme, 2001; Peter & Ekeanyanwu, 2010). The value placed on the positive or negative expectations determines the strength of the motivating or restraining factor. If one anticipates negative consequences, such as being fined for underage drinking, as a serious repercussion, then that anticipation (expectation or expectancy) will play a key role in deciding whether to engage in that behavior.

Subjective-expected utility theory is a particular version of expectancy-value theory, developed to test probabilities of risky economic decision-making (Fishburn, 1981; Savage, 1954). *Utility*, which refers to one's satisfaction (or evaluation), is combined with one's knowledge or belief in the likelihood (in statistical terms, probability) that an expected event will occur. Much like expectancy-value theories, decisions regarding a behavior ultimately depend on the relative evaluations and expectancies of the perceived consequences of a behavior (Bauman & Fisher, 1985).

Decision-making theories formalize the use of utilities and their evaluations in reaching decisions (Simon, 1959). Heuristics theory is a relevant approach to understand how problem-solving and decision-making processes occur with experience-based information. In terms of behavioral mechanisms, this approach helps in explaining the role of previous experiences in enforcing other determinants of health behavior. In everyday human contexts, trial-and-error experiences help to inform future behavioral choices. Heuristics theory posits that hardwired or learned heuristic "rules" guide individual judgments, regardless of available relevant information or certainty (Kahnemann, Slovic, & Tversky, 1982; Tversky & Kahneman, 1974).

Perhaps the most well-known social psychological theories that have applied expectancy-value concepts to health behaviors are the Theory of Reasoned Action (Fishbein & Ajzen, 1975) and its derivative, the Theory of Planned Behavior (Ajzen, 1985). In these theories, *information* influences one's *beliefs* about the consequences of a behavior (*expectancies* or expectations) together with one's *evaluation* (or valuing) of that behavior. Thus, expectancies and evaluations are derived from information and values, respectively. Information can be provided through laws and regulations (or, more accurately, by promoting them). Values may derive from one's religious background, the educational system, one's family and childhood socialization, and other broader sociocultural factors (politics, laws, mass media, and so on). However, laws and regulations may or may not be consistent with one's values—and this judgment of their fairness or legitimacy has some effect on the resulting motivation to comply with them (Tyler, 2006a; Tyler & Fagan, 2010). In these two theories, expectancies and evaluations combine to become *attitudes* toward the behavior (Fishbein & Ajzen, 1975). Aside from the costs or penalties of noncompliance, people's motivation to comply with authority or peer expectations (here a component of social normative beliefs) also plays a role in their choices.

Interpersonal Theories of Social Control

Theories of compliance with law derived from social psychology also help explain the effects of prevention and safety laws (Bilz & Nadler, 2009; Tyler, 1999). Compliance theories assume that people comply with laws because of the risk and fear of punishment. Recent research, however, suggests that perceived legitimacy of laws is a more important determinant of whether people obey laws (see Chapter 6). Studies reviewed by Tyler support the argument that people's motivation to cooperate with legal authorities is rooted in social relationships and ethical judgments, and not merely with the desire to avoid punishments or gain rewards.

As an example for how social relationships may drive behavior, social attachment theory suggests that individuals have an inherent need for close relations with others, whether it is a child–parent relationship or an intimate or romantic relationship (Ainsworth & Bowlby, 1991; Ein-Dor & Hirschberger, 2016). These close relationships almost always rely on a varying set of expectations and motivations for each other. Ryan and Deci's (2000) work on intrinsic and extrinsic motivational factors is also relevant for understanding compliance. For example, a person may be rewarded for good behavior or punished for bad behavior, or a person may wish to please others by performing a desirable behavior. Indeed, research has demonstrated that prosocial attachment and commitment is a strong predictor of behavior (Hirschi, 2002). Compliance motivations are directly affected by the degree and quality of attachment (interpersonal bonding)—people who are attached to conventional societal norms are more likely to be motivated to comply with laws and regulations that limit their behavioral choices (Gottfredson & Hirschi, 1990). Police and other authorities benefit from the more active cooperation of such people in the community (Sampson, Raudenbush, & Earles, 1997; Sunshine & Tyler, 2003a; Tyler & Huo, 2002). Moreover, evidence of integrity, legitimate evaluation, and fairness while dealing with authorities are key precursors of compliance, cooperation, or consent with laws (Tyler, 2006a).

To the extent that laws change the behavior of some people, the behavior of others might follow. Social learning theories from both psychology (Bandura, 1977b) and sociology (Akers, 1977) describe this process. According to these theories, social learning is seen to take place in the context of social structures, whereby individuals learn through interactions with different people in multiple social contexts. Application of social learning theories for understanding deviant behavior (criminal or unhealthy) emphasizes how social influences serve as either protective or risk factors (Akers, 1998; Akers & Jensen, 2007). Social situations provide the contexts for social interactions, whereby perceived norms and compliance motivations mediate legal effects. This interaction is more likely to be impactful when the individual who changes their behavior is within the close social circle or family and retains influence on others.

An extension of social learning and other theories, social cognitive theory (Bandura, 1986b) describes how learning from social role models has multiple results. First, it can influence one's beliefs (expectancies) about the consequences of a behavior together with one's evaluation of the value of that behavior. As noted earlier, expectancies and evaluations combine to become attitudes (Fishbein & Ajzen, 1975). A second result is that role models may help one to learn new skills, thereby increasing self-efficacy. Third, to the extent that role models are important to you, you will be motivated to please them (or comply with them). Motivation to comply, combined with normative beliefs (perception of others on how you behave), produces social normative beliefs (Fishbein & Ajzen, 1975), which in turn influence intentions (one's decision on whether to engage in the behavior).

Social relationships and networks clearly play an important role in determining people's behaviors, including their reactions to the law. Social network theories constitute a broad set of theories describing structural characteristics, functions, and types of social support that exist in an individual's social network (Borgatti, Mehra, Brass, & Labianca, 2009). Peer cluster theory demonstrates how small groups of peers share similar beliefs, values, and behaviors (Oetting & Beauvais, 1986). Similarly, from sociology, differential association theory (Heimer & Matsueda, 1994; Matsueda, 1988; Sutherland, 1942) proposes that individuals learn values, attitudes, and motivations for behavior within small groups. Therefore, any behavior is more probable for those with intimate exposure to others performing that behavior. Observational learning illustrates how the adoption of a new behavior is facilitated through seeing others performing that behavior reinforced by reward systems within one's social system (Bandura, 1986a; Unger, Cruz, Baezconde-Garbanati et al., 2003).

Social Impact Theory and Social Media Influence

According to the Social Impact Theory, the effects of any information source on individuals' attitudes and behaviors is a function of three dimensions: (1) strength (importance or social position of the source), (2) immediacy (time or closeness between source and target), and (3) number (quantity of sources) (Talukder & Quazi, 2011). This theory suggests the more important the source of information is the closer a group of individuals becomes and the more likely they will follow the normative beliefs of the group. Social media platforms capitalize on each of the theory's three dimensions by enhancing their impact on individuals, for good or bad, through normative informational social influence. Social media platforms may be used to promote health services, health-related information and behavior and exert pressure on policymakers shaping surrounding policies. Social media offers a ready, participatory, and cost-effective platform (Korda & Itani, 2013). It may provide a sense of social connectedness among individuals and reaches a large audience to promote or deter a health behavior in an inexpensive way across geographic distance (Ventola, 2014). While there is great potential for improving public health understanding through machine learning and natural language processing tools (Dredze, 2012), there is also growing documentation of the extent of health misinformation spread through social media platforms (Wang, McKee, Torbica, & Stuckler, 2019). For example, the role of misinformation spread through social media is evident when examining vaccine hesitancy and varying levels of COVID-19 vaccine uptake (Al-Tammemi & Tarhini, 2021; Tasnim, Hossain, & Mazumder, 2020). In another example, the deleterious effects of social media on self-esteem and broader indicators of mental health are gaining increased attention (Milmo & Paul, 2021).

According to Social Impact Theory, "when other people are the source of impact and the individual is the target, impact should be a multiplicative function of the strength, immediacy, and number of other people" (Latané, 1981). It can be assumed that as the number of people reached through social media increases, the impact on the target individual's attitude and behavior proportionally enhances. As the number of users increases who share their experiences, information, and expectations on the same issues, the impact on target users who are looking for information and recommendations on social media may increase simultaneously, either in a positive direction or negative (Mir & Zaheer, 2012). In the context of social media, all activities that actors participate in have an impact on knowledge transfer because social media interaction provides channels for information exchange and facilitates motivating actions (Wang & Chiang, 2009). Following Social Impact Theory, a wide range of changes in psychological states and subjective feelings, motives and emotions, cognitive beliefs, values, and behavior occur as a result of the actual, implied, or imagined presence of other individuals' actions (in this context, interaction is through social media) (Latané, 1981). Supporting this argument, Nowak, Szamrej, and Latané (1990) illustrate how a simple model of individual interactions, extended across individuals and across time, leads to plausible predictions of public opinion and action (Williams & Williams, 1989). Interaction, participatory dialogs, messages that are seen and heard frequently through stories, cultural practice, and audio-visual platforms (Cohen, Scribner, & Farley, 2000) all impart significance, grasping a person's attention and intensifying their values and behavior associated with the product or topic of concern (Dusseldorp et al., 2014). Naturally, these social-media-mediated social influence processes can be beneficial or deleterious to health and well-being. It is well-known that social media often facilitate the spread of unverified messages, including those that are later found to be false (Li & Sakamoto, 2014).

Moreover, effective public engagement through social media has the potential for synergistically enhancing the effects of public health laws. As far back as 2010, 74% adults were online and 80% of them reported searching for health information (Agostino & Arnaboldi, 2016; Fox, 2011). Social media are important tools for disaster management, disease tracking, and risk communication. For example, keyword content from Twitter, Facebook, and other social networks, in combination with location-tracking technologies, can be used to locate source of contamination, infections, or disease cases, and to monitor the health and welfare of populations (George, Rovniak, & Kraschnewski, 2013; Househ, 2013). While social media have considerable potential as tools for health promotion, these media, like traditional health promotion media, require careful theory-based application and may not always achieve their desired outcomes (Lipschultz, 2020). In summary, social media appear to play an increasingly important role in understanding and improving the effects of public health laws, since they can accelerate the social influence processes illuminated by the social psychological theories reviewed here.

Intrapersonal Theories

Individual predispositions and personality traits guide one's self-determination (will), skill development, and decision-making regarding a specific behavior. Important concepts within the intrapersonal dimension include self-regulation or control, social skills, and self-efficacy. One causal pathway suggested earlier involves self-efficacy, the confidence one has to engage in a specific behavior successfully. According to self-efficacy theory (Bandura, 1977a, 1986a), compliance with a law or regulation about a specific behavior will improve to the extent the rule is accompanied with specific information about how to accomplish that behavior or, better still, training and experience in how to do the new behavior. As people's skill to do the behavior (and, therefore, their confidence or self-efficacy about doing it) improves, they will be more likely to successfully perform that specific behavior.

According to the Theory of Planned Behavior, self-efficacy is the third leg directly affecting one's decision-making or intentions toward performing a behavior. Those with low self-efficacy are easily discouraged and less likely to trust their ability to perform a behavior and therefore are less likely to actually perform that behavior. In contrast, those with high self-efficacy regarding a specific behavior will likely expend the effort necessary to ensure that they achieve their expected behavioral outcomes. Theoretically, self-efficacy facilitates or buffers against compliance with laws and regulations. Self-efficacy could represent confidence either in one's ability to obey the law or one's ability to disregard or elude the law.

According to Bandura (1986a, 1986b), self-regulation is achieved by acquiring self-management skills and can be manifested in a number of ways, including goal setting, seeking social support, and self-rewards (to name a few). Self-control theory (Akers, 1991) posits that one's relative self-control forms during childhood and tends to remain stable throughout adulthood. The degree of socialization during childhood plays an important role in forming levels of self-control in individuals. Those with low self-control are more likely to engage in delinquent behaviors, including health-related behaviors such as drug use (Gottfredson & Hirschi, 1990; Miller, Barnes, & Beaver, 2011). In contrast, people with high levels of self-control are more likely to comply with legal restrictions. Therefore, one's level of self-control may mediate the effects of public health laws.

Self-esteem has been thought of as a core component of self-concept by which individuals evaluate their competence, skill, and worth in their social environment (Cast & Burke, 2002). In general, research has shown proportional associations of higher self-esteem with more positive outcomes, and of lower self-esteem with negative outcomes. Self-esteem has been conceptualized as self-motivating and as a buffer from negative experiences. Cast and Burke (2002) attempted to integrate these three conceptualizations within the context of identity theory. DuBois, Flay, and Fagen (2009) presented the self-esteem enhancement theory to help guide interventions related to self-esteem, in which self-esteem formation and maintenance processes are depicted as moderators of well-being. In the context of legal effects, self-esteem likely plays a mediating role, whereby improved self-esteem strengthens one's capacity for appropriately handling negative pressures in a manner compliant with laws and regulations.

The self-motivation conceptualization of self-esteem is related to Deci and Ryan's (1985) self-determination theory, by which intrinsic and extrinsic motivations vary in degrees according to one's goals or reasons. Intrinsic motivation is enhanced when three psychological needs—competence, autonomy, and relatedness—are met (Ryan & Deci, 2000). Levels of self-determination likely both moderate and mediate effects of laws. Those with higher levels of self-determination are more likely to comply with laws and regulations—unless such laws and regulations are regarded as illegitimate, in which case self-determination may act as a buffer to compliance. As an act of compliance, those with higher levels of self-determination contributes to leading a feedback effect on the development of laws and regulations and their perceived legitimacy through engaging in voting or other community-based activities.

Summary Comments on Social Psychological Theories

We have described numerous theories explaining various dimensions and derivations of behavior (see Table 8.1). These accounts of behavior can be organized within a *social ecological model* (Bronfrenbrenner, 2005). In this model, behavior is influenced at three main levels: within people themselves (Intrapersonal: individual's personality and predispositions), with respect to the social relationships surrounding the individual (Interpersonal), and in the broad sociocultural environment (Evaluative). Laws and regulations, of course, are part of the sociocultural environment, along with economic and political systems, the mass media, religions, and other cultural systems.

Table 8.1. Social Psychological Theories Informing Mechanisms of Legal Effect.

Evaluative Theories	Interpersonal Theories	Intrapersonal Theories

Value-expectancy theories:
  Subjective-expected
  utility theory
  Theory of reasoned action
  Theory of planned behavior
Theories of decision making:
  Heuristics theory
	Compliance theories:
	  Deterrence
	  Procedural justice
	Social attachment theory
	Intrinsic and extrinsic
	motivation
	Social Impact theory
	Social learning theories
	Social cognitive theory
	Social network theories
	Peer cluster theory
	Differential
	association theory
		Self-efficacy theory
		Self-control theory
		Self-esteem theory
		Self-esteem
		enhancement theory
		Self-determination theory
		Bounded rationality

We have described four major pathways through which laws and regulations can affect behavior and summarized social psychological theories that elaborate those pathways. The first is that laws and regulations provide information that, in turn, informs expectancies or expectations about consequences that together form attitudes toward the behavior targeted by the law or regulation.

Pathway 1: laws and regulations → information → expectancies and evaluations → attitudes

A second causal path suggests that laws and regulations have their effects through the interpersonal pathway of influencing attachment to conventional norms leading to motivation to comply.

Pathway 2: laws and regulations → attachment to conventional norms → motivation to comply

Third, we described pathways through changes in the behavior of initial compliers, thereby changing social norms.

Pathway 3: laws and regulations → change behavioral norms → normative beliefs

Finally, a pathway is made through people learning new behaviors from others.

Pathway 4: laws and regulations → modeling or training → self-efficacy

Note how each of these pathways moved from the ultimate (or root) cause of behavior, here laws and regulations, to a cause closer to behavior but still somewhat distal (for example, information, attachment to conventional norms, social norms, behavioral models), to causes even closer to or very proximal to behavior (that is, attitudes, compliance, social normative beliefs, and self-efficacy). It is immediately obvious that the proximal predictors of behavior are consistent with Social Cognitive Theory (Bandura, 1986b) and the Theories of Reasoned Action (Fishbein & Ajzen, 1975) and Planned Behavior (Ajzen, 1985)— each of these pathways are mediated by intentions or decisions to do the behavior. As intentions are a good predictor of actually doing (or at least initiating) the specific behavior, changes in any one or all of attitudes (the result of expectancies and their value), social normative beliefs (the result of motivation to comply and normative beliefs), and self-efficacy (the result of will or opportunity and skill) related to a specific behavior are likely to lead to changes in one's intentions or decisions to perform that behavior. In the Theory of Planned Behavior, behavioral control (one's perceived control over a specific behavior) replaces self-efficacy (one's actual or perceived ability to perform a specific behavior). Finally, note that using intentions to predict action/behavior has a practical benefit in legal epidemiology studies. In circumstances when direct observation of actual behavior is impossible, survey methods can be used to accurately assess intentions.

Each of these pathways sound rational, but there is wide recognition that rationality is limited. People exhibit bounded rationality, bounded self-interest, and bounded willpower (Jolls et al., 1998; Rebonato, 2014). Bounded rationality refers to cognitive limitations, such that information may have been forgotten or habits formed that limit the acceptance of new information. Bounded self-interest refers to the fact that people care about others and what those others think about them, so they may act to please others or avoid negative judgments from others, rather than act in their own self-interest. Bounded willpower refers to the limited self-control or self-determination that we all experience with some behaviors such as smoking or eating. Note the parallel of these three types of bounded rationality with the social-ecological levels in which the causes of behavior operate.

Many theories rely on intrapersonal concepts for understanding behavior, while social psychological theories posit that social contexts (interpersonal relationships) are just as important. Furthermore, social-ecological models suggest that behaviors must be understood in the broader sociocultural contexts in which they occur (Bronfrenbrenner, 2005). Clearly, none of the proposed causal pathways toward behavior operate in a vacuum—all three are strongly affected by individual (intrapersonal), social (interpersonal), and environmental (evaluative) factors. Each of these types of theories has offered important insights regarding the emergence of specific health behaviors. However, their contributions are limited to the extent that the scope of any specific single theory accounts for a limited set of influences on behavior. The Theory of Triadic Influence was developed to integrate many of the theories above and others and to provide a comprehensive explanation of the many causes of behavior. As will be seen, each of the major pathways just described, and other related ones, can be unified in this integrated, comprehensive theory (Flay & Petraitis, 1994; Flay et al., 2009).

The Theory of Triadic Influence

The Theory of Triadic Influence (TTI) represents an integration of many of the theories discussed in the previous section, as well as others. It organizes them in a coherent way that explains health-related behaviors and guides interventions for health-behavior change. We find the framework useful for explaining the effects of laws and regulations on people's health-related behaviors and population-level public health issues. As a broad ecological model, the TTI provides a metatheoretical approach both to explaining health-related behaviors and for guiding health behavior change. The TTI posits that theories and variables can be organized along two dimensions: social-ecological streams of influence and levels of causation (Petraitis et al., 1995).

The Basic Elements of the TTI

The TTI proposes that causes of behavior operate through multiple pathways from ultimate to distal to proximal levels of causation; that these pathways flow through three ecological streams, each of which has two substreams; and that experience with a behavior feeds back to change the initial causes (Figure 8.1). We discuss each of these elements in turn.

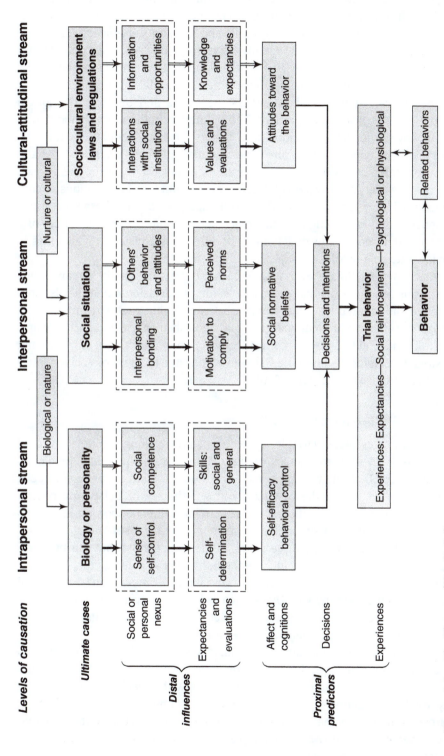

Figure 8.1. The Theory of Triadic Influence.

STREAMS OF INFLUENCE

The TTI proposes that causes emanate from and flow through three streams of influence. The intrapersonal stream flows from genetic predispositions and personality through self-determination (will) and skills to self-efficacy. The interpersonal, or social-normative, stream flows from one's social contexts and relationships (community, peer networks, family) through others' behaviors and one's level of attachment to those others, to social normative beliefs. It includes perceived norms about others' behaviors and one's motivation to comply with or please those others. The cultural-attitudinal, or sociocultural, stream flows from broad sociocultural factors (politics, economics, the law, mass media, religion) through one's interactions with these social systems and how those interactions determine one's attitudes toward a specific behavior. It includes how the social systems influence one's values and evaluations of consequences. It also considers how the information provided by these institutions influences one's expectations (i.e., expectancies) about the consequences of a behavior. All three streams end at one's intentions (or decisions), which ideally provide a reliable prediction of actual behavior.

As shown in Figure 8.1, within each of the three main streams, two substreams represent distinct processes leading to decisions: one that is more cognitive and rational (the right-hand substream within each stream) and one that is more affective or emotional (the left-hand substream within each stream). Psychologists tend to emphasize the affective or emotional aspect of the second substream; sociologists are more likely to emphasize the self- or social-control aspect (Gottfredson & Hirschi, 1990).

LEVELS OF CAUSATION

The TTI arranges these variables affecting behavior along multiple levels of causation—from ultimate causes to distal influences to proximal predictors (Flay et al., 2009). Some variables, such as attitudes toward the behavior, social normative beliefs about the behavior, and self-efficacy or behavioral control (confidence in doing a specific behavior), can have direct effects on intentions about that specific behavior and therefore are proximal causes of that behavior. Other variables are causally more distal, influencing factors that can be mediated by other variables. These include the individual's social competence, attitudes and behaviors of others, and the individual's interactions with social institutions. Finally, many variables—such as law, poverty, neighborhood characteristics, and personality—represent underlying or ultimate causes of behavior over which individuals generally have little control.

The TTI proposes that causal mechanisms generally flow from ultimate to proximal causes within each of the three streams of influence. Yet while the general flow of causation occurs predominantly within each stream, variables may also interact across streams. Thus, multiple ultimate and distal moderating and mediating factors may work together to increase or decrease the probability of a behavior occurring. For example, one's personality may moderate the effects of a law on one's values.

Experience with a behavior may produce physiological, social, or psychological reinforcements that feed back into many of the upstream variables that originally led to the behavior. Systems theories (Leischow, Best, Trochim et al., 2008; Sterman, 2006; Wiese, Vallacher, & Strawinska, 2010) describe this as forming feedback loops, while social cognitive theory (Bandura, 1986b) describes it as reciprocal determinism. The key concept of reciprocal determinism suggests that any type of environmental influence may affect the behavior of individuals and groups *and* that the behavior of individuals and groups may, in turn, affect the environment.

Application to Public Health Laws

The TTI cultural-attitudinal stream illustrates how public policies and laws affect individual health behaviors primarily by shaping social and institutional practices and structures. Institutional structures and practices influence one's opportunities and access to products and information and affects capacities for interacting with that institution. Drawing on theories reviewed earlier, the TTI proposes that attitudes toward a specific behavior are one of the key proximal predictors of intentions or adoption and is determined by expectancies and evaluations about that specific behavior. The TTI makes it clear that specific distal and ultimate causes influence many behaviors. The TTI also incorporates a developmental perspective in which all causal routes may be modified at different developmental stages (ages), and behavioral changes may affect developmental trajectories.

Interpersonal concepts are important for understanding the effects of laws and regulations on behavior. Social psychologists recognize the important role of interactions that occur within one's social context. Core concepts in the interpersonal stream of the TTI include bonding with or attachment to important others (Ainsworth & Bowlby, 1991), other's behaviors (role modeling) (Bandura, 1977a, 1986a), motivation to comply (desire to please), and social normative beliefs (Fishbein & Ajzen, 1975). The TTI suggests that family structures and dynamics and peer relations are ultimate causes within social contexts that lead to one's social normative beliefs. Laws and policies influence individual perceptions and decisions about behavioral adoption or restraint by affecting one's beliefs about social norms.

Intrapersonal dimensions, such as social skills, self-control or regulation, and self-efficacy, are important to consider when evaluating laws and policies. In the intrapersonal stream of the TTI, one's personality determines one's levels of self-control or regulation, which, in turn, moderate the influence of policies or laws. One's levels of self-esteem and self-determination not only moderate effects of existing policies and laws but also may help in the development of new policies and laws.

The TTI takes a step beyond other integrative theories, such as social cognitive theory, where it integrates a wider range of psychological and sociological theories of behavioral development and change. It conveys key concepts from many specific theories in a coherent way to explain health-related behaviors and guide behavior-moderating interventions for health behavior change. Furthermore, the TTI provides a systems perspective that includes development, feedback, control systems, and a systematic view of how multiple causes influence multiple behaviors either directly, through mediated pathways, by moderating other causes, or through feedback systems. Feedback systems may be embedded at any causal level—proximal, distal, or ultimate.

PATHWAYS OF INFLUENCE

We propose that public health laws have their primary causal action through the cultural-attitudinal stream. Laws primarily alter access to or availability of goods and information related to knowledge or expectancies of consequences. Laws also give rise to and structure interactions with government institutions; these experiences in turn influence one's view of the legitimacy of authorities or one's evaluations of the expected consequences of a specific behavior. These paths influence attitudes toward the behavior, which, in turn, influences decisions and trial behavior. A positive experience with the behavior will feed back to influence expectancies and evaluations (and information and relationships with social institutions, including the legal system) to determine future behavior. Ultimately, trial behavior that is repeatedly reinforced will lead to regular (habitual) behavior.

The paths through the cultural-attitudinal stream are similar to many rational theories of decision making and utility theories in economics (Starmer, 2000; Stigler, 1950) and to procedural justice and deterrence theories of compliance (see Chapters 5 and 6). Public health laws may also have their effects through less rational pathways that involve social relationships and emotions. For example, laws may have mediating influences on social and intrapersonal factors thereby leading oneself to change their behavior or attitudes (interpersonal stream) and ultimately change perceived norms. Then, to the extent that one is bonded with and desires to please (comply or cooperate with) others, one's social normative beliefs are altered, leading to changed intentions and behavior. Laws may also have a direct influence on one's sense of control or social competence in the intrapersonal stream. Disability discrimination law, for example, may validate a person with a disability in their efforts to get accommodations at work (Bagenstos, 2009; Engel & Munger, 2003), which will lead to changes through the intrapersonal stream down to self-efficacy and from there to intentions.

Aspects of the other streams may affect (moderate) how one responds to laws. Poor self-regulation or impulsiveness (sense of self or self-control), for example, may reduce the effects of a law on one's behavior by moderating the pathway from information to attitudes, or the path to values. Or, if everyone in one's immediate social context is not following a new rule, then one's perceived norm and normative belief will be against the new regulation and the intention behind the regulation until an enforcement is imposed, which changes a behavioral norm.

Tyler (1999, 2006b) suggests that innate human desire to cooperate is the product of an array of inter- and intrapersonal components, including trust, legitimacy, emotions, attitudes, and norms. De Cremer and Tyler (2005) have posited the importance of the "sense of social self" to the production of cooperative behavior. These views combine aspects from all three streams of the TTI: self-esteem and sense of self-control from the intrapersonal stream; social bonding (attachment) and motivation to comply from the interpersonal stream; and interactions with or involvement in social institutions and attitudes from the cultural-attitudinal stream. If compliance with law is seen as a form of social cooperation, sense of social self will largely determine one's degree of compliance with a new law or regulation. If the law is seen as having legitimate and trustworthy authorities, then compliance will be high among those with a strong sense of social self. In contrast, for individuals with a strong social self, compliance will be low if the law lacks legitimacy in the eyes of the public.

Practical Measures

The TTI identifies key measurable constructs that explain variance in behavior informing how laws change health-related behavior. We discuss measures of eleven variables that are central to understanding how legal institutions and practices affect behavior. Many resources exist for measurement development besides those we reference here (Dillman, 1991, 2007; General Accounting Office, 1993; Houston, 1997). We provide brief considerations for measurement development and identify some examples of measures of constructs from the TTI and other theories that have demonstrated good reliability and validity.

The Cultural-Attitudinal or Sociocultural Stream

In this section, we discuss measures of knowledge and beliefs, values, and attitudes toward behavior.

KNOWLEDGE AND BELIEFS ABOUT EXPECTED CONSEQUENCES

Knowledge of laws and beliefs about expected consequences is a distal factor in the cognitive substream of the cultural-attitudinal stream of the TTI. Knowledge about laws includes the important issue of comprehension of those laws and their intent. Opinion polls often contain items to assess such knowledge or beliefs. Tidwell and Doyle (1995) developed a survey to assess driver and pedestrian comprehension of pedestrian law and traffic control devices. Another example of a survey assessing beliefs is a sixteen-item measure of beliefs regarding physical activity that has shown good internal consistency (Saunders, Pate, Felton et al., 1997). Leading from an item stem of "If I were to be physically active most days it would ...", sample items include "Get or keep me in shape," "Make me tired," "Be fun," and "Be boring."

VALUES

Values are a distal component of the TTI's cultural-attitudinal stream flowing toward one's attitudes about a behavior. A popular measure of general values is the Rokeach Value Survey (Rokeach, 1973; Rokeach & Ball-Rokeach, 1989). This self-administered value inventory is divided into two parts, with each part measuring different but complementary types of personal values. The first part consists of 18 terminal value items, which are designed to measure the relative importance of end states of existence (that is, personal goals such as freedom, equality, health, national security, a world at peace). The second part consists of 18 instrumental value items, which measure basic characteristics an individual might see as helpful to reaching end-state values (for example, ambitious, responsible, honest, obedient). The scale has been used widely with Likert scales (e.g., a five-point agreement scale), generating frequency distributions amenable to conventional statistical analyses (Rokeach, 1973; Rokeach & Ball-Rokeach, 1989). Many other measures of specialized values are available (Gibbins & Walker, 1993). For example, The Culture and Media Institute conducts the National Cultural Values Survey (Fitzpatrick, 2007), which assesses cultural values such as morality, thrift, charity, and honesty or integrity (including willingness to break the law, cheat on unemployment benefits, or tolerate illegal drug use).

ATTITUDES TOWARD THE BEHAVIOR

This is the proximal predictor of behavior within TTI's cultural-attitudinal stream of influence. Ajzen (2003) provides guidance on the construction of attitude scale items specific to any particular behavior. The simplest attitude items are of the form "It would be bad for me to drive after drinking" answered on a scale of "completely agree" to "completely disagree." Fishbein, Triandis, Kanfer, Becker, and Middlestadt (2001) also suggest utilizing an expectancy-value index to indirectly measure attitudes. For example, two questions would be asked regarding a specific consequence of a particular behavior: one about one's beliefs about the probability of the consequence (expectancy), the other about one's values about (evaluation of) the consequence. The product of those two items could be summed with other paired items to create the attitude index.

Examples of valid and reliable attitude scales include Brand and Anastasio's (2006) 50-item Violence-Related Attitudes and Beliefs Scale (V-RABS) and Polaschek et al.'s (2004) 20-item Criminal Attitudes to Violence Scale (CAVS). Using a seven-point agreement scale, sample items from the V-RABS include "Trying to prevent violent behavior is a waste of time and money"; "People become violent because of their family environment"; and "The majority of violent crimes are committed by people who have mental illness."

The Interpersonal or Social-Normative Stream

In this section, we discuss measures of social attachment (bonding), observed (modeled) behaviors, and social normative beliefs.

Social Attachment (Bonding) with Family, Friends, and School

The interpersonal bonding component of the TTI's interpersonal stream is similar to Hirschi's (2002) theoretical constructs of attachment, commitment, and belief. Libbey (2004) provides a review of school attachment, bonding, and connectedness measures and items used to assess student attachment. Another example of a somewhat reliable measure of bonding (Jenkins, 1997) includes items such as, "Do you care a lot about what your teachers think of you?" "Do most of your teachers like you?" and, "Most teachers are not interested in anything I say or do."

Observed (Modeled) Behavior And Attitudes

Others' behavior and attitudes is also a distal component of TTI's interpersonal stream, directly influencing perceived norms. An eight-item measure that has shown good reliability was tested by Saunders et al. (1997), measuring social modeling for physical activity. Using the item stem "A friend or someone in the family ...", sample items include, "Thinks I should be physically active"; "Encourages me to be physically active"; and "Has been physically active with me."

Social Normative Beliefs

As a proximal predictor of behavior, social normative beliefs concern one's perception of the social influences on one's behavior. Consensus among theorists suggests that, because this measure is concerned with judging the degree to which one is motivated to comply with a particular person or social group, specific behaviors should be measured in paired items assessing both perceptions of norms (what others expect of one) and motivation to comply with those others. Ajzen (2003) provides guidelines for constructing such scales.

We could not identify any developed and tested scales for social normative beliefs using the paired-item format. However, Huesmann and Guerra (1997) provide an example of a reliable 20-item scale measuring normative beliefs about aggression. An eight-item version of this scale (Huesmann & Guerra, 1997) was found to have high reliability with elementary and middle school students (Lewis et al., 2013). Using a four-point response scale, example items include, "It is wrong to hit other people"; "If you're angry, it is OK to say mean things to other people"; and "It is wrong to get into physical fights with others." Another example concerns normative beliefs about water conservation laws (Corral-Verdugo & Frías-Armenta, 2006). Items include, "The government should pass laws banning the settlement of industries around dams, rivers, lakes, and aquifers" and "The state should impose fines on people who waste water."

The Intrapersonal Stream

In this section, we discuss measures of self-control or regulation, social competence and skills, and self-efficacy.

SELF-CONTROL OR REGULATION

In the TTI framework, self-control or regulation is seen as a distal-level variable within the intrapersonal stream. Two measures demonstrating good reliability assessing self-control are the 36-item Self-Control Schedule (Facione & Facione, 1992) and the Total and Brief Self-Control Scales (Rosenbaum, 1980), with 36 and 13 items, respectively. Sample items from the Self-Control Schedule include, "When I have to do something that is anxiety arousing for me, I try to visualize how I will overcome my anxieties while doing it"; "When I am depressed, I try to keep myself busy with things that I like"; and "When I plan to work, I remove all the things that are not relevant to my work." Response items are on a six-point scale indicating the degree to which each statement is characteristic of the respondent.

SOCIAL COMPETENCE AND SKILLS

In the framework of the TTI, skills are the distal cognitive component that flows directly into self-efficacy. This variable is important to assess, as the development of general and behavior-specific skills can be instrumental in determining one's likelihood of adopting a behavior. The 131-item Conners Teacher Rating Scale (CTRS-R), measuring six behavioral domains (Conners, Sitarenios, Parker, & Epstein, 1998), is a reliable social skills scale. Teachers rate specific behavioral items related to cognition (forgets things, avoids mental effort), perfectionism (neat, over-focused), and impulsivity (restless, excitable).

Critical thinking is an important skill domain that can affect many types of behavior. The 80-item Watson-Glaser Critical Thinking Appraisal (Watson & Glaser, 1980) and the 40-item California Critical Thinking Skills Test (Facione & Facione, 1992) have both shown good internal reliability. Subscale items measure five specific constructs: the ability to make inferences, recognize assumptions, make deductions, evaluate arguments, and make interpretations (Gadzella, Stacks, Stephens, & Masten, 2005).

SELF-EFFICACY

Self-efficacy derives from self-control or regulation (through self-determination or will) and social competence (through skills) in the intrapersonal stream. Fishbein et al. (2001) recommend that items measuring self-efficacy should be behavior-specific, be phrased in the present tense, and utilize wording from identified internal or external demands that may impose difficulty on one's ability to perform the behavior. For example, Resnick and Jenkin's Self-Efficacy for Exercise (SEE) Scale is a nine-item scale, developed for adults, and measures perceived confidence that one could continue to exercise despite various barriers. Items were prefaced with, "How confident are you right now that you could exercise three times per week for 20 minutes if …", followed by items such as "the weather was bothering you"; "you were bored by the program or activity"; and "you felt pain when exercising." Usually, these measures use a 0–100 scale, suggesting the degree to which a person feels confident enough to perform that behavior. Bandura (2006) offers a clear guide on how to construct domain-specific self-efficacy scales depending on the context of research.

Decisions, Intentions, and Feedback from Experiences with the Behavior

In this section, we discuss measures of intentions and responses to feedback from experiences with the behavior.

DECISIONS AND INTENTIONS

As the key proximal mediating variable of the TTI, behavioral decisions and intentions provide the most strongly correlated predictor of a future behavior and can be assessed with measures of likelihood or probability of occurrence. For the development of a fixed measure, it is recommended that it can be treated as a continuous variable along a response scale of likely to unlikely (Polaschek, Collie, & Walkey, 2004), although there have been issues raised as to how many points should be included (Davis & Warshaw, 1992). It is recommended that if respondents' answers are more reliable with a shorter response scale that they then be offered a two-part question (Fishbein et al., 2001). Thus, as should be noted for all measures, it is important to take into consideration the specific population for which the measure is being developed. The 19-item Scale for Suicide Ideation (SSI) designed to measure suicidal intention has shown high internal consistency and construct validity (Beck, Kovacs, & Weissman, 1979). A developed and tested intention measure for physical activity (Godin & Shephard, 1986) was used by Saunders et al. (1997) and includes a selection of five response items indicating a range of intention to be physically active during one's free time. Such statements range from "I am sure I will *not* be physically active" to "I am sure I *will* be physically active."

TRIAL BEHAVIOR PRODUCES FEEDBACK

Feedback from experience with a behavior is mostly captured through emotional reactions to the behavior. Hedonic theory focuses on affective responses to behavior as determinants of future behavior (Kahneman, 1999; Williams & Bohlen, 2019). Hedonic responses or emotional reactions (that is, good or pleasure versus bad or displeasure) can provide an index of the usefulness of behavior and its immediate consequences that may influence decisions regarding whether or not to repeat the behavior (Cabanac, 1992; Kahneman, Fredrickson, Schreiber, & Redelmeier, 1993). This tendency for humans to maximize pleasure and minimize displeasure has been examined extensively as a mechanism for various behaviors. It is a basic underlying mechanism of learning (Bandura, 1986a, 1986b).

Emotional reactions could be related to any stream of influence: in the cultural-attitudinal stream, it would feed back to attitudes, particularly evaluation of consequences and values; in the interpersonal stream, it would feed back to normative beliefs, particularly motivation to comply or social bonding or attachment; and in the intrapersonal stream, it would feed back to self-efficacy, particularly self-control or regulation and competence or skills. Fishbein et al. (2001) suggest that while no standardized measures have yet been developed, one could explore potential semantic differential terms that elicit more gut-like emotional reactions. Another approach would be to assess changes in attitudes, social normative beliefs, and self-efficacy after experiencing a behavior. For example, after first trying an illegal substance, an adolescent might have more positive or negative attitudes about drug use, depending on their physiological responses and their cognitive interpretations of those physical responses. The adolescent's relationship with peers, parents, and the law or authority is likely to change after initiating the behavior, as is, in turn, his or her motivation to comply with (or please) them; and the adolescent's sense of self-efficacy to do the behavior (or to resist it) will have changed.

Conclusion

Many social psychological theories inform our understanding of the effects of public health laws and regulations on behavior. In this chapter, we provided a review of many of these theories that contribute to understanding the effects of public health laws. We also provided an integrative theoretical framework, the theory of triadic influence, to help guide future research on the health effects of law. These theoretical perspectives make clear that laws have their effects on behavior through many pathways. The most obvious path is knowledge and values → expectancies and how they are evaluated → attitudes toward the behavior. However, many other pathways through social contexts or interpersonal relationships are also possible, involving role models (social learning) and perceived norms → attachment to or bonding with conventional values or others and motivation to comply with them → social normative beliefs. Yet other pathways occur through intrapersonal constructs, including social competence and sense of self control → skill plus will (self-determination) → self-efficacy. Attitudes, social normative beliefs, and self-efficacy each have cognitive and affective (control) components, and each contributes to the prediction of intentions to try or to adopt a particular behavior. Once a behavior is tried, the experience with that behavior feeds back in the personal, social, and cultural domains and changes the original causes or predictors. All of this occurs during life-long human development over time. Clearly, the prediction of behavior is complex, and any new law or regulation should be evaluated rigorously to assess both expected and unexpected effects.

Summary

Social psychology plays an important role in explicating mechanisms of legal effect. Social psychological theories offer theoretical constructs that help explain the web of psychological and social causes and mediators of intentions and behaviors that legal processes seek to modify. Social psychology pertains primarily to the "changes in behavior" mediator in the model of public health law research (see Figure 1.1), positing a number of possible causal pathways by which legal systems and rules may influence behavior. From a social psychological perspective, laws and regulations can be classified according to the type of causal pathway by which behaviors are modified, for example, through changing attitudes, normative beliefs, or self-efficacy concerning a specific behavior. We outline plausible pathways for many types of laws and regulations, including prevention and safety laws; environmental exposure regulations; laws regulating availability of health-enhancing and health inhibiting products and resources; and "soft" laws that prompt or inform rather than command the ultimate actor (for example, labeling laws).

Given the large number of social psychological theories and the need to structure disparate theories in relation to each other, the theory of triadic influence (TTI) is a comprehensive and integrative model that we use for describing relationships among various theoretical constructs. The TTI posits that laws and regulations influence behavior through multiple causal pathways, from ultimate causes, through distal influences and proximal predictors, all mediated by the proximal influences of attitudes toward, social normative beliefs about, and self-efficacy regarding a particular behavior. Reliable measures for these and other constructs are readily available.

Further Reading

Flay, B. R., Snyder, F. J., & Petraitis, J. (2009). The theory of triadic influence. In R. J. DiClemente, M. C. Kegler, & R. A. Crosby (Eds.), *Emerging theories in health promotion practice and research* (2nd ed., pp. 451–510). San Francisco, CA: Jossey-Bass.

Petraitis, J., Flay, B. R., & Miller, T. Q. (1995). Reviewing theories of adolescent substance use: Organizing pieces in the puzzle. *Psychological Bulletin, 117*(1), 67–86.

Tyler, T. R. (2006). *Why people obey the law*. Princeton, NJ: Princeton University Press.

Chapter 9

Integrating Diverse Theories for Public Health Law Evaluation

Scott Burris   Alexander C. Wagenaar

Learning Objectives

- Recognize how theorizing mechanisms of legal effect can support causal inference.
- Use evidence on the mechanisms of legal effect to explain the basis for legal reform and innovation to others.
- Combine concepts from various theories of how laws operate to illustrate specific hypotheses regarding legal effects on population health.

The preceding chapters have introduced a variety of theoretical frameworks and practical tools for studying *how* laws and legal practices influence behavior, environments, and, ultimately, health outcomes in a population. Theory that illuminates mechanisms of legal effect has at least three important benefits for legal epidemiology:

- *Defining the phenomena to be observed*. Theories of how law influences structures, behaviors, and environments help identify effects to measure—tell us where to look, at what point in time we might expect to see effects, how effects might evolve over time, and what sort of intended and unintended effects to look for.

- *Supporting causal inference*. Theories of how law works provide evidence of plausible mechanisms that can be used to assess causation. They help unpack a law into regulatory components that

Legal Epidemiology: Theory and Methods, Second Edition. Edited by Alexander C. Wagenaar, Rosalie Liccardo Pacula, and Scott Burris.

may have varying contributions to the overall effect and help identify dose–response relationships between specific legal components or dimensions and health-related outcomes.

- *Understanding implementation and guiding reform.* Assuming confidence that law is causing an effect, theories of how it does so provide important guidance on ways to study the magnitude of the effect, reduce unintended consequences, or produce the effect more efficiently. Implementation research in turn can suggest changes in practice or in the law itself to enhance the effectiveness of the law.

As the preceding chapters show, we draw on a rich and diverse literature to understand mechanisms of law. There is no single correct theory, and therefore no need to make an exclusive choice. Likewise, "no one causal approach should drive the questions asked or delimit what counts as useful evidence. Robust causal inference instead comprises a complex narrative, created by scientists appraising, from diverse perspectives, different strands of evidence produced by (a) myriad (of) methods" (Krieger & Davey Smith, 2016). The choice of what theory or theories to draw upon is a practical one based on research questions and designs, types of law or regulatory approach under study, and the state of current knowledge about the matter being investigated. This chapter first elaborates on why it is so important to investigate *how*, as well as *whether*, law is having an effect on health, using safety belt laws as one example. It then uses a second example in greater detail—the health effects of criminal laws regulating HIV exposure through sex—to illustrate how diverse theories of legal effect can be productively used.

The Value of Opening the Black Box

The stick-figure picture of law is that lawmakers issue a rule, and people obey it. A causal diagram for a public health law evaluation study based on this simple equation might start with no more than three boxes: one for law, one for the required behavior, and one for the health outcome. If the behavior is an established, good-enough proxy for a health outcome (such as safety belt use in relation to crash morbidity and mortality), we could even dispense with a box for health outcome. Or, if we were correlating the law with crash outcomes, we could use the health outcome as a proxy for the required behavior. In studies so conceived, the chain of events between issuance of a rule and its health outcomes is hidden within a black box. For some laws, and for some research purposes, this may be fine: the news of a law may be rapidly and widely disseminated, the rate of compliance may be quite high, or the relationship between the required behavior and a health outcome may be very strong. In some cases, local differences in the events unfolding in the black box (for example, the level of enforcement) may be small, or have little impact, so that with enough other data points they do not significantly influence the result in the aggregate. Or perhaps there is no empirical research on a particular new law, and an initial "black box" study linking the law to an important health outcome represents an important contribution. Thus, it is not always essential to know what is happening within the black box to accurately measure effects of a law on health. But the black box in which law unfolds is, at best, a placeholder for further development in a causal model, and at worst a sign of theoretical imprecision and a source of potential causal misattribution.

Defining the Phenomena to Be Observed

Law is just one of many factors that shape health outcomes. Although we often speak of a "chain" of causation, in which one event leads to another, a more apt metaphor is a causal web. As Swanson and Ibrahim explain in Chapter 10, one way to open the black box is to place the law within a simplified causal diagram that depicts one or more plausible processes through which law is expected to have its effect, and the relation of law to *other* potential causes. In quantitative studies, measurement decisions and data interpretation may depend upon assumptions concerning how quickly or evenly a law will have an effect. In these processes, the researcher necessarily states hypotheses—falsifiable propositions about legal effects—and identifies candidate variables for observation and measurement. Generating testable hypotheses is greatly facilitated by an underlying theory of how law works. And articulating a theory of the mechanism of effect makes clear underlying (and often hidden or imprecise) assumptions regarding why a given law is expected to have an effect or not.

Consider a mandatory safety belt law. A change in safety belt use after the passage of a law could be conceptualized as the result of deterrence: the causal diagram begins with the law, then proceeds through rational choices by drivers to compliance or noncompliance based on the likelihood and cost of detection. This theory would direct researchers toward an inquiry into drivers' risk aversion, or their perceptions of the likelihood and cost of detection. It is also plausible, however, that the law works by signaling the official adoption of an existing social norm of safety belt use. On this theory, the causal diagram would highlight variables related to drivers' beliefs about the legitimacy of government authority or their beliefs about what people whose regard they value would expect them to do. A researcher could then test multiple theories, by, for example, surveying drivers about both their perceptions of punishment risk and their beliefs relevant to a normative theory. Or the researcher may make a reasoned choice about which theory to investigate further. For example, if the researcher is aware that the law has a trivial fine and is not being enforced, she may elect not to prioritize deterrence as a subject of investigation. In this way, theory makes it possible to systematically generate and test explanations of how law is working.

In a quasi-experimental study of the impact of a new safety belt law, the researcher will need to decide how long to observe crash outcomes before and after the law, and at what interval (daily, weekly, monthly, annually; see Chapter 14). If we theorize that the law works solely via deterrence, we might predict a lag between the effective date of the law and increased compliance due to the time it takes for enforcement to ramp up and word to naturally spread. The expected pattern of gradual effect would shape study decisions about length of follow-up data collection and width of observation intervals. A slowly evolving deterrent effect might suggest a wider time resolution and a longer period of observation. If, on the other hand, we theorize that the law works largely by publicizing and reinforcing an existing social norm, and if the law includes funds for a substantial publicity campaign that begins even before the effective date, we might use a narrower time interval and a shorter period of observation after the law takes effect.

Supporting Causal Inference

Causal inference is both empirically and philosophically challenging. Much of the research on how law influences health is observational. Research that demonstrates a correlation between a law and a health outcome cannot always demonstrate that the law *caused* the outcome. In making causal inferences about law, we typically are confronted with a complex system, only some of the elements and outcomes of which have been or can be observed, and in which law is just one element. As we discuss elsewhere in this volume, experimental and quasi-experimental research designs can help us attain a high degree of confidence in causal inference, but in any sort of study of causation in a complex system, both observational and experimental evidence of causation is bolstered by evidence that reveals more of the system's elements. Evidence of the mechanism through which law might have caused the effects—defining and even observing a chain of events between the law and the effect—can help us decide whether an inference of causation is warranted and how confident in that inference we should be. Filling in the black box is, in legal epidemiology, closely analogous to the "evidence of biological plausibility" criterion that is a widely accepted heuristic for assessing causation in epidemiology (Hill, 1965; for a discussion of criteria approaches to causal inference, see Ward, 2009). If one has a robust association between the proposed cause and the observed effect, an inference of causation is bolstered by evidence documenting the links between them in a theory-based causal web—even more so if the association is consistent with multiple theories or causal models (Krieger & Davey Smith, 2016). Populating the causal web requires good theorizing within a solid understanding of the phenomenon and existing and analogous evidence.

We return to the safety belt question. There are many possible explanations for a correlation between safety belt use and a law requiring it. A safety belt law may have caused a change in use, but it is also possible that increasing use of safety belts changed social norms, leading to legislation as a sort of endorsement or signal of what had already occurred. Or both the rise in use and the law could be independent results of some other factor, such as a privately funded educational campaign to increase safety belt use. Research that showed that drivers who feared detection and punishment were significantly more likely to use safety belts would support the inference that law was having an effect via deterrence. By contrast, a finding that there was no connection between wearing a safety belt and knowing about the law or regarding safety belt use as the right thing would undermine the inference that law was driving the change in behavior. In neither case is the mechanism research conclusive, but in connection with other data it supports better judgments by researchers and policy actors.

Understanding Implementation and Guiding Reform

Having confidence that a law is having an effect on health outcomes is not the end of the legal epidemiology inquiry. We also need to understand what is producing the effect, through what process, so we can work to ensure the law has the largest positive effect it can possibly have, with the fewest negative side effects, and that it works optimally wherever it is adopted. Lawmakers will want to know not just whether the law works but at what cost. Along with cost-benefit and cost-effectiveness analysis, research that documents the mechanisms of legal effect can make a valuable contribution to making law work better. Explicit and implicit theories of the legal mechanism can both guide and then be tested by policy implementation research and implementation science methods to identify practices that enhance or reduce the law's impact (Nilsen, Ståhl, Roback, & Cairney, 2013). Some enforcement strategies may be better than others or may cost more than others that are equally effective. Negative side effects may be largely the result of how the law is enforced or implemented, rather than an inevitable consequence of the law's terms or design.

Safety belt law again offers an example. As states began to pass these laws, two different enforcement strategies were used. In some states, failure to wear a safety belt was deemed a *primary* traffic violation, giving police officers the authority to stop and ticket drivers for that reason alone. In other states, the enforcement was "secondary," meaning that police officers could only issue a ticket for a safety belt violation if the driver were being stopped for some other violation. We would not expect the difference in enforcement to make much difference in compliance if what drove compliance was normative agreement with the rule, or the legitimacy of the government. All states had better outcomes with safety belt laws than without. Over time, however, researchers showed that compliance was significantly higher, and crash outcomes better, in states that adopted primary enforcement. In this instance, the deterrent effect of primary enforcement seems to have made a difference to a sufficiently large number of drivers. Knowing this allowed lawmakers to make a change in enforcement provisions that improved the beneficial effects of the rule.

Also important is that different segments of the population may be differentially affected by particular legal mechanisms, and effects of particular mechanisms likely vary over time as society changes. Differential effects across groups and time reinforce the importance of theory and illustrate how selecting a single theory is often unnecessary and possibly inappropriate. In the case of safety belt laws, about 15 % of drivers used belts voluntarily when they were made available in cars (after some educational campaigns). Compulsory use (even with only secondary enforcement) then increased belt use to the majority of drivers. Once the prevalence leveled off at approximately 60 % to 70 %, more active primary enforcement was needed to reach the remaining nonusers. Apparently, normative effects of the law achieved a large part of the first major improvement in belt use and associated safety gains, while deterrence effects increased in importance for those starting to use belts later.

Keep in mind that the field of public health has firmly found that it is almost always easier and more effective to eliminate the need for individual (especially repetitive) behavior change (see Chapter 3). In the case of safety belts, public health professionals also worked on a parallel strategy to help protect car occupants from injuries without requiring individuals to engage in the behavior of using a safety belt every day—advocating for and achieving the mandatory installation of air bags in all automobiles sold in the United States. The design of airbag technology drew strongly on the sciences of physics and biomechanics, and advocacy caused regulatory tools to then be used to ensure the devices were universally installed in cars. This change in the environment around occupants of vehicles automatically protected all people in cars every day, advancing safety beyond that afforded by belts alone and providing significant protection also to those who remained nonusers of belts despite the normative and deterrence effects of compulsory belt use laws.

Integrating Diverse Theories in Public Health Law Research

As the preceding chapters have shown, there are many tools available for opening the black box. Legal epidemiology researchers can draw upon a variety of theories developed by sociolegal scholars to explain how laws are put into practice and how they influence environments and behaviors, but it is also possible to integrate laws within general social and behavioral theories. And it is in fact possible to draw on both legal and non-legal theory at the same time. Taking full advantage of available theory can substantially improve the validity, utility, and credibility of health research on effects of laws and legal practices. There is no simple single theory, no easy way to integrate all theories into a single grand theory, and no prescribed way to use theory. We now illustrate this diversity in detail by applying multiple theories to another example.

Thirty-four states in the United States have statutes that explicitly criminalize sexual behavior of people with HIV under at least some circumstances (Centers for Disease Control and Prevention, 2021). In the remaining states, people with HIV have been prosecuted under various general criminal laws for exposing others to HIV or transmitting the virus (Lazzarini, Bray, & Burris, 2002). "Criminalization of HIV," as this phenomenon is known, has been criticized on a number of grounds (Hoppe, McClelland, & Pass, 2022). There are many cases of the criminal law being used to severely punish assaultive behavior by people with HIV—spitting or biting, for example—that does not pose a significant risk of transmitting HIV. Similarly, many of the statutes are written broadly (or poorly) enough to cover sexual behavior, such as kissing, that has no realistic prospect of transmitting the virus (Galletly & Pinkerton, 2004; Wolf & Vezina, 2004). As applied to sexual behavior that does pose a significant risk of

HIV, the laws generally require disclosure, safer sex (for example, condom use), or both. Here we focus on the main question for public health law research: whether criminal laws requiring disclosure of HIV status to partners lead to fewer instances of sexual HIV exposure and a reduction in the incidence of HIV in the population.

This is a difficult question to answer, for many reasons. There is no way to randomize exposure to the treatment (law). And in this case, quasi-experimental designs are also difficult. To begin with, we lack an objective measure of the outcome. Data on incidence of HIV infection are lacking. Incidence is estimated on the basis of statistical analysis of HIV tests, which may come months or years after infection. Although technologies now exist that make it possible from a test to determine whether the person being tested was recently infected or not, generally we cannot attribute HIV infection events to specific times or places. Studies of the impact of criminal law on HIV therefore use self-reported sexual behavior as the main outcome measure (Burris, Beletsky, Burleson, Case, & Lazzarini, 2007; Delavande, Goldman, & Sood, 2007; Horvath, Weinmeyer, & Rosser, 2010). Even if a better outcome measure were available, we would be faced with the problem that many factors influence HIV infection and HIV risk behavior aside from the law. These range from population prevalence of HIV (the higher the prevalence the greater the likelihood that a given partner will have HIV) to availability and use of antiretroviral treatment (which reduces infectivity) to local norms of condom use to perceptions of risk about HIV. Widespread treatment could reduce HIV incidence even if no one practiced safer sex or disclosed infection; people in a low-prevalence population could practice unsafe sex against the law yet incidence would not change.

There are also challenges in defining the exposure to law across many jurisdictions. The laws differ from state to state, sometimes substantially; places without statutes are not places where law is absent—everywhere the same behavior may be charged as a crime under a general heading such as assault. Finally, accurately measuring whether people even know what the law is can be difficult to do in a way that does not bias later responses by prompting people to think about law. Moreover, because of the overlap between beliefs about law and preexisting social norms and beliefs, people may know about the law without knowing about it—a person who states correctly what the law is may have actual knowledge of the law, or merely assume that the law exists because of beliefs about what is the right thing to do. We end up with observational research that can correlate attitudes about what is right and legal with self-reported behavior and various demographic characteristics, but that has very limited ability to explain whether or how law is causing behavior change (Horvath et al., 2010). Or we resort to mathematical modeling that can test logical hypotheses but ultimately relies on unverifiable assumptions about behavior (Galletly & Pinkerton, 2008). This is precisely the sort of case in which theory about how law could lead to changes in health and health behavior can help us design studies that can shed credible light on the impact of law.

Compliance Models

Since we are interested in whether a law is influencing behavior, it makes sense to start with theories that explain why people obey the law. We will use the theories canvassed in the preceding chapters to generate testable hypotheses that will allow researchers to fill in the black box between an HIV-specific criminal law and sexual behavior.

KNOWLEDGE OF LAW

The threshold question in any compliance theory is whether people actually know what the law is. If they are not aware of the law at all, then their behavior can hardly be said to entail "complying" with it. The first hypothesis follows:

1. Sexually active people are aware of the law regulating the sexual behavior of people with HIV.

Generally speaking, evidence suggests that specific knowledge of the law in the general population is low. That is, most people are not lawyers and could not locate a specific provision in the code or define the elements of a crime. At the same time, people may have a pretty good idea of what is "against the law" simply on the assumption that behavior they regard as bad is also illegal. Applying this heuristic to HIV works pretty well, in that most people (including most people with HIV) seem to believe that it is right to protect or disclose to a partner (Horvath et al., 2010), and failure to do so under at least some circumstances could be prosecuted in every state in the union. Burris and colleagues used two measures in their study: the belief of the respondent that the law prohibited sexual behavior without disclosure of sero-positive status or use of a condom, and the actual law in the state of residence (Burris et al., 2007). That approach allowed the researchers to explore both objective and subjective pathways for legal effect. In contrast, Galletly and colleagues surveyed people with HIV in one state to find out not only whether they were aware of a specific law but also how well they understood its provisions and where they had learned of it (Galletly, DiFranceisco, & Pinkerton, 2008). Armed with a reasonable measure of legal knowledge or belief, we can explore compliance.

CRIMINOLOGY: DETERRENCE

In Chapter 5, Jennings and Mieczkowski explain that criminological theories of compliance—deterrence and labeling—begin with the assumption of rationality. The individual, aware of the law and having some beliefs about its enforcement, will make behavioral choices on the basis of a "utilitarian assessment of pain and pleasure." In our case, the law proposes to punish people with HIV who have sex without disclosing their status or using a condom. The deterrence hypothesis holds that a person will comply with the law if he or she believes that detection and punishment are sufficiently likely and severe enough that the prospect of future pain outweighs the attraction of current pleasure. For example, in Klitzman's qualitative study of attitudes toward these laws, one participant described "how the threat of such a law had altered his own actions after he made 'a fatal mistake' by not disclosing to a woman who later said that he was trying to kill her and that she could report him to the police. He explained that this legal threat motivated him to alter his behavior with future partners" (Klitzman, Kirshenbaum, Kittel et al., 2004).

In this model, rational choice is not a hypothesis but a premise. We assume that people who know about the law will make a rational choice. The causal diagram (see Figure 5.1) posits that these beliefs will be influenced by "direct and indirect exposure" to law—some combination of personal experience with law enforcement, such as being warned about unsafe behavior, and indirect experience, such as reading about prosecutions in the news. These experiences contribute to core beliefs about the certainty, celerity, severity, and equity of punishment for violating the law. This in turn produces two hypotheses to test:

2. People who have had more experience with the law are less likely to report sexual behavior inconsistent with the law.

3. People with positive beliefs about certainty, celerity, severity, and equity will be less likely to report sexual behavior inconsistent with the law.

Chapter 5 discusses both scenario-based and survey methods for assessing these elements. In the case of HIV criminalization, the latter are illustrated by Burris et al. (2007). To measure experience with law, subjects were asked whether they were aware of people being arrested for various acts covered by the law, and how much they knew about these cases. The perceived likelihood of being caught was measured by a set of Likert-scaled items about the likelihood of being caught for activities such as unprotected sex. The perceived severity of the sanction was measured with a set of Likert-scaled items such as "I'm not worrying about jail when I have sex or shoot drugs." The responses were then scaled to create variables for each concept. No significant relationship was found between experience and compliance, and the finding as to certainty or severity was intriguing: people who scored higher on the severity and certainty scales were more likely to report compliance with the law, but with some minor exceptions knowledge of the law was not associated with compliance. Thus people who were generally more concerned about being punished for a variety of actions were more likely to practice safer sex or disclose HIV to a partner, but this was not apparently a product of the specific law at issue.

Economics

Criminological deterrence theory is virtually identical to standard economic analysis of why people obey criminal law. Like criminology, economics assumes a rational person who will seek pleasure and avoid pain (that is, maximize utility) on the basis of an objective assessment of the probabilities of each. Following the theory, people who are "risk-neutral"—that is, who neither seek risky engagements nor prefer to avoid them—will act rationally by assessing whether the expected value of punishment is equal to the expected benefit to be gained from the behavior (Becker, 1968). These individuals will comply with the law, therefore, if the expected punishment is set higher than the expected value of benefit gained. These expectations are influenced by the probability of detection, the certainty of punishment, and the magnitude of the sanctions (Polinsky & Shavell, 2007).

Delavande, Goldman, and Sood used this assumption in a paper that also tried to account for the chances of a person actually getting into trouble. Their basic formula illustrates how economics can be used to state a set of deterrence hypotheses:

> Consider a representative risk-neutral HIV+ person who resides in a state that prosecutes HIV-infected individuals for exposing others to the virus through sexual contact. Let $\Pi > 0$ denote the disutility from being prosecuted and P (pros) be the probability of being prosecuted. The probability of being prosecuted in turn depends on the likelihood that a potential partner would report the sex act to the state and the probability that the state would prosecute conditional on receiving a report:
>
> $$P(\text{pros}) = P(\text{reported}) \times P(\text{presecuted reported}) = P(\text{reported}) \times \rho$$

The parameter ρ is a key policy of interest—states with higher values of ρ have more stringent law enforcement against HIV+ individuals (Delavande et al., 2007, p. 5).

Using this formulation of deterrence, they applied data on sexual behavior to test whether more stringent law enforcement increases safe sex, decreases disclosure of HIV-positive status, and decreases the probability of a sexual encounter. (Unlike other studies discussed here, this one found that aggressive prosecution had all these effects, which, if nothing else, reminds us that methodological and theoretical choices matter.)

CRIMINOLOGY: LABELING

Deterrence in criminology and economics assumes a rational actor calculating risks and benefits. There are plausible reasons for applying this rationality assumption to sexual behavior, but sex can also be seen as the product of social forces. Labeling theory has immediate plausibility in analyzing the effect of criminal laws governing sex because of the basic question of whether having unsafe sex or failing to disclose should be considered "wrong," or whether people who engage in unsafe sex should be considered "criminals." The labeling theory causal diagram (see Figure 5.2) suggests that some individuals with HIV may respond to the label of criminal by defining themselves as rebels or deviants, or that a social-level view of people with HIV (or gay men or sexually active people) as criminal may feed the development of an offender subculture or may deter people from disclosing their HIV status or seeking behavioral health services. Labeling theory suggests a number of interesting hypotheses, including the following:

4. People who internalize the label of criminal will be more likely to report sexual behavior inconsistent with the law.

5. People who perceive that society regards their behavior as deviant will be more likely to report sexual behavior inconsistent with the law.

6. The more people are aware of prosecutions or other negative societal reactions to the "deviant subculture," the stronger the effect of the label.

Although studies of HIV criminalization have not yet explicitly deployed labeling theory, a number of studies suggest ways these hypotheses could be tested. Dodds, Bourne, and Weait (2009) used semi-structured interviews with sexually active gay men in Britain to investigate the effects of criminalization on attitudes and behaviors. Some men, they found, reacted to the labeling of sexual behavior as a crime by, as it were, acting more like criminals, "maximizing their anonymity, and being less open about their HIV status, avoiding disclosure" (p. 141). Also using interviews, Mykhalovskiy (2011) found that the labeling of sexual behavior as criminal might influence behavior along another, unexpected pathway: HIV risk-reduction counselors reported concerns about openly discussing questions of disclosure and condom use out of fear their records might be subpoenaed in a criminal case. Social attitudes toward unsafe HIV sexual behavior, or people with HIV generally, can be measured through survey research, such as Herek's studies of HIV-related stigma (Herek, 1988, 1993; Herek, Capitanio, & Widaman, 2002).

PROCEDURAL JUSTICE

The challenge with sex is that it is usually conducted in private. Likewise, only an extremely small percentage of sexually active people with HIV are arrested or prosecuted (Lazzarini et al., 2002), so the objective chance of detection and punishment is small. Moreover, as labeling theory suggests, people's views on the "rightness" of the law or the fairness of its implementation could also influence compliance. Procedural justice theory offers a way to get to at least two important subjects: internal motivation to comply, which matters a good deal when we are talking about what is in essence an uncontrolled social behavior conducted in private, and the fact that government regulation of sex, not least gay sex, is highly contentious. It is possible that compliance of people subject to the law will be influenced by their views about whether the government should even be making these rules, or by their experiences with the "system." Procedural justice theory provides a way to understand and study these possible effects (Tyler, 1990).

Figure 6.1 is a causal diagram of the effect of procedural justice on compliance with law. For our purposes, we focus on the segment of the pathway linking the experience of procedural fairness, "legitimacy" (defined in terms of "obligation" and "trust and confidence"), and compliance. Chapter 6 explains, "[w]hen people ascribe legitimacy to the system that governs them, they become willing subjects whose behavior is strongly influenced by official (and unofficial) doctrine. They also internalize a set of moral values that is consonant with the aims of the system." Perceptions of procedural fairness—"fairness of decision making (voice, neutrality) and fairness of interpersonal treatment (trust, respect)"—are strong predictors of people's sense of governmental legitimacy.

Both legitimacy and fairness resonate in interesting ways when it comes to criminalization of HIV. It is easy to fall into the error of assuming that people at elevated risk of HIV—people who use drugs, men who have sex with men, or people who sell sex—are, by virtue of those behaviors, fundamentally different from other people in society. At the same time, it is plausible that people engaging in illegal acts such as drug use or prostitution may be more likely to have experienced what they feel is unfair treatment at the hands of authorities, and that they may not be as willing as others to accept an official view that drug use or prostitution is wrong. Similarly, gay men as a group may be more likely than others to reject a role for government in regulating sexual behavior, and to perceive laws that do so as a product of an unfair political system. The procedural justice perspective supports a number of interesting hypotheses about compliance with HIV-specific criminal laws, including the following:

7. People who have had positive experiences of procedural justice in their encounters with authority will be more likely to regard the law regulating the sexual behavior of people with HIV as legitimate.

8. People who regard the government as legitimate will be more likely to comply with laws regulating sexual behavior among people with HIV.

Qualitative research suggests that concerns about intentions behind these laws and fairness of their implementation resonate with gay men. Klitzman's interviewees had complex feelings about these laws. Some endorsed the mandate for responsibility, while others were concerned about effects on safer sex and testing. Others feared unfair prosecutions and believed that bedroom behavior was properly a private, not governmental, domain (Klitzman et al., 2004). And perceived fairness may interact with perceived effectiveness of the law—if the law does not reduce HIV transmission, it is not fair to burden certain people with obligations or restrictions that do not apply to others. The closest thing to a test of these hypotheses in the literature can be found in the study by Burris et al. (2007). The study adapted items from Tyler (1990) to investigate both the experience of procedural justice and the extent to which respondents regarded the government as a legitimate regulator of sexual behavior. As a group, respondents (a convenience sample of people recruited at high-risk sex and drug-use venues) did not have strong feelings on either issue. Most of them did believe that it was morally right for people with HIV to disclose or practice safer sex, and this belief was consistent with their self-reported behavior—but expressing these beliefs was not related to beliefs about the law or whether a specific law actually applied to the respondent. The authors inferred from these results that norms did matter to sexual behavior, but that they were operating independently of the law. Law, in other words, was not playing a major role in sexual choices (Burris et al., 2007).

PUBLIC HEALTH

There are many examples of public health laws directed at individual behaviors. In public health, however, changing the environment is often a more expeditious and effective way to promote health than intervening directly with individuals to change their behavior. Law can be a means of inducing changes in social, physical, and economic environments that change people's behavior or reduce individuals' exposure to unhealthy products or conditions (see Figure 3.1). Because law may also be a factor in exacerbating risk—for example by causing high levels of incarceration in some communities that expose many people to higher-prevalence prison environments and disrupt sexual networks—removing a law can be an important environmental intervention. A public health model of legal intervention suggests many hypotheses, including the following:

9. Laws and regulations that reduce the cost to consumers and increase ease of access to condoms will increase condom use and decrease rates of unprotected sex, unplanned pregnancy, STIs, and HIV transmission.

10. Laws that alter the physical layout and operating rules for public sex venues will reduce unsafe sex.

11. Laws that raise income among young Black and Latinx men will reduce incarceration rates, reduce HIV among the populations, and reduce subsequent transmission to others.

Law might be used to require specific locations to provide condoms at no cost to the user—for example, requiring condoms be readily available in bathhouses. Regularly seeing condoms in a sex venue could change social norms around condoms and their acceptability, as well as increasing their use simply because of ease of physical access to them at a moment when they might be needed. Such an intervention in New York City bathhouses was associated with a significantly greater likelihood of consistent condom use during anal sex in venues receiving the intervention compared to control venues (Ko, Lee, Hung et al., 2009). The basic logic applies to other locations, with regulations potentially requiring condom vending machines in rest rooms at high schools, colleges, gas stations, convenience stores, and so on. Ending legal practices that discourage condom use could also be effective. For example, police implementing laws against prostitution in some places reportedly treat a woman's possession of a condom as evidence of illegal activity, discouraging sex workers and other women from possessing them (Blankenship & Koester, 2002).

Law may also promote safer sex by requiring changes in the layout or operating rules of establishments that cater to people looking for sexual encounters. Courts and city councils have taken this approach over the course of the HIV epidemic, issuing orders and ordinances variously requiring public sex venues to remove doors from cubicles, enhance lighting, post safe-sex rules or warnings, and eject patrons having unsafe sex (Burris, 2003). William Woods and colleagues (Woods, Binson, Pollack et al., 2003; Woods, Euren, Pollack, & Binson, 2010) surveyed 75 gay bathhouses and sex clubs across the United States and reported that all were engaged to some degree in offering HIV prevention, and that most clubs that allowed sexual behavior among patrons had instituted one or more environmental interventions. Unfortunately, there are no published studies of the effectiveness of these efforts.

Thinking about how environments influence behavior tends to shift the focus from the way individuals cope with a given set of stimuli (that is, promoting "good choices") to promoting environments that maximize good options. Thus, in a public health framework, a researcher might be less likely to ask whether criminal law encourages safer sex than to investigate the "social determinants" of HIV transmission. For example, unemployment and lack of opportunities for full participation in society (along with other related factors) result in very high incarceration rates among US Black young men. In prison, many of those men acquire HIV—prisons appear to be a major "hot spot" for HIV transmission (World Health Organization, United Nations Office on Drugs and Crime, & UNAIDS, 2007). Social networks are important factors in the spread of HIV (Ward, 2007). Incarceration disrupts networks as those left behind in the community form new relationships (Khan, Wohl, Weir et al., 2008). A variety of laws and regulations affect employment, business investment, and education and skills development in ways that increase or decrease employment opportunities for this population. A quasi-experimental study of 73 metropolitan areas over 8 years estimated that a $1 higher minimum wage at baseline was associated with a 27% lower rate of new HIV cases among heterosexual Black residents (Cloud et al., 2019). Such economic policies, targeting the social determinants of health rather than a specific prohibition of unsafe sex, may be the most important focus of legal epidemiology.

Modeling Law Within Broader Social and Behavioral Theory

Our discussion thus far applies well-developed theories about how law works. They are quite rich and provide many insights for public health law researchers. At this point, however, the reader may notice the bias in the foregoing inquiry: we have implicitly assumed that law is a significant, or at least detectable, driver of behavior. Rather than construct the question in a framework of how law influences behavior, a researcher could start with a general behavioral theory in which law is simply added as one of many factors and not treated as the preeminent effect to study.

THE THEORY OF TRIADIC INFLUENCES

The theory of triadic influences (TTI) presents a detailed scheme for understanding the many factors that produce an intention to behave in a certain way and, ultimately, the behavior itself (see Chapter 8). It integrates and expands upon other theories that have shown the importance of three proximal factors to a behavioral intention: the individual's attitudes toward the behavior, the individual's perception of social norms and beliefs concerning the behavior; and the actor's sense of self-efficacy or behavioral control in reference to the behavior. Figure 8.1 highlights main pathways along which law may be hypothesized to influence these constructs.

A law can influence an individual's attitudes toward a behavior along two substreams. In the "cognitive-rational" substream, law provides information about the behavior society expects or regards as desirable. This information may also be experienced more emotionally or affectively in interactions with social institutions. In both instances, the streams lead to an attitude toward the behavior composed of both conscious/rational elements, and more emotional/ affective ones. And of course, the legal inputs in this process are interacting with other ones as well, such as information about safe sex and HIV.

Law may influence behavior via self-efficacy or behavioral control if it makes a behavior easier to adopt. In our example, a law requiring universal condom use the first-time people have sex with one another, as Ayres and Baker (2004) have proposed, could in theory reduce the emotional and social barriers to proposing condom use when approaching sexual relations. Here, too, the broader behavioral science framework easily accommodates other possible influences on condom use, such as sex education or the provision of condoms in sex venues.

Finally, law can work via the social-normative stream. The theory posits that people will be influenced by how others perceive their behavior. We are sensitive to general social norms and the values of our important associates. Law may be taken as a reflection or reinforcement of social disapproval of unsafe sex, bolstering the norm of safer sex or disclosure. The innate desire to please others in relationships and to avoid conflict may promote safer behavior or disclosure, though of course the social milieu may send quite contradictory signals. A perceived norm of disclosure may be blunted in its effect on behavior by the perception that people with HIV are not considered desirable sex partners.

A great variety of hypotheses about HIV criminalization and sexual behavior can be generated and tested within this framework. One strategy is to embed standard compliance theory within the TTI. For example, one can conceptualize deterrence as operating via knowledge and expectancies; certainty, celerity, severity, and equity become variables within the pathway of rational responses to the environment. Or one can treat law as a distal influence on the social-normative stream, influencing others' behaviors and attitudes and the actor's perceived norms. The richness of the model makes it possible to test hypotheses about direct legal effects or to link tests of law to broader behavioral questions. Examples include the following:

12. People who know about the law are more likely to perceive a norm against having sex without disclosing HIV status or using a condom.

13. People who perceive a norm requiring safer sex or disclosure of HIV status are more likely to disclose or practice safer sex.

Hypotheses of this sort can be explored in interviews. Several of the respondents in the study conducted by Dodds et al. (2009)

> feared condemnation from their local gay community should it become known that they had engaged in unprotected sex as a diagnosed man … . A criminal prosecution case had the potential to make public such behaviour and raised the fear of judgment from peers and the negative social consequences of being identified as morally reprehensible. As a result they were particularly cautious about avoiding the

circumstances that might lead to such an accusation. "I'm very, very acutely aware of kind of where the law is on it, you know? And although I could say that he knew I were positive there, [pause] I could possibly still be ostracized if it came out in the community that I was the one who infected him and all of this sort of stuff. I didn't want that really and I didn't fancy being prosecuted" (Late 30s, diagnosed 18 years) (Dodds, Bourne, & Weait, 2009, p. 140).

An advantage of the TTI and several of the theories it integrates is that there are well-developed measurement approaches to eliciting information, scaling, and quantifying the results for purposes of predicting behavioral intentions and behavior. The survey designed by Burris and colleagues drew on the theory of planned behavior (Burris et al., 2007). In addition to a variety of items that explored people's own attitudes toward safer sex and disclosure, items probing perceived behavioral control used true-false statements such as, "If I am sexually aroused I can stop before sex to use a condom." Perceived social norms were investigated with true-false statements such as, "People I know best expect that I will always discuss my HIV status with partners before having sex." The integration of behavioral theory and legal compliance avoids the assumption that law is a primary driver of behavior while allowing law to be investigated along the many plausible pathways of effect.

Economics

Economic theory rests on "rational actors" who seek to maximize their own well-being subject to constraints, such as income and time, thereby naturally weighing the perceived benefits and costs of different actions. Chapter 7 offers a more complex account of the operation of law in an economic framework. For most economists, a perfectly competitive market generates the most efficient allocation of society's resources and is therefore optimal, and the sole (or at least predominant) rationale for legal intervention in the market is to ameliorate market failures that prevent a perfectly competitive market from operating. Some might feel uneasy about applying market language to choices and actions involving intimate encounters between individuals, but a longstanding closely related theory in sociology does exactly that. Social exchange theory (Blau, 1964; Cook, Cheshire, Rice & Nakagawa, 2013; Homans, 1958) deems all social interactions (not just economic transactions) to be characterized by persons attempting to maximize their gain for a given investment, and has long been applied to human mate selection processes (Goode, 1970, 1971). The theory is not without its critics (Rosenfeld, 2005), but our purpose here is merely to illustrate application of such theory to the example before us.

Assuming that individuals seeking sex and other dimensions of an intimate relationship attempt to maximize their return on investment, for this "market" to work well everyone must have full information about the relevant dimensions under consideration in the transaction. Information on HIV status of potential partners is one such datum, and laws requiring disclosure of seropositivity are attempting to improve the operation of this market by improving information availability. The objective could be furthered by related regulations, such as requirements for regular automatic HIV testing at all preventive health care visits. As always, possible side effects of such efforts to improve information in this market must be considered, such as the risk that disclosure of HIV status, and reliance on that (potentially incorrect) disclosure by others might increase risk of HIV spread by reducing condom use, an outcome suggested by some recent studies (Butler & Smith, 2007). Likewise, fear of prosecution may influence the decision to be tested by raising the "cost" of knowing one's status (Kesler et al., 2018).

"Law and Society" Research

The theories we have seen so far all tend to treat law as a distinct thing, a piece of information with an objective set of characteristics that acts, in a causal chain, on environments and people who are separate and distinct from the law. The law and society tradition moves beyond how people "use" or "obey" law to bring critical empirical attention to how the rule of law is socially constructed, enacted, contested, and perpetuated in social fields (Cooper, 1995). While there is certainly a body of evaluation research in the law and society literature, "the unique contribution of the law and society approach," Robin Stryker writes in Chapter 4, "is to suggest mechanisms of legal effect emphasizing *meaning-making*." This literature provides powerful theoretical and research methods for getting at how both legal agents and legal subjects understand their roles, their ability to act within a legal framework, and indeed the nature of that legal framework itself (Yngvesson, 1988).

The law and society approach doesn't just allow researchers to ask about the effect of laws in different ways, it suggests different questions. If law is within society and inside people's heads—a way of thinking, a form of meaning—the question is not so much how law influences individual behavior as how law shapes the meaning of acts and the identities of people, from which behavior flows. Law isn't just a set of expressed rules that instruct people specifically how to act in particular situations. "Law" is a repertoire of strategies for getting by, or an alien intrusion to be contested, or just one possible script for understanding one's situation (Ewick & Silbey, 1998). Laws more broadly contribute to the social structuring of expectations of what should and will happen, and how all that can be explained. So, for example, Musheno (1997) used case studies of people with HIV at the margins of society—welfare beneficiaries, drug users—to show how "[p]revailing ideologies and belief systems serve to codify what a person in a given position is likely to perceive or expect to accomplish when confronted with trouble ... ." (Musheno, 1997, p. 103).

Law and society research, with its focus on meaning, often draws upon qualitative methods, including interviews and participant observation, that allow people the opportunity not simply to explain law in their own words but to come to law when they are ready to see it. The concern that the researcher not define the law for the subject has produced some interesting methodological refinement. In their work on how law was influencing the lives of people with disabilities, for example, Engel and Munger (1996) used an "autobiographical" approach in which subjects told and repeatedly edited their life stories. Rather than starting with knowledge of law, or even asking specific questions about law, the researchers waited for the law to emerge on its own in the stories. Law, they found, was not just important when a formal claim or command arose. "Rights may be interwoven with individual lives and with particular social or cultural settings even when no formal claim is lodged. Rights can emerge in day-to-day talk among friends and co-workers; their very enactment can subtly change the terms of discussion or the images and conceptual categories that are used in everyday life. Such subtle yet profound effects may be overlooked in traditional studies of legal impact, yet they can be detected through the analysis in depth of life stories" (Engel & Munger, 1996, p. 14).

Law and society methods are well-suited to understanding how law operates as a meaning-making and meaning-expressing social activity. Public health generally has had its greatest success in interventions that work by changing the social and physical environment, which can both influence individual behavior and reduce exposure to toxic unhealthy conditions (see Figure 3.1). A sociolegal perspective could be deployed to investigate how the legal classification of homosexual behavior as a crime, or the long exclusion of gay people from marriage, might be shaping sexual relationships and the risk of HIV (Burris, 1998a; Chauncey, 1994). Here we consider two narrower hypotheses in the law and society vein:

14. The meaning and implementation of HIV criminalization laws and court decisions will be mediated by how HIV service organizations interpret them and integrate their interpretations into behavioral counseling.

15. Court proceedings and decisions in HIV criminalization cases will be shaped by underlying beliefs about race, nationality, class, and gender.

Working in an interpretive tradition, law and society research often is not framed in terms of testing a specific hypothesis. Nonetheless, researchers pursue specific questions within clearly stated theoretical parameters. Mykhalovskiy (2011) studied HIV criminalization as a case of "the social organization of knowledge," focusing on how criminal law shaped the environment of HIV testing and counseling organizations and the people within that environment. He used interviews and focus groups "designed to elicit experiential narratives in which participants reflected on the topic of criminalizing HIV nondisclosure in ways grounded in their actual, day-to-day experiences" (p. 3). His "[a]nalysis of interview data was focused on bringing into view how an abstract criminal law obligation is made meaningful and expresses itself in people's lives through multiple social and institutional channels" (p. 3).

The work added insights into compliance. Mykhalovskiy (2011) found a great deal of confusion among his subjects about the meaning of the legal concept of "significant risk," which the courts in Canada used to create the dividing line for criminal liability in a sexual encounter. People with HIV seemed to have fairly precise knowledge of the rule—but didn't understand what it meant for actual behavior. For their part, counselors interviewed were equally confused, and for them the problem was compounded by having to offer guidance based on some resolution of the legal and public health advice on risks. Many felt that what they would endorse from a public health point of view as "safer sex" might be criminal under the "significant risk" approach used by courts. But beyond the difficulties of "counseling with an eye on the law" (p. 5), Mykhalovskiy found signs of a process in which law changed the purpose and contents of risk reduction counseling, which in turn seemed to be changing the law: counselors were starting to promote disclosure as a way to avoid legal trouble, beyond its utility as a risk-reduction strategy, and in turn lawyers were noting that prosecutors and judges were "citing to the fact that this person was counseled by public health nurse X on these three occasions to disclose and use a condom and then that becomes used to sort of bootstrap the criminal law obligation into you have an obligation to disclose and to use condoms, which in fact is not what the Supreme Court said. ...." (p. 7). In this instance, law was not just influencing compliance—compliance was influencing law.

Law and society approaches can be used to explore in a richer way how law is shaping meaning and behavior. It can also be deployed to understand how a variety of social factors and processes influence how law is made and used. Matthew Weait (2007), who conducted close textual analysis of court opinions, found that notions of risk and responsibility interacted with gender roles, race, and nationality to shape how judges applied legal rules in HIV exposure cases. His work illustrates how a public health law may actually be doing very different kinds of work, policing moral and ethnic boundaries. Many of the most influential social analyses of HIV have explored law's role in the mediation of HIV's shame, stigma, and inter-group conflict (Altman, 1986; Bayer, 1989; Patton, 1990). Social theory can help researchers explore the many legal influences on health and health behavior that do not work through specific behavioral rules directed at individuals.

Conclusion

This chapter illustrates the use of theory and tools from a range of social and behavioral sciences and legal research traditions to study mechanisms of legal effect in legal epidemiology research. Such theory largely addresses how law shapes health-relevant behaviors, but theory also guides investigation of legal mechanisms that influence health by changing institutions and environments. Scientists and legal scholars can and should draw upon theory to clarify and guide research questions, shape the design of studies, increase specificity of hypotheses to investigate, and improve the data collected or used to directly test those hypotheses. Results from such studies then can better illuminate what happens between the passage of a law and changes in institutions, environments, and behaviors that enhance the health of the population. Better understanding of mechanisms of effect in any specific case, that is, confirming a theory in one situation, also substantially improves the generalizability of a successful public health law in one area to other times, places, settings, and other public health problems.

Summary

Theory illuminating mechanisms of legal effect has at least three important benefits for public health law research and practice: defining the phenomena to be observed, supporting causal inference, and guiding reform and implementation. The choice of what theory or theories to draw upon is a practical one based on research questions and designs, types of law or regulatory approach under study, and state of current knowledge about the matter being investigated. Legal epidemiology researchers can draw upon a variety of theories developed by sociolegal scholars to explain how laws are put into practice and how they influence environments and behaviors. Similarly, it is possible to integrate laws within general social and behavioral theories. And it is in fact possible to do both at the same time. These methods make it possible to substantially improve the validity, utility, and credibility of health research on effects of laws and legal practices.

Compliance theories explain why people obey the law. The threshold question in any compliance theory is whether people actually know what the law is. Both deterrence theorists and economic theorists posit that people will behave rationally (i.e. optimize their own net gain) given what they know about the law and the consequences of disobedience. Labeling theory posits that criminal law works by defining proscribed behaviors as "wrong" and people who engage in it as "criminals." Procedural justice theory focuses on the internal motivation to comply and how it is influenced by the perceived fairness of legal authorities. In the public health tradition, law is often used to change social and physical environments to reduce exposure to risks, rather than to directly regulate individual behavior itself.

Rather than construct the question in a framework of how law influences behavior, a researcher also could start with a general behavioral theory in which law is simply added as one of many factors, and not treated as the preeminent effect to study. The theory of triadic influences (TTIs) presents a detailed scheme for understanding the many factors that produce an intention to behave in a certain way and, ultimately, the behavior itself. Economics places the law and the phenomena it regulates within a framework of markets. Finally, research in the law and society tradition provides powerful theoretical and research methods for getting at how both legal agents and legal subjects understand their roles, their ability to act within a legal framework, and the nature of that legal framework itself.

Further Reading

Dean, K. (1996). Using theory to guide policy relevant health promotion research. *Health Promotion International, 11*(1), 19–26.

Hedstrom, P., & Ylikoski, P. (2010). Causal mechanisms in the social sciences. *Annual Review of Sociology, 36*(1), 49–67.

Hill, A. B. (1965). The environment and disease: Association or causation? *Proceedings of the Royal Society of Medicine, 58*, 295–300.

van Rooij, B., & Fine, A. (2021). *The behavioral code: The hidden ways the law makes us better ... or worse*. Boston, MA: Beacon Press.

Part Three

Identifying and Measuring Legal Variables

Now that we have seen the wide range of theory that can be applied to legal epidemiology research and perhaps gained a vision of hundreds of specific research questions representing studies waiting to be done, we turn to the steps necessary to conducting high-quality legal epidemiology studies. Before collecting and analyzing data, there is an intermediate step that involves drawing on theories of how law affects population health to specify the exact causal paths that will be the focus of a particular study. No single research project can study all possible causal links—all the ways that a law can affect health. Each study of necessity pulls out a few of those links for evaluation. Any study is subject to limits arising from current knowledge regarding theory, the degree to which particular laws vary in ways that facilitate study, the availability of implementation and outcome data, and the willingness of funders to support the research.

Swanson and Ibrahim begin this section with a practical guide to using causal diagrams. Causal diagrams clarify the specific theories and concepts that are the focus of the study; make explicit often implicit hypotheses about how the law works; shape the ways laws are measured for a particular study; reveal key implementation characteristics, mediators, and moderators that need to be measured; and point to the set of

Legal Epidemiology: Theory and Methods, Second Edition. Edited by Alexander C. Wagenaar, Rosalie Liccardo Pacula, and Scott Burris.
© 2023 John Wiley & Sons, Inc. Published 2023 by John Wiley & Sons, Inc.

health outcome indicators best suited for the study. The causal diagram for any particular study illuminates expected patterns of legal effect over space and time, and therefore guides more than the measurement and data-collection features of the study. It also shapes the basic design of the study, the number and time spans of baseline and follow-up observations, and the composition of experimental and comparison groups. Causal diagrams can help reduce study bias, by forcing research teams to carefully consider and clarify their causal assumptions, identifying otherwise overlooked mediators and confounding factors. Finally, causal diagrams often surface clusters of causal pathways that are poorly understood by primary investigators, opening up the need for collaborators in other disciplines. The result is more broadly transdisciplinary teams, and better integration and advancement of knowledge.

The second and third chapters of Part Three focus on identifying and measuring characteristics of law. The complexities of coding laws into categories and assigning numeric values to register the amounts of various dimensions are addressed for statutory law and regulations by Anderson, Thomas, Treffers and Wagenaar in Chapter 11, and distinct issues that arise with coding case law are discussed by Hall in Chapter 12. Measuring law for evaluation is quite different from the way lawyers measure law in traditional legal research. Legal research typically is focused on assessing the idiosyncrasies of a law and using methods of legal interpretation to predict how it can be applied to a single, particular situation considering the law at that moment in time. In contrast, scientific research is focused on accurately measuring what the law says, and relating those measurements to other data measuring implementation and effects in society. And, to more validly assess legal effects, scientists usually study effects of changes in law over time.

Theory and practice of legal measurement also varies between legal epidemiology and other traditions of policy research. While it is common in policy research to define "policy" in terms of a range of examples—including statutes, administrative rules or court cases, and organizational practices or norms—legal epidemiology understands "policy" strictly speaking as a rule-based or rule-like mechanism for generalizing a desirable behavior or standard in an organization, community or society. This view supposes that a policy always starts with a text of some kind that delineates the practice to be adopted and by whom, and thus makes identification and measurement of the policy the presumptive first step in any research process. Typically, the policies considered in legal epidemiology research are set out in statutes, rules, and court decisions, but they may also be found in legally informal or entirely unofficial documents, such as an organizational memo, handbook, or standard operating procedure. Measurement begins after a research team has clarified the research question and theories underlying the study, specified causal diagrams, and selected specific hypotheses for study.

Chapter 11 also makes an important point about the distinction between measuring the apparent features of a policy text and creating variables or scales that attribute qualities or weights to the law or particular elements of the law. Anderson and colleagues distinguish two phases of legal measurement. In phase 1, researchers collect and measure observable characteristics of the legal text that have been identified as important to assess (does it include provision A, yes/no; provision B, yes/no; what is dollar amount of statutory fine for first offense, etc.). In this phase, the coding protocol is designed to minimize interpretive judgments and achieve highly accurate recording of apparent features in the law. This phase of work creates a transparent, reproducible, and substantially objective data set capturing the attributes of the policy. In the second phase, specific provisions may be combined, summed, ranked, or weighted to create indicators that represent theory-based concepts (e.g., "stringency" of a law). By distinguishing phase 1 from phase 2, legal epidemiology methods ensure that the analytic steps and judgments required in phase 2 are transparently based on the measurements made in phase 1. The collaboration between lawyers and scientists throughout this process produces more reliable and valid measures of law, better research, and improved public health practice.

Chapter 10

Picturing Public Health Law Research

The Value of Causal Diagrams

Jeffrey W. Swanson   Jennifer K. Ibrahim

Learning Objectives

- Describe ways that conceptual models can be used to understand a phenomenon in public health law and translate that understanding into research designs.
- Construct a causal diagram, including inputs, mediators, moderators, outputs, and outcomes.
- Compare and contrast different applications of a basic causal diagram across a range of disciplines.

In 1927, New York publicist Frederick Barnard published a misattributed "Chinese proverb" that captured an obvious, yet profound idea: "One picture is worth ten thousand words." Barnard was trying to sell advertising space on streetcars, but the phrase aptly expressed a core truth about human cognition and learning: that we naturally use symbolic pictures to apprehend, organize, summarize, remember, and convey complex information.

Whether it is worth 10,000 or 1,000 words (as today's shortened version of Barnard's adage has it), the reason we can trade all that language for "a picture" is that we understand the world around us largely through a process of simplifying representation (Dansereau & Simpson, 2009). We organize complex information into small chunks that can be visualized and recalled. We build mental models of the world—of what the chunks stand for and how they fit together and causally affect each other—and we unconsciously test and adapt

Legal Epidemiology: Theory and Methods, Second Edition. Edited by Alexander C. Wagenaar, Rosalie Liccardo Pacula, and Scott Burris.
© 2023 John Wiley & Sons, Inc. Published 2023 by John Wiley & Sons, Inc.

such models to accommodate new, corresponding observations and experiences over a lifetime.

These images of our surroundings and of "how things work" are useful for what they include but also for what they leave out; they enable us to ignore a vast amount of distracting information and to focus our attention on what is most relevant for a particular purpose. Models also allow us to understand a larger context, as they provide an overall orientation and a "place to stand," from which we can focus on smaller sections of the picture.

The use of images to represent concepts and mechanisms also creates opportunities for interpretation and evaluation from diverse perspectives. Given the multidisciplinary nature of public health law research and the wide range of topics included in legal epidemiology, the use of commonly understood pictures to illustrate ways in which law and health interact can be invaluable (Burris, Wagenaar, Swanson et al., 2010). The depictions also facilitate conversation between policy makers, practitioners, and researchers in developing, implementing, or evaluating public health law. Ranging from laws that prohibit individual behaviors to laws that provide authority to act to laws that regulate organizational practices, legal epidemiology seeks to understand the mechanisms by which laws can improve health; visualizing these mechanisms in diagrams is an important tool for achieving such an understanding. The purpose of this chapter is to review some basic conventions used to create visual models, evaluate relevant examples of models in published studies, and offer recommendations for constructing clear and informative models.

Varieties of Visual Representation

Academic disciplines—from the sciences to medicine, law, engineering, business management, and education—have long used formal schematic pictures to efficiently represent complex processes and to articulate theories about phenomena of interest (Coryn & Scriven, 2008; Ellermann, Kataoka-Yahiro, & Wong, 2006; Hamilton, Bronte-Tinkew, & Child Trends Inc., 2007; Jordan, 2010; Misue, Eades, Lai, & Sugiyama, 1995; Recker, Rosemann, Indulska, & Green, 2009; Wright, 1934). Various knowledge enterprises have given many names to their pet graphic images, as schematic pictures have become a key currency of technical information. Molecular diagrams depict basic structures of matter in chemistry (Daudel & Daudel, 1948). System flow charts illustrate how computer programs, court proceedings, and organizations work (US Bureau of Justice, 2011). A business process model can show how a particular firm produces goods and services, sells a product, and makes a profit (Recker et al., 2009). Logic models illustrate plans for public health or policy interventions and lay out criteria for evaluating whether these interventions function as designed and produce desired outcomes (W. K. Kellogg Foundation, 2004). Concept mapping or concept webbing can elicit and clarify culturally divergent views of health and disease (Novak & Cañas, 2008). Statistical path analysis schematizes and guides empirical testing of theories of the component causes of social-behavioral phenomena in populations, drawing out ways in which causal factors sometimes interact or may take meandering detours in route to their effect (Duncan, 1966; Land, 1969; Wright, 1934). Regardless of the specific type of model and the associated discipline, all of these approaches are working to do the same thing: tell a story in a single image.

For their part, public health law researchers can use representational diagrams to derive specific research questions and hypotheses from a relevant theoretical framework and then design an appropriate study to test such hypotheses. An overarching model may encompass a broad agenda for research on a legal epidemiology topic, thus allowing the investigator to locate and sequence particular research questions and projects while understanding how they fit into a "big picture." Diagrams can also be used to help policy makers understand or refine a complex legal epidemiology topic. By viewing a diagram that clearly depicts a law's effect in, for example, modifying individual health behaviors or risks in the environment, stakeholders can understand how law is supposed to work or where there may be unintentional consequences. Moreover, this becomes a key communication tool for the media or advocates to explain the policy to public audiences.

Our purpose in this chapter is not to comprehensively review all the various graphical devices that have been used to corral knowledge across fields of human inquiry. Neither is it our purpose to endorse one discipline's particular modeling conventions or to propose some new iconography unique to legal epidemiology. Rather, in what follows, we set forth a few general principles—suggest modest guidelines—for drafting graphic models that are likely to prove useful in conceptualizing, implementing, and critically evaluating innovative legal epidemiology projects. We describe and illustrate several specific purposes that causal diagrams may serve, as they guide research on the effects of law and legal practices on population health.

What do we call these pictures for legal epidemiology? Without taking it too seriously, we use the term *causal diagram* (CD). We suppose that *causal* is a key element, insofar as the depiction of determining relationships between variables is a main point of these devices; if nothing else, they show how one thing leads (or could lead) predictably to another. Second, the word *diagram* seems to work because its Greek meaning is, roughly, "to mark out by lines."

Elements and Conventions of Causal Diagrams

What are the basic components and rules of causal diagrams? Novak and Cañas (2008) provide a useful description of "concept maps" that applies generally to CDs at the simplest level: "graphical tools for organizing and representing knowledge. They include concepts, usually enclosed in circles or boxes of some type, and relationships between concepts indicated by a connecting line linking two concepts.... We define concept as a perceived regularity in events or objects, or records of events or objects, designated by a label" (p. 1).

For the most part, the concepts represented in CDs are variables—characteristics or quantities with changeable values, which may be either observed, observable in principle, or theoretically postulated. CDs have a dynamic quality, using arrows to depict temporal processes, relationships, and sequences of events. Figure 10.1 adapts the main ideas of traditional statistical path analysis (Duncan, 1966; Land, 1969; Wright, 1934) to illustrate some of the key components and representational conventions that are common to many CDs.

CDs of this kind can be read "chronologically" from left to right in the manner that one might read a complex grammatical sentence. The diagrams "tell a story" with a beginning, middle, and end; there are things that happen first (causes, inputs), things that happen last (effects, outcomes), and a variety of things that happen in the middle (mediators, pathways, interactions, arguments). The "middle" involves a sequence of smaller steps or stages. Thus, depending on the focus of a particular study or analysis, the "dependent variable" may also function as an intervening output in the overarching legal epidemiology model.

In Figure 10.1, the boxes labeled X1 through X4 could be considered antecedents or hypothesized component causes of Y. In turn, Y is the consequence, the thing to be explained, or the problem to be solved by an intervention. Boxes depicted on the left edge of the diagram are often referred to as "exogenous" or independent variables, meaning "of outside origin" and not affected by anything internal to the system. Variables configured to the right, within the system, are termed "endogenous." In some CDs, a double-headed arrow is drawn between two independent variables, as with the arrow connecting X1 and X2 in Figure 10.1. Here the arrow represents a preexisting correlation—a reciprocal association between two exogenous causes.

To put some flesh on the skeleton, let us consider a hypothetical CD depicting the effects of state firearms laws on the rate of gun-related fatalities. If we were to assign relevant labels to the boxes in Figure 10.1, variable X1 might

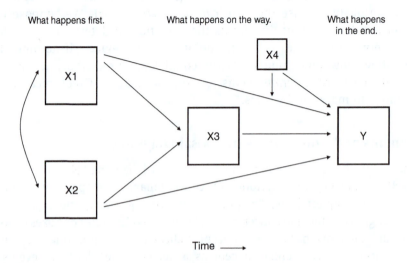

Figure 10.1. Some Conventions of Causal Diagrams.

represent the household gun ownership rate while variable X2 might stand for the restrictiveness of a state's gun laws. In a test of a legal epidemiology theory of gun control effectiveness, these two variables predictably would be correlated with each other, as indicated by the arrow connecting X1 and X2, and both would be expected ultimately to affect the risk of gun violence in the community (Y).

The box labeled X3 in the diagram is a *mediator*—a variable that comes between the main cause(s) and the effect in question (Edwards & Lambert, 2007). To qualify as a true mediator, a variable must be related significantly both to the preceding cause and to the effect that follows, and must thereby explain some of the bivariate association between the first cause and its ultimate result; the mediator explains how it happens. In our gun laws example, X3 might capture a key mediating variable such as the frequency of crimes involving handguns. Logically, if there are more guns in the population (X1), then whenever a crime occurs it may be more likely to involve a gun (X3); in turn, when guns are used in crimes, it is more likely that a fatal injury will occur (Y). Exogenous predictor variables are also sometimes referred to as "distal" causes while mediating variables that immediately precede the outcome of interest are termed "proximal" causes (Greenland & Brumback, 2002). In the current example, an intervention aimed at a distal cause of firearm fatalities might focus on reducing the number of guns in the population, while an intervention targeting a more proximal cause might focus on reducing violent crime.

Finally, the box labeled X4 represents both a moderating variable and one that interacts with another causal factor in the system. As depicted, this variable exerts a direct effect on Y but also modifies the pathway between X1 and Y (that is, is also a *moderator*); hence, the arrow leads to another arrow, rather than to a box. In our gun control example, X4 might stand for a variable measuring implementation of firearms laws, such as the extent to which states report disqualifying records to the National Instant Criminal Background Check System (NICS). The diagram would help us show that we expect NICS reporting to exert a direct effect in lowering the risk of firearm fatalities (Y), but also to potentiate the effect of the law itself (X1)—interact with the law to produce a larger impact than the sum of each of these component causes' single effect. Another important way in which a moderating variable can operate is when a causal effect is stronger in one group than another, or when it works only in one group and not another. For example, Ludwig and Cook (2000) found that the Brady Handgun Control Act significantly reduced suicides, but only in people over age 55. Thus age was found to be a "moderator" of the law's effect.

It is important to recognize that building a CD is an iterative process; as an evolving model confronts new theoretical ideas or evidence, new mediators or moderators may be added, blocks may change position or be removed, and the direction of arrows may even reverse. The descriptive example here is just one way in which to create a CD. Ultimately, the CD should provide a one-to-one correspondence between the theoretical constructs and a testable empirical model. CDs are helpful to evaluate how well constructs in the model are operationalized with available data. Next, we move on to review a range of different options for constructing CDs and note the strengths and weaknesses of each approach in relation to legal epidemiology. However, all of these models proceed from the same basic idea of working through time with the inputs on the left and the outcomes on the right.

Variations on the Theme

Several different types of causal diagrams may be useful in legal epidemiology. These serve distinct but complementary purposes, and some of them follow the conventions we have just described more closely than others. There is no one-size-fits-all approach, and it is important for the researcher to modify the CD according to the features and complexity of the specific study, as well as the intended audience(s).

A Common Understanding

The first purpose of CDs is descriptive classification, addressing the need for a specific, common understanding of the thing to be studied. For example, suppose we wish to examine whether involuntary outpatient commitment laws improve population health and safety. As a general definition, outpatient commitment is a civil court order requiring that a person with mental illness meeting certain criteria participates in outpatient psychiatric treatment.

However, there are several types of legal outpatient commitment (Swartz, Swanson, Kim, & Petrila, 2006); without understanding these types and distinguishing them from each other, it would be difficult to proceed with an informative study of outpatient commitment. Figure 10.2 illustrates how a CD can be used to define and graphically describe the different types of outpatient commitment laws (OPCs), showing the pathways by which someone in a mental health crisis may qualify for each type.

A Process Blueprint

A variation on the descriptive purpose of CDs is process modeling for a specific legal intervention, policy, or program. The goal of process modeling in legal epidemiology is to provide a detailed blueprint of a given legal intervention and how it is designed to function. By analogy, if a generic descriptive CD defines an automobile and distinguishes generally between cars and trucks and buses, a process model CD would "lift the hood" of a particular vehicle and show how the engine works.

Figure 10.3 illustrates such a diagram for a program of legal outpatient commitment, New York's Assisted Outpatient Treatment Program (AOT) (New York State Office of Mental Health, 2011). This type of model can also be used as an action map or decision guide for system actors who are involved with the AOT program. The CD moves from referral to investigation to assessment and service delivery, highlighting the range of potential mechanisms involving clinical and legal actors. The CD also provides context for how the

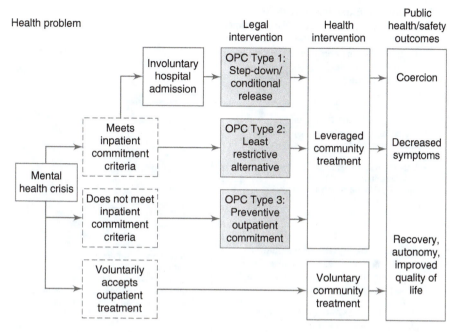

Figure 10.2. Types of Involuntary Outpatient Commitment.

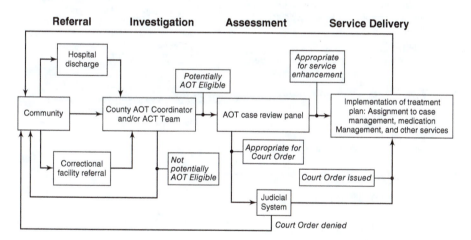

Figure 10.3. Schematic Representation of AOT Processes in Nine Areas of New York State.
Source: New York State Office of Mental Health (2011).

individual moves through different institutions, which is important to consider when formulating or revising policy interventions.

Sometimes the same information can be conveyed using different types of CDs to reach different audiences. While graphical boxes labeled with different types of actors and organizations may be useful for program administrators, these images may be meaningless to the general public or policy makers. As an alternative, Figure 10.4 presents a CD on the same New York AOT program, but directed toward a general lay audience (Pataki & Carpinello, 2005); this CD is centered on the perspective of an individual trying to navigate the system.

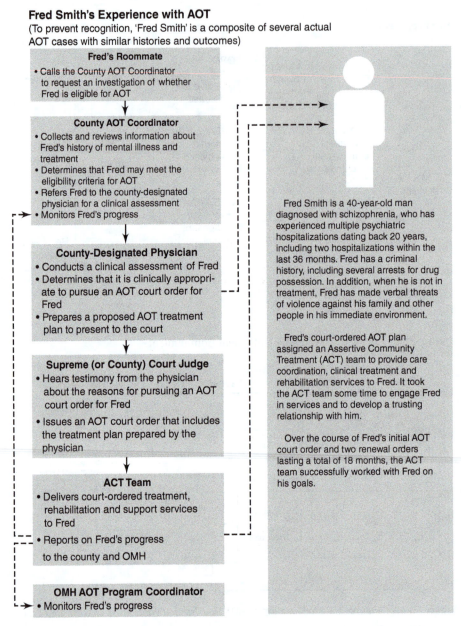

Fred Smith's Experience with AOT

(To prevent recognition, 'Fred Smith' is a composite of several actual AOT cases with similar histories and outcomes)

Fred's Roommate
- Calls the County AOT Coordinator to request an investigation of whether Fred is eligible for AOT

County AOT Coordinator
- Collects and reviews information about Fred's history of mental illness and treatment
- Determines that Fred may meet the eligibility criteria for AOT
- Refers Fred to the county-designated physician for a clinical assessment
- Monitors Fred's progress

County-Designated Physician
- Conducts a clinical assessment of Fred
- Determines that it is clinically appropriate to pursue an AOT court order for Fred
- Prepares a proposed AOT treatment plan to present to the court

Supreme (or County) Court Judge
- Hears testimony from the physician about the reasons for pursuing an AOT court order for Fred
- Issues an AOT court order that includes the treatment plan prepared by the physician

ACT Team
- Delivers court-ordered treatment, rehabilitation and support services to Fred
- Reports on Fred's progress to the county and OMH

OMH AOT Program Coordinator
- Monitors Fred's progress

Fred Smith is a 40-year-old man diagnosed with schizophrenia, who has experienced multiple psychiatric hospitalizations dating back 20 years, including two hospitalizations within the last 36 months. Fred has a criminal history, including several arrests for drug possession. In addition, when he is not in treatment, Fred has made verbal threats of violence against his family and other people in his immediate environment.

Fred's court-ordered AOT plan assigned an Assertive Community Treatment (ACT) team to provide care coordination, clinical treatment and rehabilitation services to Fred. It took the ACT team some time to engage Fred in services and to develop a trusting relationship with him.

Over the course of Fred's initial AOT court order and two renewal orders lasting a total of 18 months, the ACT team successfully worked with Fred on his goals.

Figure 10.4. New York State Office of Mental Health Diagram Explaining AOT to the Public.

Source: Pataki and Carpinello (2005, p. 6) / US Department of Health and Human Services.

Mapping Multiple Interventions

The CD can also be used to map the cumulative and interacting effects of a range of interventions that address a specific health topic. Figure 10.5 provides an example of a model depicting ways to curtail youth consumption of alcohol, such as reducing economic and physical access to alcohol, enforcing societal norms, and exercising other social control mechanisms. The model combines

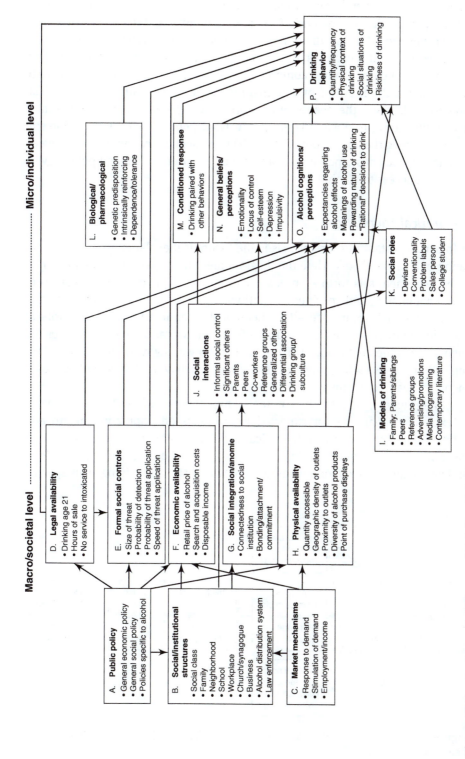

Figure 10.5. An Integrated Theory of Drinking Behavior.

Source: Wagenaar and Perry (1994, p. 322) / Taylor & Francis.

theoretical elements from several disciplines, including social and behavioral sciences and economics, and engages the issue of underage drinking from the perspectives of several key actors, including the minor who would consume alcohol, the retailer who would sell alcohol to minors, and the law enforcement officer who would detain the minor (Wagenaar & Perry, 1994). While this is a complex model, it represents an inherently complicated set of interconnecting phenomena and does so in a comprehensible way that provides an opportunity to consider multiple points of potential modification to existing laws and legal practices. However, the beauty of a complex model such as this one is that it allows the viewer to trace different pathways depending upon need while still acknowledging the larger context. The CD may facilitate collaboration between a behavioral scientist and an econometrician to better understand policy levers to restrict access to alcohol.

Theoretical Foundations

A fourth important purpose of CDs is the theoretical explanation or the articulation of a causal theory. Here the diagram identifies a particular phenomenon to be explained, sets forth a proposed cause or multiple component causes of the phenomenon, and specifies the pathways of association—patterns of common, sequential occurrence—that theoretically connect the causal factors to the effect of interest. Figure 10.6 draws from behavioral theory and applies the theory of planned behavior (TPB) to explain how a law restricting or prohibiting cell phone use while driving can result in a behavior change and improvements in health outcomes.

In this model, we offer three potential hypotheses for how TPB can be used to explain mechanisms for expected legal effects on population health and safety. The diagram clarifies theoretical mechanisms by which legally restricting cell phone use while driving can be expected to change driving practices, and potentially reduce mortality associated with distracted driving. This specific

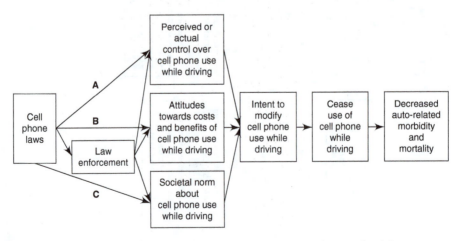

Figure 10.6. Use of Theory of Planned Behavior to Frame Distracted Driving Behaviors.

example demonstrates the integration of a classic behavioral sciences theory with classic legal theory on deterrence.

First, a "fear hypothesis" (path A in Figure 10.6) would posit that fear of being caught and punished—deterrence, in legal terms—inhibits the individual's independent action of using a cell phone while driving. A second option is the "guilt hypothesis" (path B), which posits that negative social sanctions attached to the behavior of using cell phones while driving affect the actor's attitude toward these behaviors and persons who engage in them. Finally, the "shame hypothesis" (path C) posits that laws and law enforcement activities can induce in the actor a sense that others look down on the sanctioned behavior, in this case, that fellow drivers will be annoyed and irritated by someone using a cell phone while driving. These attitudes determine the intention to use a cell phone while driving.

If the law is working, one or more of these mediating mechanisms will modify the subjects' intention and behavior, and eventually, the risky practice of driving while using a cell phone will decrease across the population. Given valid measures and sufficient observations of data from a representative sample, such an effect would be detected as predicted by the model. We could also expand the model to include mediators and moderators of the relationship between the intent to modify the behavior of using a cell phone while driving and actually stopping the behavior. However, it is best to keep the CD focused on a few elements that are both theoretically relevant and empirically testable, rather than to include any number of extraneous variables that might co-vary with the law and correlate with its outcome.

Moving from Pictures to Measures

A fifth purpose of CDs in public health law research is to guide tests of direct and indirect causal effects of laws on public health outcomes (Rothman & Greenland, 2005). To illustrate, Figure 10.7 articulates testable mechanisms by which various tobacco control policies could modify smoking behavior (Fong, Cummings, Borland et al., 2006). Any policy's effect is likely to be moderated by individual characteristics—from sociodemographic descriptors to personality features and previous smoking behaviors—and mediated by psychosocial factors such as shared beliefs and attitudes, group norms, and perceptions of risk. The model allows us to think about the specific measures and sources of data that would be necessary to test alternative and complementary hypotheses. While the model was created mainly as a general framework for tobacco control policy efforts, it also provides a useful catalogue of mediating variables that specific policies might target and which could be measured to test these policies' effects. The CD could also help identify variables that have not yet been operationalized and may therefore be included in future data collection.

A final purpose of CDs in public health law research is to depict and guide the process of research or evaluation itself. An extensive literature exists that explains the use of "logic models" in public health program evaluation (W. K. Kellogg Foundation, 2004). The main distinguishing feature of these types of

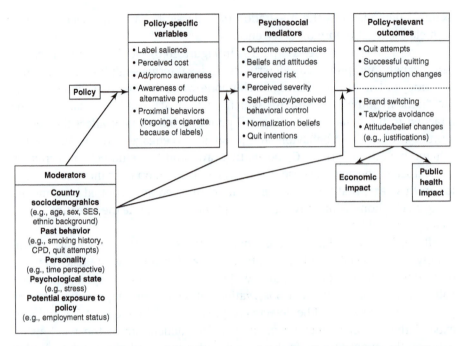

Figure 10.7. Conceptual Model of the Impact of Tobacco Control Policies Over Time.
Source: Fong, Cummings, Borland et al. (2006, p. iii5) / BMJ Publishing Group.

CDs is a depiction of programs' "theory of change," including inputs, activities or strategies, outputs, and impact or outcomes in order to demonstrate and evaluate effectiveness. Beyond use for research or evaluation, CDs may also be deployed as a tool for program development, policy making, and analysis, particularly in cases when policy makers must make decisions without the benefit of strong evidence for the likely effectiveness or adverse consequences of a course of action. By graphically unpacking a policy's potential requirements, goals, and expected pathways of effect, the CD provides an opportunity to consider hidden assumptions, barriers, or unintended "side effects" that might not otherwise be debated. Figure 10.8 is an example of CD that was used to develop and monitor strategies to minimize the spread of COVID-19 when there was rapidly changing science around the disease and a lack of evidence on the effectiveness of different interventions (Centers for Disease Control and Prevention, 2020a,b).

What Makes a Good Causal Diagram?

Scholars have described several criteria to evaluate the adequacy of representational diagrams used in process modeling, particularly in the context of business and information sciences (Recker et al., 2009). The ideas underlying several of these criteria can be adapted to evaluate CDs for public health law research and to identify specific problems that may arise with these models. We propose related criteria that can be summarized as the "Three C's": correspondence, comprehensiveness, and clarity.

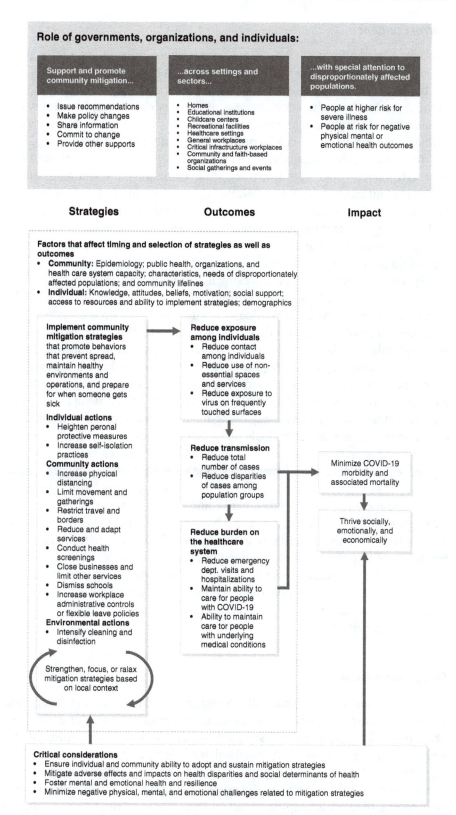

Figure 10.8. Logic Model for Monitoring and Evaluating Community Mitigation Strategies for COVID-19.

Source: Centers for Disease Control and Prevention (2020a,b).

Correspondence

The first criterion for evaluating CDs is *correspondence*, meaning that a given concept or construct in the model must correspond in a valid, specific way to the particular phenomena or set of observations that it purports to describe in the real world. Since the basic premise of the model is to explain real-world phenomena to facilitate research, it is important that each box has a clearly defined connection to some element directly or indirectly observed in reality.

To illustrate this criterion, consider a CD that is designed to illustrate a test of whether states' laws against driving while using a mobile communications device prevent motor vehicle crashes and injuries. Imagine that the CD depicted in Figure 10.6 had included separate boxes labeled "distracted driving laws" and "laws against texting and driving." The first problem with such a model would be a *poor correspondence* between at least one of the constructs and the real-world phenomena of interest.

Specifically, the box labeled "distracted driving laws" would suffer from what Recker et al. (2009) call "construct overload." As they explain (in the context of business process modeling), construct overload occurs when a term "provides language constructs that appear to have multiple real-world meanings and, thus, can be used to describe various real-world phenomena. These cases are undesirable, as they require users to bring to bear knowledge external to the model in order to understand the capacity in which such a construct is used in a particular scenario" (p. 349). In short, "distracted driving laws" could refer to distractions such as eating, doing make-up, reading, and a whole host of other activities that individuals may do while driving, rather than the intended focus on the use of mobile communications devices while driving.

Second, the inclusion of two boxes labeled with slightly different definitions of the law, and with varying degrees of specificity, would also show poor correspondence. The logical deficit here could be called *concept redundancy*. A legal epidemiology model containing constructs with overlapping meanings and real-world referents is difficult to understand, impossible to test, and hopeless to apply to policy making. As mentioned earlier, it is possible to create a CD that includes multiple legal interventions to address a particular public health issue, but it is imperative that each box has a mutually exclusive definition within that model, and that hypothesized interactions are depicted with appropriate precision.

Comprehensiveness

A useful CD should incorporate all necessary elements to achieve its specific purpose—whether description, classification, explanation, testing, or evaluation. Thus the model must include sufficient detail to adequately represent the hypothesized legal causes, hypothesized mediators, and health effects to be examined in a legal epidemiology project; it should not omit relevant variables and pathways. At the same time, the model should not be made more complex than necessary in an attempt to "represent the whole world." Just as a figure

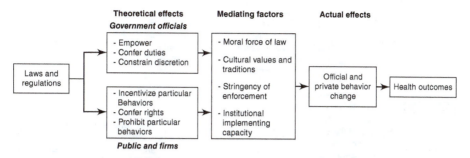

Figure 10.9. Conceptual Model of the Effect of Law on Public Health Outcomes.

that is too basic invites misinterpretation, a diagram that is too complicated may create confusion. The goal is to construct a model that strikes an appropriate balance between the bare bones and the byzantine.

Figure 10.9 is a CD designed to explain how laws and regulations influence the behaviors of the public and government and private entities, resulting in a change in health outcomes (Mello, Powlowski, Nañagas, & Bossert, 2006). The model provides an example of a CD that avoids the clutter of irrelevant details, yet does not oversimplify its relevant constructs and connections. The model is thus able to achieve its goal of visually representing, and therefore illuminating, the link between theoretical and actual effects of law on public health outcomes. Moreover, while the model provides an overall picture, it is possible to segment out one section of the model—for example, government actors only—and create a more granular version that elaborates on the mediating and moderating factors. The comprehensiveness criterion is also related to the term *parsimony* as used to evaluate theories in philosophy of science: all things considered, the simplest explanation is the best.

Clarity

The final CD criterion that we will mention here is clarity, which refers to both visual intelligibility and conceptual lucidity. Clarity means, in essence, that a CD's images and accompanying labels should be easy to read, and they should make the concepts they stand for easy to understand. While this is related to considerations of correspondence and comprehensiveness, the clarity criterion expresses the model's intuitive logical appeal and the extent to which it conveys an intended message with sufficient detail in definition—the elements in sharp focus with a minimum of surrounding "fog." The diagram must also be visually appealing and easy to follow; the reader should spend time thinking about the ideas, not figuring out how to interpret the boxes and arrows. It is possible for a model to be relatively simple, even to have good correspondence between constructs and their real-world referents, and still not be clear. For example, consider a model designed to depict the population health effects of regulatory action on pharmaceutical companies' innovation in developing new antimicrobial medications. Imagine a series of boxes labeled "regulation," "innovation," "incentives," "overutilization," "resistance," "effectiveness," and

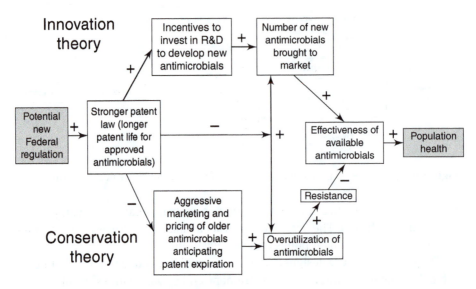

Figure 10.10. How Stronger Patent Laws Could Improve Antimicrobial Effectiveness.

"population health," with multiple arrows connecting the boxes. The main problem with such a model would be a lack of clarity: What does it mean? How do these elements fit together according to some logical scheme?

Figure 10.10 presents a model of clarity using the same basic concepts, but lays out the logic for two different approaches to solving the public health problem of antibiotic resistance—innovation and conservation—and shows how strengthening patent law could plausibly work through both mechanisms simultaneously (adapted from Outterson, 2005). The picture is clear and it is easy to see potential research questions, hypotheses to be tested, and measures to represent each box. This is the ultimate goal of CDs.

How to Create an Effective Causal Diagram

An informative and effective CD begins with careful preparation. The creative activity of sketching boxes and arrows should follow from, not precede, a solid understanding of the substantive topic at hand. Thus, the first step should be to selectively review the current academic literature on several facets of the subject: the basic dimensions of the public health problem at hand; its established or putative causes; contours of the law, policy, or regulatory scheme whose possible effects on health are the subject of inquiry; and what may already be known about the mechanisms of these laws' effect on health. It may also be valuable to review the literature on parallel topics to glean lessons from other applications of the law. A selective literature review should be carried out to extract key constructs, ideas, and causal relationships that recur in the literature across relevant fields of study, or that seem to bridge parallel understandings in diverse disciplines—from the health sciences to social sciences and the law.

The selective literature review should be driven by several basic theoretical questions that could also become research questions: What are the major causes of this public health problem? How could law, policy, or regulation conceivably affect the problem? What factors could modify or strengthen the law's effect on the health problem? Are there reasons to posit a fairly direct link between law and health in this instance? Or is it more likely that complex processes—environmental change, structural change, behavioral change, or all three—would intervene as foreseeable mechanisms of effect?

Armed with a basic understanding of key concepts and how they might fit together, there are many ways to actually draw a CD. Here is one: start by sketching a box that represents the health problem—the main outcome to be affected—on the right-hand side of a sheet of paper (or its computer-screen equivalent). Next, sketch a box representing the legal intervention on the left of the drawing space. Connect the two boxes with a long arrow from left to right; keep in mind, the diagram "moves" chronologically from left to right. Next, stop and ponder: What other important variables could influence the health problem, and how might they be affected by the law as well? Add these variables to the diagram in the form of labeled boxes positioned above or below the central horizontal arrow, and suspended between the legal intervention on the left and the health outcome on the right. Connect these middle boxes with diagonal arrows coming from the law and proceeding to the health outcome.

The final step involves revising the diagram with an eye to the whole picture—repositioning boxes, adding or subtracting arrows—until the CD begins to form a clear, legible, and intelligible portrait of a health problem and its potential legal solution, along with any necessary "scaffolding" to make it work. While described here in a few steps, in practice this is an iterative process. The final result should be a CD that is sufficiently detailed to convey all the information that is necessary to represent the theoretical mechanism or research problem at hand without extraneous conceptual or visual clutter.

Conclusion

Causal models have become increasingly common in the presentation of theory-driven research schemes across a variety of disciplines. However, there are few clear conventions in the current practice of graphic representation of variables, associations, interactions, and time that allow such pictures to be understood across disciplines. In this chapter, we have described a set of simple conventions for using causal diagrams as heuristic models to visually represent key independent and dependent variables, hypothesized mediators, moderators, and direct and indirect pathways of effect. The use of these models in legal epidemiology can yield powerful insights into the intended and unintended effects of laws on population health, as well as the social and institutional contexts in which they occur.

Causal diagrams can do important work in legal epidemiology, insofar as they answer several kinds of questions. They can help to describe ("how things are now"), classify ("why things go together"), explain ("how things really work"), predict ("what will happen if"), and decide ("what you should do now"). As conceptual models, CDs not only map the steps by which law may impact health but also allow a researcher to more carefully consider the set of measures to be used in developing a methodologically rigorous study. Models that exhibit valid correspondence and are appropriately complex yet clear will help legal epidemiology researchers plan and carry out their work. Images that accurately represent the topic at hand may also be useful for policy makers in understanding new evidence for the many ways that laws may improve population health.

Summary

Given the multidisciplinary perspectives of public health law research and the wide range of topics included in legal epidemiology, the use of commonly understood pictures to illustrate the ways in which law and health interact can be invaluable (Burris et al., 2010). Ranging from laws that prohibit individual behaviors to laws that provide authority to act to laws that regulate organizational practices, legal epidemiology seeks to understand the mechanisms by which laws can improve health; visualizing these mechanisms in diagrams is an important tool for achieving such an understanding. The purpose of this chapter is to review some basic conventions used to create visual models, evaluate relevant examples of models in published legal epidemiology studies, and offer recommendations for constructing clear and informative models.

Causal diagrams can do important work in legal epidemiology, insofar as they answer several kinds of questions. They can help to describe ("how things are now"), classify ("why things go together"), explain ("how things really work"), predict ("what will happen if"), and decide ("what you should do now"). As conceptual models, CDs not only map the steps by which law may impact health but also allow a researcher to more carefully consider the set of measures to be used in developing a methodologically rigorous study. Models that exhibit valid correspondence and are appropriately complex yet clear will help legal epidemiology researchers plan and carry out their work. Images that accurately represent the topic at hand may also be useful for policy makers in understanding new evidence for the many ways that laws may improve population health.

Further Reading

Coryn, C. L. S., & Scriven, M. (2008). The logic of research evaluation. In C. L. S. Coryn & M. M. Scriven (Eds.), *Reforming the evaluation of research (New Directions for Evaluation)* (Vol. 118, pp. 89–105). San Francisco, CA: Jossey-Bass and American Evaluation Association.

Dansereau, D. F., & Simpson, D. D. (2009). A picture is worth a thousand words: The case for graphic representations. *Professional Psychology: Research and Practice, 40*(1), 104–110.

Ellermann, C. R., Kataoka-Yahiro, M. R., & Wong, L. C. (2006). Logic models used to enhance critical thinking. *The Journal of Nursing Education, 45*(6), 220–227.

Krieger, N., & Davey Smith, G. (2016). The tale wagged by the DAG: Broadening the scope of causal inference and explanation for epidemiology. *International Journal of Epidemiology, 45*(6), 1787–1808.

W. K. Kellogg Foundation (2004). *Logic model development guide: Using logic models to bring together planning, evaluation*. Battle Creek, MI: W.K. Kellogg Foundation.

Chapter 11

Measuring Statutory Law and Regulations for Empirical Research

Evan D. Anderson   Sue Thomas   Ryan D. Treffers

Alexander C. Wagenaar

Learning Objectives

- Describe the concept and value of systematic measurement of law.
- List the steps in a systematic process for measuring law and creating a numeric legal data set.
- Identify important logistical challenges in legal measurement projects.

Measuring law, as the term is used here, means determining dimensions or components of an area of law relevant for particular research studies and using the resultant categorization schema to produce accurate representations of the law in terms of counts and numeric indicators. The process for measuring law relies on techniques that are common in both quantitative and qualitative social science research. Although few of these techniques are conceptually challenging, their application to the law can be difficult. The bulk of this chapter is devoted to providing a step-by-step guide for reflecting variation in laws across time, space, or both. To provide context and make clear the importance of these steps, the chapter begins with a short section explaining some of the basic principles underlying the process. A final section describes common challenges and offers suggestions for addressing them.

Legal Epidemiology: Theory and Methods, Second Edition. Edited by Alexander C. Wagenaar, Rosalie Liccardo Pacula, and Scott Burris.

The Impetus Behind Measuring Law

Supreme Court Justice Louis Brandeis famously remarked that "it is one of the happy incidents of our federal system that a single courageous state may, if its citizens choose, serve as a laboratory; and try novel social and economic experiments without risk to the rest of the country" (*New State Ice Co. v. Liebman*, 1932, p. 311). Innovation by states and other political units is vital to having an effective regulatory system. This policy experimentation is frequently a necessary step to identify effective public health laws. Consider the problem of motor vehicle crashes for teenagers and graduated driver licensing (GDL) laws. In the mid-1990s, a few states began experimenting with laws that restrict when and under what circumstances teenage drivers could operate a motor vehicle. As these laws proliferated in number and type, researchers evaluated their effects, first in studies comparing crash rates in single states before and after the adoption of a GDL restriction, and then in studies comparing changes in crash rates in states adopting GDL laws of varying restrictiveness. As these studies accumulated, it became clear that restrictive laws saved lives. Now most states have adopted similarly restrictive laws, though important variation in the law across states remains. Teen crash rates have declined continuously since, marking GDL laws as one of the great modern examples of how policy innovation, rigorous evaluation, and evidence-based dissemination save lives (Preusser & Tison, 2007).

Two factors made GDL research possible. First, there was variation in both state laws and state motor vehicle crash rates. Second, there were methods for measuring that variation that enabled statistical comparisons. Measuring crash-related harms is accomplished by generating counts through police reports, hospital records, and other administrative data. But how does one measure and quantify something textual like the law? The answer is not too difficult using one or more experienced legal researchers, careful consideration of a handful of persistent sources of error, and attention to the usual basic principles of science. As any qualitative researcher can attest, characteristics of texts are observable and these observations converted into numeric indicators, or *coded* as it is often called. At its core, the task of coding law is not altogether different from coding an open-ended interview transcript. In each instance, researchers strive to measure the features of the texts in ways that are consistent with scientific standards of reliability and validity.

There are two primary sources of difficulty in the process of measuring law. The first is typical of almost all research that involves analyzing the meaning or contents of texts. Law is, by its nature, an abstraction with at best an uncertain underlying empirical foundation. For this reason, measurements of law themselves cannot be directly validated against observable phenomena in the natural world. The method for measuring law offered in this chapter is more like observation than traditional legal interpretation, because the method emphasizes observing the text (what the law says) and minimizing interpretation (what the law means). But few observations can be made of laws that do not require some predicate legal decision-making based on assumptions about the nature of the legal text being examined. The types of observations of laws that are defensible regardless of context or purpose—like the number of words in a statute or whether it includes a specific term—tend not to provide much value in public health law evaluations. Researchers' decisions that shape the laws that are collected and how they are understood increase the importance of reporting how and, in some instances, why specific legal measures were adopted to represent a particular construct.

The second primary source of difficulty in measuring law is identifying the correct legal texts to collect and examine. Unlike the qualitative researcher who creates a file of transcripts for coding by, for example, interviewing a defined group of people, the legal rules that regulate life in the United States are distributed over space, time, levels of government, and types of law. Determining the prevailing law governing the sale of sugar-sweetened beverages in a selection of cities, for example, might necessitate gathering laws from different sources (legislative, executive, judicial, electoral, and constitutional) and at different levels of government (federal, state, and local). In addition to difficulties finding the relevant legal provisions, researchers also must consider how provisions interact within a broader legal framework. In most instances, lawyers are needed to help determine which laws are relevant, how to find them, and, in some instances, how they are to be interpreted—which means that for empirical researchers embarking on an evaluation of law, collaboration with legal colleagues is usually necessary.

Although legal expertise is essential to measuring law, it is not sufficient to generating valid data. The bulwark against error in legal measurement is a deliberate commitment to standard principles and practices of good science. The method described here provides steps for operationalizing those principles and practices in legal research. Some standard scientific practices—such as the creation of a detailed research protocol that enables replication and updating of data—might seem odd at first to legal colleagues who are accustomed to the more normative and interpretive world of traditional legal research in which the process for doing research is idiosyncratic to each practicing lawyer, and closely guarded as the lawyer's stock in trade. But our experience is that legal researchers can and do quickly internalize these rules and procedures drawn from scientific research; indeed, they often find them valuable in other areas of their work.

Projects that blend legal and empirical research fall into two primary categories. In the first, legal research measuring the features of law is driven by the goal of testing a specific hypothesis. An hypothesis-driven project might be, for example, investigating whether increasing the age at which individuals can drink will reduce fatalities from motor vehicle crashes (Wagenaar, 1983b). In such instances, decisions about measurement are guided by, and typically limited to, the question of interest. Suppose that state law bans use of cell phones by bus drivers and novice drivers. Researchers evaluating the effect of the law on novices will typically exclude legal information in these laws pertinent to the bus-driver ban. In the second category, what we refer to as *legal mapping studies*, the purpose is to survey the legal terrain in a policy domain capturing all major characteristics that vary in ways related to health. When conducted with appropriate rigor and transparency, legal mapping studies yield data sets that can be used in empirical evaluations examining many different hypotheses. These data sets are also the basis of ongoing policy surveillance (Burris, Hitchcock, Ibrahim, Penn, & Ramanathan, 2016). This chapter focuses on measuring law for hypothesis testing, but the same principles and practices are, with exceptions, required for legal mapping studies.

The Process for Measuring Law

As is the case in all scientific research, questions of interest and availability of data define measurement objectives. The types of legal data pertinent to evaluation research vary widely depending on, among other things, whether legal measures are used as independent or dependent variables, and the research design chosen for the study. Notwithstanding these differences, the process for measuring law depicted in Figure 11.1 is composed of steps that are essential in all legal measurement projects. The process is generally iterative, with one or more steps being repeated as discoveries at one stage expose inadequacies of constructs developed at a previous stage. The following sections describe each step in the figure except the first, which is addressed in other chapters.

Establishing the Legal Framework

The first step in any legal measurement project is to identify the legal framework of interest. It is seldom practical or feasible to study every possible law related to a health issue. Consider the problem of distracted driving. It is clear that using a mobile communication device while operating a motor vehicle is a dangerous behavior. Many states and localities have responded by prohibiting activity with such devices for different groups of drivers. For empirical researchers interested in understanding the relationship between law and this high-risk behavior, these interventional laws have obvious importance. But they are not the only or even necessarily the best place to start. The tort system could exert an equal if not greater influence on drivers' tendencies to answer a call or send a text message, if those drivers expect that injuring someone while using a device is likely to result in a successful lawsuit against them. Or it could be that law regulating insurance or employer liability is a plausible factor affecting distracted driving. Decisions about the type of law to study depend on the purpose of the study and theorized relationships of interest.

Assume that a researcher decides to focus on state laws that specifically prohibit activity with mobile communication devices. These laws exist at the local and federal levels too (for example, those that apply to long-haul truckers). Choice of legal framework is in this way also a choice of at which level or levels of government law will be studied. Table 11.1 displays a familiar categorization of law by level of government and by source, with the most common type of law in each cell. Statutes enacted by Congress or state legislatures are generally the easiest source of law to measure because they are readily

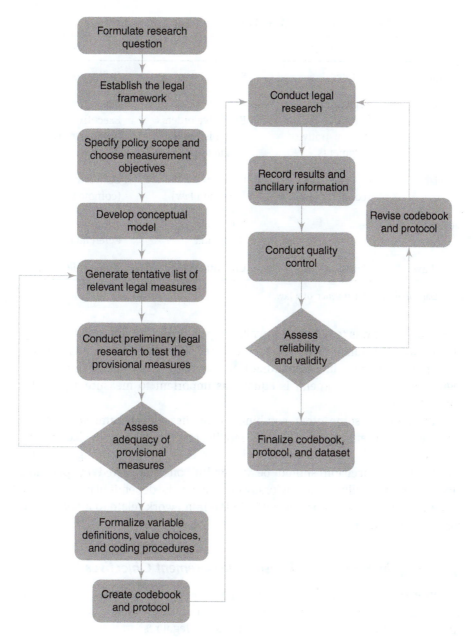

Figure 11.1. Process for Measuring Law.

Source: Adapted from Tremper, Thomas, and Wagenaar (2010).

accessible and—compared to common law created by courts—relatively straightforward. The ordinances of cities, counties, and other units of government below the state level offer similar advantages, although they may require more effort to locate. Bills under consideration by a legislature may also be of interest. For example, Wagenaar et al. (2006) used measures of bill introductions as an intermediate outcome in a national evaluation of statewide coalitions

Table 11.1. Types of Law by Level and Source.

	Federal	*State*	*Local*
Legislative	Statutes	Statutes	Ordinances
Executive	Regulations Executive orders Administrative judgments	Regulations Executive orders Administrative judgments	Regulations Executive orders Administrative judgments
Judicial	Case law (common law)	Case law (common law)	Case law (common law)
Electoral	—	Initiatives Referenda	Initiatives Referenda
Basic Law	Constitutions	Constitutions	Home rule charter

Note: Dash indicates the absence of a law.

whose objective was to reduce the availability of alcohol to youth. In this study, bill introductions functioned as one indicator of policy attention to an issue. For some policy domains, law emanating from the executive branch (for example, regulations, executive orders) is equally as important to measure as statutes and ordinances.

All, none, or some other combination of these legal frameworks might yield levers for effectively reducing mobile communication device use by drivers. In choosing a legal framework, there is no right or wrong answer a priori. But the decision should be a mindful one supported by plausible theories—both legally and behaviorally or biologically, depending on the nature of the exposure—about how laws within the framework relate to a health outcome of interest.

Specifying the Scope and Choosing Measurement Objectives

To conserve resources and ensure that legal measures generate data capable of illuminating the hypothesis of interest, it is important to define measurement objectives at the start even if they change during legal research and preliminary coding. In a study of distracted driving, for example, one might begin with the objective to capture how laws prohibiting driver activity with mobile communication devices have evolved over a 10-year period in regard to covered activity, devices, and classes of drivers. The preceding sentence is deliberately vague on one point: What is the right unit of analysis? Is it state statutes, federal motor vehicle regulations, local ordinances? The answer depends on the purpose of the measurement.

In most evaluations, the unit of analysis is a rule that applies to a certain population of organizations or individuals. That rule is defined in one more legal provisions (perhaps across bills and statutes). Each record—or row in a two-dimensional table—represents observed and recorded characteristics of that rule during a designated time period or at a specified point in time. Measuring these characteristics sometimes involves multiple provisions set out in numerous statutes. For example, one state might classify texting while driving as a Class A offense while another might classify it as a simple misdemeanor. Understanding the fines associated with those offenses—which might be important to understanding their effect—would then require reading the statute that defines those categories of offenses and associated penalties. A data set reflecting variation in law for all US states and the District of Columbia would therefore have 51 rows excluding headings (and leaving aside the issue of data encompassing changes in the policy over time). The columns in the table would represent variables and the characteristics of state law those variables describe. Although that is generally the intended structure of the final data set, seldom it is the easiest way for organizing and making sense of laws in the early stages of research. This is especially true in instances in which there are many related or similar provisions in a single state.

Periodic discussion by the research team (including scientists and lawyers) clarifying the unit of analysis ensures that different ways of organizing the search for legal data in early phases of the research do not muddle the purpose of the legal measurement and therefore its ability to inform the hypothesis of interest. Casual and shorthand descriptions of the legal research increase the chance of confusion; it is easy to describe the example in this section simply as a study of "distracted driving laws." A truer articulation of the project and the underlying measurement objective is to determine which activities with mobile communication devices are prohibited for specified drivers under state statutory law, how those prohibitions are enforced, and what the fines are for associated violations.

The primary goal is objective measurement of observable features in the law. The design of the measurement protocols and creation of a legal data set should seek to eliminate both legal and conceptual interpretation during the data collection and coding process, with the necessary exception of a precise definition of the laws of interest and what legal terms used to represent it. It is essential to avoid conflating primary observations with subsequent, secondary analytic steps. For example, a research plan might be heading toward a classification of distracted driving laws as weak and strong, or broad or narrow, or some other underlying theory-based conceptual differentiation. Assuming that such a second-phase classification system can be devised and defended conceptually and empirically, such classifications are based on the previously observed and consistently coded observable characteristics of the legal text. Thus, in the distracted driving example, the first-phase coding of observable provisions should start with a broad definition of what might be construed as "distracted driving," so that nuanced differences in definitions across states might be captured; such definitional differences might be important later when observed provisions are combined in various ways to represent underlying theory-based constructs. First one observes that the fine for violation in state A is $100 and in state B is $1000. It is a second analytic and conceptual step, independent from the coding of observed provisions, to classify A as a weak state and B as a strong state based on size of the fine (Burris, 2017). A third step is conceptually grappling with whether the larger fine is 10 times "worse" or 10 times more important than the smaller fine. Separating the first phase of coding of the observable characteristics of the text from later classification, scale building, or other forms of measurement development makes the development of measures more reliable and the analyses more transparent and reproducible—a *sine qua non* of good science.

Developing a Causal Diagram

Having defined the scope of laws to be collected, the next question is which provisions of the laws are to be measured. Causal diagrams—as described in more detail in Chapter 10—are valuable tools for this purpose. By forcing researchers to identify and clarify plausible links between law and health outcomes, causal diagrams help flush out the legal inputs relevant to the research question. In the distracted driving context, for example, researchers might suspect that the primary legal mechanism mediating reductions in device use is deterrence. In other words, laws that are easier to enforce and carry higher penalties result in the greater reductions in high-risk behavior. In that instance, provisions specifying whether police officers can enforce prohibitions as a primary offense—that is, without needing another pretext to make stops—have obvious relevance. Also important in that scenario are provisions specifying fines or other penalties such as suspensions for drivers on learner's permits. A causal diagram based in part or entirely on theory positing different mechanisms would suggest measurement of different legal provisions.

Generating a Tentative List of Relevant Legal Measures

In hypothesis-driven research, causal diagrams limit the laws to be studied on the basis of theories about how those legal inputs relate to some other outcome. The legal inputs themselves are often until this point understood as concepts such as manner of enforcement, scope, and severity. To capture how these conceptual legal inputs vary, the important components of each must be identified—specific legal provisions that must be coded to later be combined to best measure a theory-derived concept. Operationally, this is the point in the process to start creating variables, one for each specific provision coded. For the case of distracted driving laws, a sufficient set of preliminary measures to describe the scope of the laws might be categorical variables reflecting activities prohibited (for example, only texting, only talking, talking and texting, other), classes of drivers covered (for example, all drivers, bus drivers, inexperienced drivers, other), and devices (for example, cell phones, personal digital assistants, laptop computers, other) subject to the law.

Conducting Preliminary Legal Research

Whether the tentative measures align with relevant variation in extant laws is an empirical question that should be tested on a sample of the jurisdictions to be studied. If little is known about the variation in the law across jurisdictions, examining a random sample of jurisdictions increases the value of a preliminary review. If the structure or operation of law on the topic of interest is known to vary systematically across jurisdictions in terms of a small number of major characteristics, purposely sampling jurisdictions across such strata is best (e.g., urban versus rural states). The size of the sample depends on the law being studied and the a priori knowledge that the research team possesses about legal variation in the area. In addition to examining a handful of jurisdictions, surveying literature that describes the policy environment, whether in legal journals or other social science research, sets the research on firmer ground moving forward. Preliminary research illuminates relevant dimensions of the law and provides the research team with a basis for estimating the breadth and complexity of the legal provisions being studied and the resources needed to systematically collect and analyze.

Assessing the Adequacy of Provisional Measures

Pausing to test the adequacy of provisional measures reduces the likelihood of wholesale recoding that would be necessary were the coding scheme to be found later in the research process to be incapable of reliably and validly capturing relevant variation. At this stage in the process, insights about important dimensions of variation in the law and how to elicit variation through coding questions should be crystallizing in the minds of the research team. For the distracted driving example, researchers might decide that the provisional measure describing classes of covered drivers is insufficiently specific. Rather than lumping all inexperienced drivers into one group, the variable could be refined to distinguish between laws that cover drivers by age (that is, at ages 16, 17, 18, 19, and above) and laws that apply to all new drivers regardless of age. It might also become apparent that a handful of exceptions reduce the scope or enforceability of prohibitions, such as exceptions for hands-free device use or exceptions in statutes banning texting that permit typing keys to start or end a call.

Formalizing Variable Definitions and Coding Procedures

It is in coding that measurement of law differs most significantly from traditional legal research. Traditional legal research typically produces narrative descriptions of how one or more laws differ in both their text and their meaning; measurement of law for empirical research employs precisely defined and documented procedures used to represent each legal provision. From an operational perspective, this means first identifying all relevant ways that laws vary and then finding numeric schemes (or preliminary textual ones such as "yes" and "no") to capture that variation. Although it is counterintuitive and may strike legally trained staff as odd at first, coding questions and the variables they define must be precise and strive to eliminate human judgment. Precision means each item coded should be an elemental record of observation of a specific provision: is the provision present (yes/no)? Coding questions requiring interpretation undermine reliability because of ambiguities in legal interpretation and innate differences between coders. Consider a coding question asking whether a law prohibiting communication on wireless telephones by drivers applies to talking over an internet connection through a headset attached to a laptop. Different coders could reach entirely defensible but different conclusions depending on how they interpret the operative terms and ultimate meaning of the rule (that is, "a computer is not a wireless telephone" versus "anything that allows electronic transmission of oral communication is a telephone even if embedded in something that has other purposes").

Adding a "not sure" category to the coding choices for a variable provides an important safety valve, especially in early stages of coding. The "not sure" category gives coders an option for handling ambiguity that may or may not be resolved by additional research or subsequent developments such as a court ruling during the course of the study. Regular review of "not sure" cases by the entire research team often leads to revision of the coding protocol, increasing reliability, precision, and comprehensiveness. Sometimes a "not sure" or "unsettled" code will remain in the final data set so that those records can be excluded from analyses or addressed separately in a sub-study.

The use of blanket dichotomous "law or no law" variables to code the presence or absence of a particular type of law is useful only in rare situations of limited research questions and study designs (Burris, 2017). This is distinct from the recommended practice of using simple dichotomous measures for each specific relevant provision or feature within a law. Without careful specification of provisions, dichotomous variables representing overall presence/absence of a law can easily obscure a great deal of legal variability and hence limit the value of a data set for evaluating legal effects. Consider the example of underage alcohol purchase data set from the National Institute of Alcohol Abuse and Alcoholism's Alcohol Policy Information System (2021). A dichotomous law or no law variable initially might seem adequate for indicating whether a state prohibits people under age 21 from purchasing alcoholic beverages. Most states have such prohibitions, and most of the laws on the topic are clear and simple. Several jurisdictions, though, permit purchases by youths in some situations, such as acting in conjunction with law enforcement, or drinking in some situations, such as in the presence of parents. New York and Delaware do not prohibit underage purchase, but they do prohibit obtaining alcohol in connection with making a false statement. Rather than trying to shoehorn these laws into a dichotomous law or no law variable, a polychotomous variable could be created, in this case with four codes to include an absolute prohibition, a prohibition with exceptions, a prohibition against purchase in connection with making a false statement, and no restrictions. Better still, the categorical variable should be separated into four dichotomous variables, each measuring one dimension, an approach adhering to the principle that a coded variable should always concern a single distinct, unitary attribute.

One of the preliminary measures identified for distracted driving defined the possibilities for regulated activity as (1) only texting, (2) only talking,

(3) talking and texting, and (4) other. A simpler approach is to create two dichotomous variables that respectively answer the questions "Does the law prohibit texting?" and "Does the law prohibit talking?" Unidimensional variables can later easily be combined to reflect instances when both activities are prohibited or combined with other variables defining the existence of exceptions (for example, exception for hands-free use yes/no) to represent regulatory permutations.

For the coding of legal texts, classifying features of laws into categories—that is, using categorical variables—is the most common way to reflect variance. The categories—or attributes—of a categorical variable have no natural numeric ordering or quantitative relationship. In contrast, the attributes of ordinal variables have a natural ordering (for example, low, medium, high). Interval variables are a special type of ordinal variable in which the difference between attributes is meaningful and assumed to be equal across the distribution (for example, separation into first, second, third, and fourth quartiles). Some features of the law can be measured at ordinal or interval levels, thereby enabling dose–response analyses, possibly enhancing statistical power to detect the law's effects, or more closely matching the analytic model to theory. Penalty type, for example, can be coded as an ordinal variable, with civil infractions, misdemeanors, felonies, and capital crimes as values representing ascending severity as defined by law.

Continuous variables, which can take any numeric value (for example, temperature in Celsius), provide even more analytic benefits than ordinal variables. Attributes such as length of jail terms, maximum fines imposed, appropriation amounts, and legal thresholds (for example, alcohol-impaired driving in terms of blood alcohol content) are often measurable with continuous variables. Careful definitions and coding protocols can also produce continuous variables based on a law's nonnumerical features. For example, researchers might use primary observations of the length of jail sentence, the magnitude of fine, and the availability of defenses to create a composite measure of "stringency." Such composite measures are designed to represent concepts that come from a theory that underlies the research. It is critical for reliable and valid measurement to maintain a careful distinction between the "phase 1" coding—finding all instances of relevant laws and accurately coding the elemental observable provisions of each law—and "phase 2" measurement development, which combines the coded variables created in phase 1 to create measures of concepts derived from a theory underlying a particular study.

Creating a Codebook and Protocol

Creating a codebook and a well-defined, precise coding protocol to capture the decisions made during the design phase facilitates both the initial legal research and any subsequent attempts to replicate or update the data. The codebook should reflect the standards of any good data-collection documentation as well as the special considerations for coding laws. Elements include a description of the study; scope of data collection; variable definitions; values (codes and their definitions); algorithms for constructing scales; technical information about files—tables, records, relationships, number of records for each case (some jurisdictions have multiple related laws); and details about the data (columns, text, numeric, Boolean).

A codebook alone is inadequate for any but the simplest study because critical decisions about coding conventions and procedures for legal data are rarely apparent from examination of a codebook alone. A comprehensive protocol includes information about how the laws were collected (for example, exact legal text databases searched, exact search terms and syntax used); inclusion and exclusion criteria for defining the body of legal texts to be coded; precise rules for coding the variables (which legal terms support classification into a specific category); conventions used regarding effective dates or other determinations about a law's operation; and standards for collecting legal citations.

For teams composed of social scientists and legal researchers, up until this point, most activity should have been a joint effort with a lot of dialogue. In the next phase, however, the distribution of labor shifts considerably. Collecting the relevant laws requires legal training. Especially if legal researchers have not been integrated into the earlier steps, but even if they have, this is an ideal time for training all of the coders. It is imperative that law students and other legal researchers understand not only what they are looking for but also why, so that they can report on unanticipated nuances in the law. Legal researchers must follow good legal research practices such as reading provisions in context by carefully locating and considering legal definitions of all operative terms. Relevant provisions are often located by keyword searches; without explicit instruction some legal researchers will not inspect other provisions in the same part of the statutory code. The use of statutory tables of contents is not always emphasized when training law students but is indispensable for making sense of statutory schemes, especially across jurisdictions. Being observant for court decisions that influence status of the law is also essential. Key points of emphasis in discussions with attorney or law student coders include keeping records of any needed modifications in the research protocol, erring on the side of over-inclusion in the collection of law, and raising questions for discussion with supervisors. The training of legal researchers naturally coincides with collective review of the protocol and codebook. Whether the legal researchers are students or experienced lawyers, from this point forward, the protocol and codebook should provide a high degree of clarity to guide the location, organization, and eventual coding of legal texts.

Conducting Legal Research

Having tested and refined the coding scheme, a project team can then proceed to the task of systematically collecting and coding the relevant law. Available resources to perform original legal research include Westlaw and Lexis, both comprehensive proprietary online legal research services. HeinOnline is another proprietary source that provides access to state session laws going back in some instances to the 1840s. Alternatives to these tools that can suffice for some studies include the commercial service Fastcase and publicly available online sources such as the Library of Congress website (www.congress.gov) for federal material. The commercial service StateNet (www.statenet.com) offers access to recently enacted statutes and pending bills. An excellent resource for studying legislative activity is LexisNexis Advanced Legislative Service, which catalogues bills eventually adopted. The returns provide a valuable picture of how law has evolved in a particular area and can be used for updating or checking established legal data sets. Conducting searches in these databases and making sense of returns requires legal training in most instances. For large projects, and given the continued development and expansion of features and products offered by the many legal services available, consulting with legal librarians and database vendors—which typically offer assistance free of charge for law students and many other legal researchers—can increase efficiency of research even for experienced lawyers.

Finding legal materials at the city and county levels is often difficult. There is currently no comprehensive or authoritative collection of local laws. Lexis, Westlaw, and FindLaw maintain partial collections of municipal ordinances, and many jurisdictions publish their own materials directly online or through local law publishers and repositories including www.municode.com, www.amlegal.com, and www.statelocalgov.net. If the research goal is limited to one or a few local jurisdictions, finding the relevant ordinances is often feasible. As the number of jurisdictions expands, the task can become unwieldy and require extensive investment of researcher time to search multiple databases and, on some occasions, query local governments directly (Sanner, Grant, Walter-McCabe, & Silverman, 2021). As Natural Language Processing, a branch of artificial intelligence, improves and becomes more widely available, searching many local governmental websites may become routine.

Recording Results and Ancillary Information

Well-designed data-collection software for gathering legal source material is crucial for a smooth process. An adequate data-collection system for coding the law stores much more than the final resulting codes for each variable. The system must retain ancillary information supporting the coding, typically in the form of extended blocks of legal text. The software should allow for changes to variables and codes as the project progresses, knowledge is gained, and previous decisions are updated, as well as keep a record of such changes. At a minimum, all relevant statutory, regulatory, and case law citations must be collected and recorded. Because coding of a single variable may depend on several sources of law (for example, three regulations, two statutes, and a court case), a data field with no character limit is generally best for citations. Ideally, citations should be stored in records that have a many-to-one relationship with the coding record so that each citation can have its own field and be stored together with additional notes.

Along with citations, collecting relevant text facilitates subsequent review of coding decisions. Microsoft Access, which permits up to 60,000 characters of text in each data field, can be used for cataloguing small- or medium-sized laws. Custom-designed databases can also be purchased from commercial vendors for large legal measurement projects, and software specifically designed for legal coding and measurement are also available, for example MonQcle (Center for Public Health Law Research, 2022). Rigorous and consistent coding decisions are enhanced by recording rationales for coding in the data-collection system, especially in instances when there is latent ambiguity. In addition to storing legal information, retention of the coders' notes, comments, and questions offers a big advantage not only to the current research team but also to future users of the data set. Maintaining records of each coding decision is essential. Although coding decisions should always have a solid basis in the observable features of the legal text, there may remain instances when the text of a law is explicit but important extrinsic information exists that changes the effect of the legal text. Law enforcement agencies may choose not to enforce a law through an organizational policy that is not included in the data such as, for example, widespread refusal to prosecute cannabis possession offenses in many cities. There may also be instances when the answer to a coding question is clear, but some feature of the legal text is noteworthy. For example, consider a study measuring whether states include syringes within the definition of prohibited drug paraphernalia. Every state that defines a class of such objects refers to it as drug paraphernalia except Georgia, which uses a different term, drug-related objects. Noting this sort of nuance in terminology is another appropriate use of comment boxes and can reduce inaccuracies and confusion during later analyses.

As with all tasks that require repeated actions and fine-tuned manual manipulations, random human error is an inevitable threat to data integrity. The traditional model of coding texts involved three objects: a codebook describing the coding question, a datasheet in which coding decisions were placed (typically an Excel file or other sheet with lots of rows and columns), and the text to be coded. Moving between the three objects provides coders with many opportunities to make mistakes. This sort of error can be reduced through the use of coding platforms that integrate codebooks, datasheets, and the legal text. Data entry forms designed in Microsoft Access or MonQcle, for example, enable researchers to create templates in which the legal text to be coded is visible next to the coding questions that drive data to an underlying data table.

Clear coding roles for each person and adherence to rigorous implementation procedures reduce both outright errors and subtle distinctions that might otherwise go unnoticed. Regardless of how many coders work on the project, each will need to scrupulously follow clearly defined protocols and adhere to all coding guidelines. This is true for all types of research, and no less so when measuring law. Coders not only must be thoroughly versed in conventions adopted at the design stage of the research project, they also must be empowered to alert the principal investigator to oddities that arise in the course of coding that may require modification of those conventions, or the use of caveats and elaborations in subsequent descriptions of the research.

Quality Control

Quality control measures are intended to test how well legal researchers have applied the protocol and coding scheme. Even perfectly executed protocols and codebooks can generate errors. It is important to have two researchers redundantly and independently compile and code the laws. Comparing the two resulting data sets for inconsistencies reduces the likelihood of undetected random or careless error and points to possible areas of underspecified coding conventions. Such double-coding also provides a direct assessment of inter-coder reliability. But sometimes even independent coders share similarities that bias their treatment of the law. Being systematically integrated into a research project can subtly influence how the coder collects or codes law; likewise, coders often share characteristics that predispose them to similar patterns of observation or analysis, which could bias resulting data. A final important step to address these concerns is to have a third legal researcher who is totally naïve to the project recode a randomly selected portion of the records. If desired, the rate of divergence can be reported as a crude rate or as a rate that adjusts for the probability of randomly selecting the correct answer. The statistical metric for assessing inter-rater reliability, Cohen's Kappa, provides a more conservative estimate of the reliability of a test than the crude rate of divergence by accounting for the fact that, for example, on a dichotomous variable, independent coders picking randomly will get the same result half of the time simply by chance. Unlike with survey research, there are no clear thresholds for deciding when divergence rates are too high. Generally speaking, anything more than the occasional discordance (that is, divergence rates of greater than 1 or 2%) is cause for concern.

After assessing inter-coder reliability, the codebook and protocol specifications typically are revised to improve coding of some of the measures. The research team then cycles back to conducting legal research with the newly revised protocols, repeating the quality control procedures and assessing reliability. The research team advances only when the highest practically achievable levels of reliability are attained, which often requires multiple rounds of revisions and testing.

A complementary approach to quality control avoids routine double-coding of all records by random sampling codes and double coding those sampled. This is done early in the process to identify ambiguous coding instructions or lack of clear specification of the elemental observable legal provisions the coding is intended to include. Rounds of revisions to the coding instructions are made and evaluated via double coding, until error rates are acceptably low. In this approach, a more-experienced coder or senior attorney is typically used for the second coding, to better identify errors by regular coding staff and better point to effective ways for improving the coding instructions. At that point, final production coding is completed; achieved error rates are always documented and published with the final data set.

When concluding the legal data collection and coding phase, the codebook and protocol documents should be carefully reviewed to ensure that they reflect all changes in definitions, coding conventions, or other matters that occurred during the legal data collection and coding process. The final codebook and protocol should be sufficiently specific to enable exact replication of the data set if those procedures are implemented by a separate team at a later time. The codebook and protocol facilitate future updates and ensure comparability of the data collected at different times and by different teams. Norms of scientific publishing require final codebooks and protocol documents be publicly available to other researchers for verification and replication studies.

Challenges and Next Steps

Challenges unique to measuring law for empirical research arise in the process we have described and deserve additional discussion.

Comparing Law Across Jurisdictions

Jurisdictions have considerable authority to create law. This independence extends not only to the substantive features of law but also to the way in which policies are drafted as provisions and organized as statutory code. As a result, statutory regimes vary considerably across states and even more drastically across countries (Kavanagh, Meier, Pillinger, Huffstetler, & Burris, 2020). States can accomplish identical policy positions through a variety of legal strategies and mechanisms. In some states, for example, a single comprehensive statute specifies different options for mental health care directives (Swanson, McCrary, Swartz, Elbogen, & Van Dorn, 2006); other states have a legal arrangement that creates a functionally equivalent policy through provisions that are scattered across probate codes, health and safety codes, and civil practice and remedies codes. In the distracted driving example, some states define the regulated activity, the fine for violations, and the manner of enforcement in one statute; others specify these details in multiple statutes. Some laws are detailed; in others a broad mandate is filled in by executive agency regulations.

It is not just that the text of provisions varies across states. Even if texts are identical, laws operate within regulatory structures, and those structures differ, sometimes markedly, between jurisdictions. Failure to account for the broader legal context in which a law exists can produce misleading comparisons. Consider, for example, a researcher interested in determining whether states where syringe exchange programs are legal have lower incidence of HIV/AIDS. For that researcher, a reasonable way to start might be to collect all the laws that explicitly authorize syringe exchange programs. If the collection of law stopped there, however, the resulting findings would present an incomplete and inaccurate picture of the relevant state law. In some states, syringe exchange is legal under state law simply because no laws forbid it; categorizing such states as prohibiting syringe exchange because they have not explicitly authorized syringe exchange would be legally invalid. Accurately measuring how states vary with respect to the legality of syringes requires collecting not only public health laws that explicitly authorize syringe exchange but also criminal paraphernalia laws regulating possession and distribution of syringes, pharmacy statutes and regulations defining restrictions on the delivery of syringes, and criminal laws banning drug possession that could apply to residue in used syringes that are possessed prior to exchange (Fernández-Viña, Prood, Herpolsheimer, Waimberg & Burris, 2020). Challenges like this highlight the need for project teams to incorporate legal expertise early at the stages of conceptualization and design of the study, as well as during implementation.

Tracking Change Over Time

The weakness of purely cross-sectional comparisons for inferring causal effects is well known. Evaluations of *changes* in law, best with longitudinal data over many years, are much stronger. This chapter takes as given the necessity of determining when a law was enacted or became effective and whether subsequent legislative or judicial action nullified it or modified it in ways relevant to the research—the question is which dates and how. In most states and at the federal level, except for emergency legislation, there is a lag between the date of enactment of legislation and the date it legally takes effect. For evaluation research, the effective date of a law is usually the most appropriate measure for the law's onset, because many studies assume that a law cannot affect health outcomes until it legally takes effect and is therefore enforceable or assumes any anticipatory effects of a law before it legally takes effect are small and conceptually distinct. For some studies, such as those examining correlates of policy choice in legislatures or those evaluating the relationship between legislation, public attention, and social norms, the date of legislative passage may be more appropriate.

Effective dates are usually determined either by a specific clause in legislation or by the jurisdiction's legislative rules, which to the uninitiated can be quite abstruse and confusing. Identifying changes in the law over long periods can be time and labor intensive. Lexis, Westlaw, and a few specialized services such as HeinOnline compile archived statutes and other legislative materials, which can make coding and validation easier. However, these historical materials tend to have more anomalies and interjurisdictional variations (for example, differences in years of coverage for archived statutes across states) than collections of current law. To perform historical legal research, coders typically need additional training. Effective dates often do not appear in the text of legislation or statutes, or the legislation might refer to an extra-legal event, for example "60 days after the end of the legislative session." StateScape's free online 50-state chart is invaluable (https://www.statescape.com/resources/legislative/bill-effective-dates/), although only for current, not historical, practices. Retrospective research in some cases may be impossible at the local level or for state regulations because of the inaccessibility of historical records.

Amendments or other changes that occur after a law has been enacted and takes effect also require attention. Subsequent legislation that either directly amends a statute or repeals it entirely is the most obvious example of a modification. A sunset clause in a bill that nullifies it after a period of time is another important source of possible change. The judiciary, too, can invalidate a statute either in whole or in part. Such legal changes must be examined carefully to determine relevance to the research topic. Very high accuracy in coded effective dates is essential for legal evaluation research because errors in effective dates can invalidate studies.

Reliance on Secondary Sources

At the start of a public health law evaluation project, discovering that someone else has already produced a summary of applicable laws might seem like a windfall that obviates the need for painstaking legal research. Many advocacy and think-tank websites and publications offer authoritative-looking fifty-state lists and similar compendia of "the law." These secondary sources can be useful for getting an overview of the law at a particular time and for use in the quality assurance process, but they are rarely sufficient sources of legal data for research projects. With few exceptions, these lists have one or more serious flaws, including that they do not result from rigorously defined protocols and verification processes; lack effective dates or other indications of the period during which a law is in effect; provide data only for one point in time, which often is not specified; lack documentation of the research process and coding conventions used to produce them (preventing replication); and often contain significant errors.

Another seemingly sensible shortcut is to use key informant interviews or surveys, perhaps targeting agency staff presumed to know the law they are charged with administering. Experience has repeatedly demonstrated, however, that agency staff members do not always have the right answers. Surveys or other instruments addressed to an appropriately knowledgeable official at an under-staffed agency may be completed by a subordinate and returned without review by the expert. A study by LaFond et al. (2000) found that original legal research produced more accurate results than key informant interviews or surveys of agency directors and staff. Error rates for some data collected by surveying agency personnel exceeded 50%.

There are few high-quality sources of legal data available. One of these, the Alcohol Policy Information System (APIS, alcoholpolicy.niaaa.nih.gov), developed by the National Institute on Alcohol Abuse and Alcoholism, relies on research attorneys to classify legal data on alcohol and recreational cannabis policy topics for all 50 states, the federal government, and the District of Columbia. The Prescription Drug Abuse Policy System provides data on state laws related to prescription drug abuse (pdaps.org). The LawAtlas portal (lawatlas.org) provides data on wide range of public health laws and allows users to interact with the data by creating custom charts and maps. Notwithstanding these examples, obtaining accurate legal data for an evaluation research project almost always entails conducting original legal research, which requires specialized legal and conceptual expertise beyond simple familiarity with a particular policy. Especially for multistate studies, anyone conducting research without considerable legal training and experience will seldom produce sufficiently reliable and accurate data sets.

Creating Composite Measures

After reliable coding of observable legal provisions, individual provision indicators are often then combined in the construction of indices and scales, thereby creating measures of theory-based constructs. Novice researchers can damage the reliability of the original legal coding by having coders make judgments to code levels of higher-level constructs such as breadth, stringency, or strength of laws. The objective is to always have lawyers and law students as coders tasked only with reliably and accurately coding *observable* provisions or characteristics of the law. Then, the scientists, based on theory and proposed study hypotheses, create measures (ranks, scales, combinations, continuous variables) that match the concepts desired in a way that is suitable for the planned statistical analyses. Thus, the scientists take the elemental codes produced in phase 1 and build measures in phase 2. Imagine a law is reliably coded on a dozen provisions each as present or absent. Based on theory, the scientific team then designs a composite measure: if at minimum the law has provisions A and C, then it gets score 1 = low, if it has three or more other provisions from the list as well along with A and C then score 2 = medium, and if in addition to A and C the law has five or more of the other provisions then score 3 = high. The legally trained coders do not make judgments on whether a law is low or high on such a dimension; they code the elemental provisions, and the scientist team specify combinations (summing, ranking, weighting) to create measures of concepts needed to test a particular theory or hypothesis.

Adding such composite variables to data sets often increases the value of empirical legal data sets to other users. The data set for distracted driving laws (https://lawatlas.org/datasets/distracted-driving-1470663668) includes well over a hundred variables. Granular coding of legal features into separate variables provides the basis for classifying a jurisdiction's laws in many ways, matching divergent theories on the law's mechanisms of effect. Starting with granular coding not only enhances reliability and accuracy of legal coding. It also allows much more diverse sets of analyses later.

Developing good scales for legal measures remains particularly difficult, and few flawless examples exist (Moxham-Hall & Ritter, 2017). Among the best are rating systems such as the Naimi et al. (2014) alcohol policy environment scale. The development of the tobacco policy scale by Chriqui et al. (2002) bears several hallmarks that distinguish well-developed complex measures. First, the scale is firmly grounded in a causal diagram that links its components with tobacco use outcomes. Second, both legal and social science experts collaborated in constructing the scale. Third, a Delphi panel or other structured process was used for proposing, testing, and revising the scales. Because scales are by nature synthetic measures that encode assumptions along with observations, clarity and transparency regarding exactly how scales are constructed are essential to a study's integrity. All coding conventions and scaling procedures as well as the scale's limitations must be documented and reported. If data for the scale are to be analyzed using statistical techniques that require interval-level data, it is important to, in addition, specify how increments between scale values are equalized.

Creating simple scales based on the number of statutes in a jurisdiction or otherwise treating all laws as equally important may be useful for certain purposes, but simple counts may be misleading because of omnibus legislation and interjurisdictional variations in codifying bills (for example, three statutes in one state may be equivalent to one statute in another or equal to a combination of statutes and regulations in a third). In addition, some laws are likely to have much more effect than others. For example, a researcher might identify a dozen different state laws pertaining to child safety and use them in a study of childhood injuries. This design may mask the reality that a single law or combination of very few laws accounts for all of the influence of law on injuries; moreover, some of the specific laws in the scale may be inversely correlated with the outcome measure. How a scale is constructed is necessarily shaped by the underlying theoretical model, and a scale that is appropriate and useful for one purpose may be quite inappropriate for a different purpose.

Reliability and Validity

The design and creation of reliable and valid empirical legal data sets requires following the same principles of measurement developed in the social sciences over the past half century (Nunnally, 1978). We have already emphasized the need to clearly specify simple observable provisions in legal texts, avoiding the need for coders to make conceptual or interpretive judgments, to achieve primary legal coding with high levels of *inter-rater reliability*. Following the same coding procedures on the same law at different times should also produce the same result—*stability reliability*. Subtly changing norms of legal interpretation over time might threaten stability reliability if coding procedures are not sufficiently specific. After construction of the primary legal data set, the elemental variables are typically combined to create measures of higher-level constructs, and those composite measures should have high levels of *internal consistency reliability*—items purportedly measuring the same underlying construct should be highly correlated with each other and with the overall scale score.

Reliability is about getting the same result each time a procedure is followed. It is a prerequisite for a valid measure, but not sufficient. Validity is about making sure the procedures produce a measure that actually measures the concept intended. *Face validity* is simply whether the measurement procedures "on the face of it" appear to reflect the intended construct. More usefully, *content validity* addresses whether the procedures produce a measure that reflects the full domain of intended dimensions. Consider an intended measure of law's overall "strength" that only includes fines and jail time, missing dimensions of "strength" that reflect celerity (speed of penalty implementation), another key dimension from deterrence theory. At this point in measurement development, one also assesses *construct validity*—does the measure correlate well with other measures the theory states it should be correlated with (convergent validity), and is it not correlated with other measures theory states it should not be correlated with (discriminant validity). Finally, *criterion validity* is whether the constructed measure is highly correlated with a "gold standard"—an available measure widely accepted as the most accurate and valid. Unfortunately, such gold standard measures are rarely available in legal epidemiology. But the notion is still helpful—comparing new measures of law with existing measures, to help understand validity and accuracy of each.

Making Sense of Preemption and Federalism

The interplay among laws at the federal, state, and local levels adds another dimension of complexity to determining what the law "is" in any particular place. Sometimes the law being studied—say, state law aimed at regulating sugar-sweetened beverages—is contingent on law at other levels of government. At least two federal laws (the Child Nutrition Act of 1970 and the Child Nutrition and WIC Reauthorization Act of 2004) address this issue, as do statutes or regulations in at least 34 states (Mello, Pomeranz, & Moran, 2008). Moreover, some municipalities have their own ordinances, and many school districts have adopted rules as well. Evaluations of state limitations on sales of sugar-sweetened beverages in schools may be influenced by federal law and may show different results depending on whether local law is included or ignored.

Conflicts among laws at different levels of government generally are resolved by their hierarchy, with federal law being supreme and state law trumping anything at the local level. This seemingly straightforward arrangement is more complex than it initially appears, however. In some situations, federal law and state law may conflict. For example, as of January 2022, 18 states have legalized adult recreational cannabis use, which remains illegal under federal law. Although federal officials could enforce federal law in these states, they have chosen not do so as a matter of discretion. The varieties of preemption—a term that encompasses different arrangements of authority between levels of government—present some of the most interesting and complex legal questions. Here again, the need for collaboration with legal experts is essential.

Research Design, Assumptions, and Inferences

Although this chapter is devoted to measurement, a few comments about inference and analysis bear mentioning. For legal epidemiology studies there is an analog to the "If a tree falls in the forest" question: What if a law exists but no one follows it? Low compliance by relevant populations, varying enforcement by police or administrative personnel, unwillingness of prosecutors to bring charges, differing interpretations across jurisdictions, and inadequate funding for implementation can create misleading evidence about whether the law "on the books" could produce different health outcomes "on the street." Although the existence of a law supports an inference that it is being enforced, the possibility of nonenforcement or inconsistent enforcement can make a critical difference to compliance and assessments of a law's effect (see Wagenaar & Wolfson, 1994). Laws often have both deterrent and norms-shaping effects, and the latter can occur independently of enforcement. Research designs that include measures of enforcement and compliance better isolate the effects of laws as written.

Even when a mandate is clearly stated, implementation may not necessarily follow. Particularly in studies of laws that require resources for implementation—such as those that create systems for providing treatment or give citizens a right to receive governmental services—another factor looms: whether adequate funds are available. Legislatures are more apt to pass authorizing legislation for a program than to pass appropriations to fund it. Executive agencies, which are charged primarily with implementing and enforcing laws, may divert or delay funds with little recourse for policy makers. This chapter demonstrates that law is measurable for scientific study like other phenomena. Collecting and coding legal texts, however, is only the start. One also needs to measure a range of implementation factors and other features of jurisdictions to fully understand how law and health relate.

Conclusion

This chapter describes methods for measuring law and creating data sets for use in legal epidemiology research. The aim is to generate scientifically consistent and defensible measures that reflect in quantitative forms how laws vary over space and time. In addition to adding rigor to the study of legal texts, it provides a method for increasing the efficiency of studying legal change over time, a key requirement for evaluation research. Although these legal coding methods are still developing and uniform standards and best practices are evolving, measurement and coding issues are an essential if underappreciated element of public health law research. Implementing the procedures offered in this chapter advances the field of evaluation research by increasing the utility and accuracy of research using legal data, ultimately improving public policy and its effectiveness in achieving important goals advancing population health and well-being. By blending the knowledge and skills of social, statistical, and health scientists with those of legal experts, scholars can produce more accurate and more useful policy evaluations. As the field continues to advance, adopting minimum measurement standards along the lines suggested here will elevate the threshold of acceptable quality for designing, funding, and conducting evaluations of public policies embodied in law.

Summary

Effectively studying the relationship between law and population health requires variation in both the law and health outcomes over space as well as time, and reliable and valid methods for capturing variation and representing it in forms that allow comparison and analyses. A rigorous method for measuring law generates numeric data representing variation in law. The key feature of the method—and that which distinguishes it most from traditional legal research—is that it relies on careful and consistent observation of the apparent features of legal texts. This approach produces data that is replicable through a process that is transparent. Transparency and replicability are essential attributes of scientifically defensible data.

There are many challenges in measuring law. Relevant legal texts can be hard to find and rife with ambiguous and conflicting meanings. Formulating reliable and valid ways of reducing complex bodies of law into numeric data can be difficult. There are also cultural and logistical hurdles to forming teams that combine legal scholars and social scientists, blending a full range of legal and scientific expertise. These challenges can be overcome by a methodical process of design, data collection, and analysis that adheres to scientific standards. Steps include the careful delineation of the scientific and legal questions to be addressed and the scope of the research; the iterative development and refinement of coding schemes; an intense focus on quality control; and the production of a transparent research protocol and codebook to accompany the resulting legal data set.

Further Reading

Burris, S., Hitchcock, L., Ibrahim, J. K., Penn, M., & Ramanathan, T. (2016). Policy surveillance: A vital public health practice comes of age. *Journal of Health Politics, Policy & Law, 41*(6), 1151–1167.

Kavanagh, M. M., Meier, B. M., Pillinger, M., Huffstetler, H., & Burris, S. (2020). Global policy surveillance: Creating and using comparative national data on health law and policy. *American Journal of Public Health, 110*(12), 1805–1810.

Policy Surveillance Program. (2022). Learning library. Retrieved from http://www.lawatlas.org/page/lawatlas-learning-library.

Chapter 12

Coding Case Law for Public Health Law Evaluation

Mark Hall

Learning Objectives

- Describe strengths and limitations of content analysis in legal epidemiology.
- Identify steps in the systematic identification and coding of case law.
- Design an analysis plan for coded case law.

This chapter explains how the research method of content analysis can be applied to study legal decisions. Content analysis is a method for systematically reading and analyzing "texts" of any kind. Developed by sociologists and political scientists, the method is also used widely in the communications field (Krippendorff, 1980; Neuendorf, 2002). It can be applied not only to conventional written material but also to images or audio content. Written texts abound, of course, in the legal sphere, including statutes, regulations, hearing transcripts, and court filings. But our sole focus here is one especially important example: judicial opinions.

The content of judicial opinions merits careful study not simply because opinions reflect or respond to the law, but because they *are* the law. Legal researchers are correct to recognize that it "is almost impossible to study law in a meaningful way without some attention to the [content of] opinions that contain these justifications" (Friedman, 2006, p. 266). For instance, a researcher wanting to know what effect the First Amendment's protection of speech, religion, and association might have on enforcement of various public health laws would need to analyze Supreme Court opinions as a primary source of legal rules.

Legal Epidemiology: Theory and Methods, Second Edition. Edited by Alexander C. Wagenaar, Rosalie Liccardo Pacula, and Scott Burris.

But more than this, judicial opinions are detailed repositories that show what kinds of disputes come before courts, how the parties frame their disputes, and how judges reason to their conclusions. For example, Haar et al. (1977) coded for the presence or absence of 167 different factors in each of 79 zoning dispute cases decided by one state's Supreme Court over a 25-year period, to determine which factors appear to influence the outcome of these cases. It is this factual and analytical richness of judicial opinions that establish both their substantive legal importance and their utility as instruments for public health research of various designs.

On the surface, content analysis appears simple, even trivial, to some. It boils down to three steps: (1) selecting cases, (2) coding cases, and (3) analyzing (often through statistics) the case coding. The method comes naturally to legal scholars because it resembles the classic scholarly routine of reading a collection of cases, finding common threads that link the opinions, and commenting on their significance (Hall & Wright, 2008). But content analysis is much more than a better way to read cases. It brings scientific rigor to the collection and analyses of case law, which could create a distinctively legal form of scientific empiricism. This approach to reading cases can be used profitably in three distinct types of studies: those that identify determinants of judicial decision-making, those that measure consequences of judicial decisions, or those that document how the judicial system operates.

What Content Analysis Can and Cannot Tell Us

Content analysis has certain advantages, but also substantial limitations, compared with conventional legal analysis. At best, the method generates objective, falsifiable, and reproducible knowledge about what selected courts do and how and why they do it. It works best when each of the judicial opinions in a collection holds essentially equal value, but not when what is needed is a deeply reflective understanding of a single pivotal case. Content analysis therefore does not displace traditional interpretive legal scholarship. Nor does it reveal how all aspects of a legal system function (Hoffman, Izenman, & Lidicker, 2007). Instead, it offers distinctive insights that complement the types of understanding that traditional legal analysis can generate or that could be obtained by direct observation of legal systems.

How Content Analysis Complements Conventional Legal Analysis

Traditional legal scholarship relies, like the interpretation of literature, on the interpreter's expertise to select important cases, draw out noteworthy themes and identify potential social effects. Readers depend on the author's judgment about which are the "leading cases" that best illustrate the matter in question. Interpretive legal scholars read opinions closely, looking for themes running through several opinions. They ponder the meaning of a decision for future cases by asking how the outcome in the current case relates to its facts, procedural posture, and the court's reasoning.

Although legal writing in this mode may make assertions about how judges think or act, it is not a scientific form of empiricism. These legal analysts report what they see in key cases and how they interpret these observations, not unlike how a literary critic might interpret poetry. Establishing some plausible basis for the minimally empirical claims in such work is usually done simply by citing relevant sources that readers can verify if they wish.

Although content analysis has different epistemological aims, it can be seen as a logical extension of the school of jurisprudence known as Legal Realism. Over a century ago, Justice Oliver Wendell Holmes, Jr., famously proclaimed that "prophecies of what the courts will do in fact, and nothing more pretentious, are what I mean by the law." This credo, once revolutionary, is now so widely accepted that it is sometimes said in the legal academy that "we are all legal realists." Content analysis seeks to use accepted scientific methods to support the verifiable claims that legal researchers frequently make about what judges do and say.

Content analysis can augment conventional analysis by identifying previously unnoticed patterns that warrant deeper study, or correcting misimpressions based on ad hoc surveys of atypical cases. Once detected, these previously unnoticed and unexpected features of the law, observed only on the surface, can be explored more deeply through other, richer methods. Scientists speak in terms of "triangulating" different methods—that is, exploring whether different approaches offer similar conclusions, each approach rigorous in its own way, but each illuminating different dimensions and potentially overcoming their respective shortcomings. Quantitative description can tell us the *what* of case law; other methods may be better suited to understanding the *why* and *wherefore*.

Neither type of scholarship standing alone is as strong as the different types combined. Content analysis reaches a thinner understanding of the law than that gained through more subjective interpretive methods. The coding of case content does not fully capture the strength of a particular judge's rhetoric, the level of generality used to describe the issue, and many other subtle clues about the precedential value of the opinion. Or, as an example to put the point more bluntly, the "legal and cultural salience of Roe *v.* Wade far outruns its statistical significance" (Goldsmith & Vermeule, 2002).

Content analysis is valid if it accurately and reliably measures the particular components of the decision that the researcher wants to study. Using systematic defined coding protocols improves measurement by removing elements of researcher bias, enhancing thoroughness, precision, and accuracy. However, to the extent that content analysis cannot reach important aspects of legal interpretation that are impossible to code objectively (such as nuance related to infrequent or highly complex factual and procedural patterns), content analysis alone is not capable of measuring what lawyers or scholars would consider to be a full and accurate statement of the law.

Counting Case Outcomes

One basic use of content analysis is simply to document the bare outcomes of cases. Measuring who won and who lost differs fundamentally from measuring the law of a case. Case outcomes are much narrower and more objective questions, requiring much less legal judgment, than what legal principle a case embodies. One might, for instance, want to simply tote up the number of cases in which the authority of local public health laws was challenged, and who won and lost, either in one jurisdiction or many, over a period of time.

Counting case outcomes in this fashion is best done when each decision should receive equal weight, that is, when it is appropriate to regard the content of opinions as generic data. Coding and counting cases usually assumes that the information from one opinion is potentially as relevant as that from any other opinion. Because content analysis tends to regard all cases, judges, courts, and jurisdictions in the same way, it should be used only with great caution when any of these have a great deal more status or influence than the others, for the question addressed. Differential influence is often true in legal analysis because precedent and persuasiveness depend on various qualitative judgments about the reasons given or the source of the decision. A US Supreme Court decision, for instance, obviously carries a great deal more weight than a state's intermediate appellate court.

Taking this limitation into account, scholars have found that it is especially useful to code and count cases to document the *absence* of some element that is thought to be present in case law. "Proving a negative" is much harder than simply pointing to what is present in case law because the nay-saying researcher needs to demonstrate that he or she has looked exhaustively for all likely instances of the missing element.

Counting cases can also be useful in studying a wide range of social and economic phenomena that might affect judge-made law. Treating case outcomes as the dependent variable, the range of potential influences on judicial behavior that might be studied statistically is limited only by the bounds of a researcher's imagination. One study, for instance, explored whether the political makeup of Congress or changes in the presidential party in power affected the outcome of federal appellate cases in which health and safety regulations were challenged, over a 25-year period (Revesz, 1997, 2001).

Case law can also be used as an independent variable, by asking how it influences various social and economic conditions. Law's effect on society is obviously a rich field of inquiry, but most such studies trace the effects only of statutory or regulatory law. Researchers have neglected the possible effects of judge-made law, including statutory interpretation. For instance, social host and bar owner liability for alcohol-related injuries is determined by both judicial decisions and statutory enactments, which vary widely by state and over time. These differences might contribute to a variety of public health effects of interest. With its diverse laboratory of states, the United States offers boundless opportunities to learn from the natural experiments created by the inevitable differences in case law among jurisdictions and over time.

Evaluating Legal Doctrine

Opinion coding is not suited, however, to evaluating the legal correctness of judicial opinions. Certainly, many content analysts draw normative implications from what they observe, but their coding of cases aims only to document what judges do rather than to evaluate in a formal empirical manner how well they perform. Without an independent "gold standard" for what the law should be in any particular case or jurisdiction, who is to say its judges are legally wrong, in an empirical sense? After all, what judges say is the law. Therefore, normative evaluation of legal doctrine ordinarily can be done convincingly only through some form of traditional legal analysis.

But beyond documenting merely the bare outcomes of legal disputes, content analysis might be used to study the legal principles one can extrapolate from those outcomes and the facts and reasons that contribute to those outcomes and principles. Such analyses raise important epistemological and jurisprudential issues.

"JURIMETRICS"

The most ambitious use of content analysis is to study the legal factors that determine the outcomes of cases, using sophisticated statistical methods to model or predict the behavior of judges. This general approach at one time was called "jurimetrics" (Loevinger, 1961). This kind of study might attempt to predict the likely result in a case when the parties present the judge with a particular combination of legally relevant factors. Often the stated purpose is to help practicing lawyers make better-informed decisions about handling particular cases. Other times, the purpose is more scholarly—to test various claims on the basis of legal theory.

An especially interesting subgenre uses content analysis to find some order and logic in a body of case law that, by conventional analysis, appears chaotic or haphazard. As Fred McChesney (1993) notes, "the academic history of American law generally is replete with instances in which scholars have proclaimed traditional common-law modes of distilling 'the law' from cases unworkable." These conventional legal analysts, throwing up their hands, conclude that the law on the topic is hopelessly confused and inconsistent, or, less pejoratively, dependent on individual facts. Nuisance law might be one relevant example. Are public nuisances solely "in the eye of the beholder," or are there patterns of factors that are associated with the likelihood of finding or not finding legally actionable public nuisance? Content analysis is well suited to answering this question in a body of case law that otherwise might appear unfathomable.

THE CIRCULARITY OF FACTS IN JUDICIAL OPINIONS

Judges marshal the facts and reasons that support the outcome of the case. Therefore, their opinions might not fully or accurately describe the real-world facts or the true nature of the judge's decision process. Indeed, there is every reason to think just the opposite. This limitation entails two distinct problems: factual incompleteness and factual distortion. Incompleteness results because judges' presentations are meant only to explain as much of the facts as are necessary to justify the out-come. This judicial parsimony can severely distort analysts' measurement of facts that might be important across a range of cases. An apt example is the study of racial factors. Whites might be identified in only a fraction of cases in which race is mentioned, but most likely this is because courts usually do not consider it appropriate to mention race unless they think this might be legally relevant in a particular case.

The second problem is the possibility that judges distort the facts they report to justify the results they reach. This is a highly contentious charge, but distortion does not have to amount to outright misrepresentation. Instead, distortion arises simply from the inevitability that courts select and filter the facts as relevant to the explanation of their decision, but doing only that creates a serious methodologic challenge, since it is circular to predict judicial outcomes from facts that reflect rather than generate the result.

ANSWERING THE SKEPTICS

There are four possible responses to concerns about the usefulness of legal content analysis. First, scientific data aim only to be a reasonable approximation of underlying reality. As a probabilistic endeavor, they can tolerate a degree of imprecision, especially when such imprecision is randomly distributed, not reflecting biased measurement (for example, when the measurement of a particular dimension of law systematically underestimates or overestimates). Similarly, for facts reported by judges, even though they may not be a full account of the "real facts," they may be as close an approximation as is reasonably available to study a particular question. This assumption is not heroic. Lawyers and law professors who stake their life's work on believing (by and large) judges' renditions of facts are, on the whole, hardly naive idealists.

Second, researchers specifically can examine the fidelity of reported facts, looking for indications of distortion or incompleteness, to determine if the facts are close enough to reality for use in statistical analysis. One such technique is to compare facts reported in an appellate opinion with those reported in either the trial court's opinion or a dissenting opinion.

Third, the "bias" created by courts' justifying their decisions may be precisely what a researcher wishes to study. After all, the facts and reasons the judge selects are the substance of the opinion that creates law and binding precedent, so they merit careful study for this very reason. This justification calls, however, for precision in setting the goals of study. Instead of predicting outcomes, content analysis can aim simply at studying judicial reasoning itself, retrospectively.

Finally, the fact that content analysis may not provide definite answers to factors affecting judicial decisions does not mean the method lacks all value. Even if doubts remain about cause-and-effect relationships with judicial decisions, identifying apparent or possible associations of interest can merit further study using additional, and perhaps more experimental, methods.

Exploring the Landscape of Case Law

Rather than trying to predict or explain case outcomes, content analysts can take advantage of the factual, rhetorical, and legal details in judicial opinions simply to describe or explore a body of case law. Observing and documenting what can be found in case law is more akin to mapping than to testing. Like a naturalist exploring new (or familiar) terrain, researchers can code cases to document trends in the case law and factors that appear important to case outcomes, such as the apparent effect of a new precedent, statute, or legal doctrine.

Wright and Huck (2002), for instance, code and analyze 440 decisions regarding milk production and purity standards during the 80-year period starting in 1860, exploring the historical question of whether courts were hostile or receptive to state legislatures' progressive public health agendas. They conclude that judicial hostility was greater than legal and social historians frequently recognize.

The primary criticism of some descriptive or exploratory studies is that they can draw conclusions about features of the legal landscape that cannot be observed fully from judicial opinions. As discussed more further on, win-loss records from published opinions do not necessarily tell us about legal disputes that were never filed in court, or those that the parties settled, or those that judges resolved without written or published opinions. Nevertheless, even if judicial opinions offer a skewed view of what occurs elsewhere in the legal system, they are a highly valuable source for systematic study because they reveal the portion of the legal world that in many ways is most important. It is published opinions that set legal precedent and that guide lawyers.

Published opinions are especially probative of questions about the spread of ideas within the legal system or the types of information that judges appear to rely on. A number of studies analyze courts' reliance on different types of social science evidence (Hall & Wright, 2008). Naturally, caution is warranted in concluding that a mention of a source in an opinion indicates actual importance judges place on this type of evidence and argument. Still, with appropriate caveats on the claims being made, systematic study of how judges reason in their written decisions is perhaps the most compelling application of case content analysis because it best fits the method with the type of question that researchers are asking.

Finally, because published opinions represent "law," the amount, nature, and legal influence of particular dimensions of such law may well affect a diverse set of public health outcomes. To advance empirical study of the public health effects of law, we need counts, weights, scales, and other numeric indices of such law. Precise and specified procedures, and consistent implementation of such protocols, are required to meet scientific standards for reliable measurement.

Guidelines for Identifying and Coding Case Law

Assuming the decision has been made to conduct content analyses of case law (in contrast to traditional legal analysis), we next consider how best to design and implement such a content analysis. In brief, a content analyst selects a set of opinions on a particular subject via a predefined set of search-and-inclusion criteria; reads the documents systematically, recording features of each one in a consistent and reliable manner; and then draws inferences about the use and meaning of those documents.

Selecting Cases

The first decision in any case-coding project is which cases to select. There are two components to consider: sampling frame and selection method. The sampling frame is the theoretical universe of all relevant cases, and the selection method determines which cases will actually be sampled and studied. For both dimensions, researchers should specify exactly the protocol used (databases, search terms, repeated review and correction cycles, and so on) so that it is fully understood and reproducible by others.

SAMPLING FRAME AND BIASES

Frequently in empirical studies, it is not feasible to observe all or most members of a relevant population. The potential biases introduced by sampling method ordinarily are a topic of considerable methodological attention, so that a study sample accurately represents the true population of interest. Fortunately, most studies of legal decisions can avoid this concern because the sampling frame contains a small enough number of cases that *universal* sampling of *all* relevant cases is often feasible. When the total population is too large to be manageable, however, sampling techniques might include true random sampling (best done by computer-generated list of random numbers); systematic sampling, such as every fifth case; quota sampling, such as all cases up to 200, per jurisdiction per year; or purposive sampling, such as cases that are cited by leading treatises and casebooks or cited by other cases.

The more troubling question is the relevant sampling *frame*. What are the boundaries of the subject matter in question? Obviously, this depends critically on the study's central questions and purposes. Study questions can be narrowed to fit the sample frame that is available, or a theoretical sample frame can be imagined that is unrealistically broad but that fits a more interesting or important set of questions the analyst wishes to pursue. Political scientists, for instance, often study political and institutional influences on judicial decision-making by looking not at *all* Supreme Court cases or a random selection, but instead at a particularly controversial or value-laden set of decisions, such as those involving freedom of speech or unreasonable searches and seizures.

Whenever the actual cases selected do not fully match the sampling frame that theoretically applies to the questions posed or studied, an issue of sampling bias exists. For example, studies that sample cases until a certain date cannot, necessarily, claim with confidence that their findings reflect what happened after that date. (This is true as well for studies that sample from certain jurisdictions.) Researchers should at least reflect on these potential distortions or limitations, and mention in their reports those that merit explanation.

One scholar, for instance (who happens to be the author of this chapter), explored how courts determine effectiveness of medical treatment in health insurance disputes by studying all *published* judicial opinions resolving such disputes (Hall, Rust Smith, Naughton, & Ebbers, 1996). That universe of observations is most relevant to understand how appellate courts reason their decisions on such issues, but the sample frame of all published opinions does not fully reflect what all courts do or how state trial courts actually make their decisions.

There is potential selection bias at each of many points in the litigation process. Only some human interactions produce disputes, only some disputes result in legal claims, many claims are settled, and many trial decisions are not appealed. Appellate courts regularly dispose of cases without opinions or decide not to publish some opinions, and computer databases inconsistently include cases that are not officially published. At each of these junctures, there are a variety of factors that potentially distort what one stage can reveal about the other. These biases can fundamentally threaten the validity or generalizability of a study's findings. In these situations, careful consideration of selection biases may lead to major redesign of a study as originally conceived.

Sometimes, however, agonized handwringing can be minimized or avoided. No concern arises if the researcher defines the research question in terms that match the population of cases actually sampled. For instance, if it is precedential law that one wants to study, rather than simply the generalized behavior or attitudes of judges, then unpublished opinions are irrelevant and so excluding them requires no justification. In other situations, when excluded cases are theoretically relevant, the exclusion can easily be justified if the likely direction of bias or distortion is considered. When the bias runs in the same general direction as the study's findings (that is, the excluded cases are even more likely to exhibit the observed pattern), then including the additional cases would likely only strengthen the findings. The only major harm from excluding them is potentially to have missed some additional findings of interest or to have produced a false observation of no effect.

In other situations, likely differences between studied cases and omitted cases are sufficiently inconsequential that the omission should create no more a concern than other limitations obvious and inherent in the sample frame itself, such as one date range rather than another. All empirical studies are imperfect—observational (non-experimental) studies especially. The realistic standard for selecting cases is not a perfect match between sample frame and research objectives, but only a strong connection between the two.

SELECTION TECHNIQUES AND REPLICABILITY

An essential attribute of scientific objectivity is the ability to reproduce a project's findings using the same methods. Replicability is the overriding reason for using systematic content analysis with a detailed protocol. Both the selection of cases to be included and their coding must be described with sufficient transparency in the protocol to be replicable.

Transparent case selection usually consists simply of specifying the search terms used to locate candidate cases in the Westlaw or LEXIS databases. However, these Boolean searches rarely return only or mostly relevant cases. Cases that mention a topic of interest often do so only in passing. Those that decide an issue sometimes do so on technical or procedural grounds that are not relevant to a particular study. Therefore, further narrowing is usually needed in order to reduce an initial selection of candidate cases to those that are directly relevant to the research question.

Most legal researchers do so using somewhat subjective criteria of relevance that cannot be fully replicated, but should be described as fully as possible in a list of inclusion and exclusion criteria. Another option is to refine the initial search strategy. Useful strategies include searching case digests or headnotes rather than the full case itself or searching a sample of cases selected initially because they cited particular statutes, or because they appear in a subject-matter classification drawn by someone else, such as West's Key Numbering System or the publisher of a subject-matter-specific reporter. In effect, such researchers are relying on case selection criteria employed by someone else to establish probable relevance of cases.

Verifying the replicability of case selection is essential for a rigorous study, eliminating the possibility that a researcher subconsciously chose cases according to whether he or she appeared to support the researcher's preliminary hunches. Either formal reliability testing or case selection by someone who is otherwise uninvolved in the study is a way to guard against this potential bias.

Coding Cases

Once cases are selected, a defined coding scheme focuses attention systematically on various elements of cases, and is a check against looking, either consciously or not, for confirmation of predetermined positions. This effort to articulate beforehand the features of a case worth studying also allows researchers to delegate some or all of the reading to assistants. More important, coding cases, even for just qualitative description and analysis, strengthens the objectivity and reproducibility of case law interpretation. Experts in content analysis outline four basic steps that should be followed in coding any material (Krippendorff, 2004; Neuendorf, 2017):

1. On the basis of questions most germane to the study, create a tentative set of coding categories a priori. After thorough evaluation, including feedback from colleagues, study team members or expert consultants refine these categories.

2. Write a coding sheet and set of coding instructions (called a "codebook"), and train coders to apply these to a sample of the material to be coded. Pilot test the reliability (consistency) among coders by having multiple people independently code some of the material, and calculate the correlation across coders (that is, inter-rater reliability).

3. Add, delete, or revise coding categories according to this pilot experience, and repeat reliability testing and coder training as required.

4. When the codebook is finalized, apply it to all the material. Then, or during that process, conduct a final, formal reliability test. This section elaborates on each of these steps.

Coding Categories and Instructions

Categories used to code content of judicial decisions are tremendously diverse, owing to the wide range of questions that researchers pursue. Commonly used factors might be sorted into four general groups: parties' identities and attributes, types of legal issues raised and in what circumstances, basic outcome of the case or issue, and bases for decision. Coders often do not distinguish the "facts" of a case from various arguments that are made. Instead, they usually code simply for whether a variety of factual or legal factors are present in the case in some fashion. Coders should consider whether it suffices if these factors are merely alleged, realizing that the allegations may be sharply contested. If mere allegations are not sufficient, what is? Obviously, the procedural posture of a case (summary judgment versus post-trial) can complicate this evaluation.

Regarding the bases for decision, coders frequently distinguish between procedural and substantive rulings, and they record the various types of authorities that courts cite or rely upon. Some researchers also code for the degree of importance that various factual or legal factors have in the court's analysis or holding. A common focus of coding is also the court's style of analysis or approach to statutory or constitutional interpretation, categorized in various ways.

Coding is not restricted to manifest variables that are explicit in the text; it has been shown to work well also for some "latent" variables that require inference or evaluative judgment. For instance, Johnson (1987) demonstrates the ability of law students to code cases with some degree of reliability for the clarity, complexity, and completeness of their discussion of facts, issues, holding, reasoning, and the law.

Coding experts advise researchers to create more coding categories, and to make coding more fine-grained, than the categories they may ultimately use. Even though this produces more information than the project will eventually require, the advantage is allowing the researcher to test different categorization schemes to learn through trial and error which work best. Ultimately, the goal is to maximize the exhaustiveness of coding while keeping mutually exclusive categories—in other words, to capture all the relevant information, but to avoid having categories that duplicate or overlap each other. This does not mean, however, that a coding category must be devised for each possible nuance of relevance. Instead, categories should be used only if they occur with some frequency, or if the objective is to document their absence. Rare or unusual features can be coded simply with a miscellaneous "other" option.

A good example of exhaustive and mutually exclusive coding is categorizing case outcomes. It is usually not a simple matter to define what counts as a win or loss across a range of cases. Appellate cases arise in a variety of procedural postures, they usually involve multiple issues, and each issue can be resolved in several different ways. Case coding projects often have to devise complex categories to capture all the relevant detail. The United States Court of Appeals Database (http://www.wmich.edu/nsf-coa/), for instance, defines all possible case outcomes using nine categories. This illustrates that it is a better practice to be over-inclusive at the coding stage, waiting until the analysis stage to collapse the various categories into discrete win-loss columns.

When categories are finalized, it is essential to good coding practice to record their description and specific instructions for their application in the protocol or codebook. Obviously, this is necessary if coding is done by someone other than the researcher, such as student assistants. Even if authors do their own coding, the scientific standard of replicability requires a clear written record of how categories were defined and applied, permitting other research teams to correctly replicate the procedure in future studies.

Experienced coders advise that errors will be reduced if coding forms are designed to minimize writing. For instance, a form might provide a checklist of factors to indicate presence or absence by ticking boxes rather than having to write in a number or letter. Also, while the objective is to reduce the need for coder judgment, detailed instructions can be conveyed either through the coding form itself, or in a supplemental manual. A balance should be struck between a form that is so spare it offers almost no on-the-spot instructional information for coders, forcing them to refer frequently to the detailed coding manual, and a coding form that is overlong because each form contains a full set of instructions. Thus it typically does not help to extensively revise succinct, well-written coding categories simply to satisfy the whim of each coder who might ask for more detailed instructions. It is inevitable that some measure of ambiguity will remain in how coding categories apply to atypical cases, and a residual notes file should be included to record unusual situations.

CHOOSING AND TRAINING CODERS

A major dilemma in coding cases is whether principal investigators should do this work themselves, or supervise students (or others). In theory, the most scientifically rigorous method is for researchers to train others to do the coding and for coders to work completely independently once they are trained. Using generic coders helps ensure that the researchers' preliminary hypotheses and personal views do not bias the coding. Also, this can save researchers considerable time and effort in large coding projects. Moreover, the imposed discipline of training and supervising coders ensures that coding instructions are written in a way that others can follow. Training and using multiple coders promotes the reproducibility that is essential for good science. Coding by law students is appropriate when some general legal knowledge is required but it is not necessary to be an expert in the field of study. Still, coding reliability improves the more that coders are trained. Researchers should describe how training was done in sufficient detail that others can replicate all of the steps.

Other considerations might counsel doing one's own coding, however. Training coders to achieve accurate and reliable results can be a difficult and time-consuming undertaking, one that may require considerably more resources and effort than would researchers simply doing their own coding, especially in smaller projects. A relevant selection of cases is often sufficiently small that a single reader can handle the coding alone. Also, even trained coders can make a surprising number of mistakes, even on seemingly simple and objective criteria such as dates. Although delegating coding may promote reliability, this can threaten the validity of results if the information that coders record is not accurate or is too "dumbed down" to be meaningful. It may be that student coders lack the level of expertise needed to code reliably the more complex or subtle, yet more meaningful, aspects of judicial opinions. If so, researchers will be sorely tempted to do their own coding. When this is done, however, it is especially important to conduct reliability tests by recruiting a colleague with similar expertise to independently double code at least a subset of cases. Resulting reliability estimates should always be recorded and published along with the substantive findings.

Testing Reliability

Demonstrating the reliability of coding is an essential aspect of good content analysis. If coding categories are so objective and straightforward that it is obvious they can be applied consistently, then perhaps this step is not necessary, though that is rarely the case. If there are significant elements of subjectivity or uncertainty in applying coding categories to legal decisions, scientific rigor requires evaluation of whether different people would code the documents consistently. This is essential because the theory of coding—the reason systematic content analysis is done at all—is the implicit claim of reproducibility, that other researchers using the same methods will achieve approximately the same results. This claim is undermined if coding reflects primarily the subjective, idiosyncratic interpretation of the particular individuals who read the cases, or if coding has large elements of error or arbitrariness.

It is true that even without any reliability testing it is perfectly possible that a coding scheme in fact is reliable. But this cannot be ensured unless investigators test coding reliability in some fashion. The best method is to conduct formal reliability tests during (at least) two stages in the process: initially, while piloting the draft coding process, and later, once coding categories and instructions are optimized. Formal testing calls for at least two coders independently to code a sample of cases and to compare their results statistically.

The most common statistic is simple percentage of agreement. However, a simple percentage does not account for the level of agreement that would be expected purely by chance. Because chance agreement varies according to the type of coding scheme (that is, a variable with two possible answers will naturally produce more agreement than a variable with eight possible answers), the best practice is to report one of several coefficients that reflect the extent of agreement beyond what is expected by chance. There are several such statistical tests, the most common of which is known as "Cohen's Kappa" (after its inventor) or simply the Kappa statistic. Ranging from 0 to 1, Kappa indicates the proportion of observed agreement that exceeds what would be expected by chance alone, with 0 indicating agreement entirely by chance and 1 indicating perfect agreement.

If statistics such as these are used, they must be employed correctly. One mistake is to test the overall reliability of all variables combined. The correct method is to test and report each variable's reliability because reliability can vary widely across items and aggregate statistics can mask serious problems with key variables. Also, when the response pattern for a variable is highly skewed (one of several available responses occurs much more frequently than the others), this should be noted or taken into account in the statistical measure used. Otherwise, the nominal level of agreement can be deceptive. If one were to code for the presence or absence of one hundred factors in each case, most likely only a dozen or so will appear in any one case. Testing for coding reliability may find a very high percentage of agreement then, but only because most factors are not present in most cases. The key question, though, is whether coders agree when they indicate a factor is present.

When reliability testing reveals discrepancies, as it almost always will, this will usually point to unresolved questions in the coding instructions, problems that can be corrected if the error appears after the pilot phase rather than after the completed coding. Also, poor reliability in the pilot round of coding often reveals conceptual ambiguity that can be clarified to more accurately measure the dimensions or their components that are actually most relevant to the particular research question.

After final coding, compulsive researchers might try to get to the bottom of remaining disagreements and resolve all discrepancies, both in the reliability testing sample and across the entire selection. When there are large numbers of cases being coded, resolving every discrepancy may be unnecessary and impractical. Disagreements sometimes arise from overt errors, but often they result simply from judgment calls or inevitable ambiguities that may be virtually impossible to eliminate without compromising the independence of individual coders. Perfect reliability is the goal, but rarely fully achieved. A key requirement of science is transparency—reporting the exact levels of reliability of the resulting data.

Refining coding rules to eliminate all elements of ambiguity is usually not possible, no matter how prescriptive the rules. Plus, each time the rules are rewritten, the best practice would be to retest the refined rules for reliability, producing a never-ending cycle in search of elusive perfection. Therefore, coders should learn to live with a certain degree of imperfection once coding is found to be reasonably reliable and draw appropriately modest conclusions when relying on variables with weaker levels of inter-coder reliability. Although there is broad agreement on the desirability of testing for reliability, and some agreement on the methods for doing so, there is not firm agreement on what *level* of reliability is the minimum that is acceptable. The goal is aspirational—to achieve high levels of agreement—rather than merely to rise somewhat above purely random agreement. One suggested rule of thumb is that a reliability coefficient of 0.8 (that is, data agree 80% more than mere chance agreement) is good, with indices from 0.67 to 0.8 being sufficient for "tentative conclusions" (Krippendorff, 1980). Others claim that this is too demanding, especially for coding categories that produce highly skewed responses, since even small levels of disagreement can cause the statistical index to drop rapidly. Therefore, other methodologists provide a more lenient classification for the Kappa statistic (Lombard, Snyder-Duch, & Campanella Bracken, 2005): ≤0.00 is poor; 0.01–0.20 is "slight" agreement; 0.21–0.40 is fair; 0.41–0.60 is "moderate"; 0.61–0.80 is "substantial"; and 0.81–1.00 is "almost perfect." Keep in mind that these recommendations are for agreement levels beyond what is expected by chance. For a raw, unadjusted percentage, agreement levels below 70 to 80% are usually not considered to be good.

If coder agreement is not acceptable, researchers must either retrain coders, revise their coding categories, decide not to use the data, or use the data but with appropriate caveats. Following best practices, the first two options call for retesting of reliability. One convenient remedy is to combine marginally reliable detailed coding into a more aggregated category that has better reliability.

ALTERNATIVE CODING TECHNIQUES

Researchers might consider alternatives to independent coding by assistants. One is to have a group of assistants code each case and then assign the value that is coded by the majority. Group coding creates the impression of greater objectivity, and may in fact improve reliability, but this is not necessarily the case. Resolving split votes with whatever the third person thinks might be as arbitrary as using a single coder. The only way to find out for sure is to test the reliability of panel coding by coding a sample of cases independently with a different panel.

Similarly, some researchers have coders confer when they disagree in order to seek consensus, or the researchers use their own expertise to resolve disagreements. Again, this may or may not improve reliability, but it does not *establish* reliability. The process of reaching consensus might be arbitrary, or the lead investigator's expert view might not be objectively reproducible.

A variation of these techniques is expert panel consensus. Developed for evaluating medical judgments, this has not been used so far for legal judgments but it is worth exploring. Following what is known as the Delphi technique, each expert first rates a case independently, then learns how peer experts have rated it, and then, following discussion, each expert gives an independent final rating, with the majority controlling when there is not unanimity (Shekelle, Kahan, Bernstein et al., 1998). This has been shown to be a fairly reliable method for rating highly complex and judgmental aspects of medical decision-making (Park, Fink, Brook et al., 1986). It combines elements of "gold standard" expertise with consensus building and majority rule.

Finally, there is an innovative technique that avoids altogether the vagaries of training coders and demonstrating reliability: using completely mechanical forms of content analysis that can be done by computer or simple computation. For instance, some studies count the number of words or paragraphs devoted to discussing particular factors as an indication of the factors' relative importance. Also interesting is research that analyzes judicial texts entirely by computer, looking for revealing patterns in syntax or semantics (McGuire, Vanberg, Smith, & Caldeira, 2009; Wahlbeck, Spriggs, & Sigelman, 2002).

Analyzing Cases

A credible content analyst does not necessarily need to use complex or sophisticated statistics—or, indeed, any statistics at all. Often, researchers simply report counts and frequencies to show how commonly a given feature appears in the cases. Quantitative descriptive analyses may be sufficient to document trends in the case law, to challenge conventional wisdom, or to raise provocative questions meriting further study. Because many case-counting studies code the entire universe of relevant cases, statistics are not essential for analyzing the probability that the sample cases reflect the reality in a larger population.

Moreover, content analysis need not involve numbers at all. Instead, it can employ rigorous methods of purely qualitative analysis that focus on themes and patterns that are best understood through conceptual description and narrative illustrations rather than numbers. Empirically evaluating public health effects of case law, however, requires the use of counts and numeric indices and scales, and so statistical analyses are often essential.

One danger in using statistical testing in exploratory studies is that, without a tightly controlled analytical focus, such as a predefined set of theory-based hypotheses that are being tested, it becomes too easy to find associations and patterns of apparent significance entirely by chance. If enough variables are examined and enough comparisons are made, odds are that statistically significant findings will emerge, but some or all of these apparent findings could be due entirely to chance without additional statistical adjustments for the number of possibilities that were explored.

Potentially more revealing is multiple regression analysis, which can uncover hidden relationships among multiple factors, both internally within court decisions or between decisions and external factors. In attempting to explain the legal outcomes or health-related effects of a set of cases, for example, several factors may each appear significant by themselves, but when each is held constant, only one or two factors may emerge as the most important predictors of decisions. Sometimes, factors that legal analysts thought were dominant or important turn out to be red herrings. Alternatively, factors that, standing alone, may not appear significant might emerge as such once the influence of other factors is controlled statistically. It is advisable, however, to use regression analysis only for cases that are relatively homogenous, focusing on a single or narrow set of legal issues. Otherwise it may become too difficult to measure and control for all the relevant variables.

Another aspect of statistical analysis worth considering in broad perspective is whether each case (or part of a case) should be given equal weight. It is possible to weight each case according to an objective measure of its significance, such as how often it has been cited or followed, or where it stands in a line of precedent. The difficulty with this approach, however, is deciding how much weight to assign. Nascent efforts to apply network analysis to the citation patterns among cases may eventually prove fruitful in assigning appropriate weights to different cases (Smith, 2005). But, absent any objective means to assign different quantitative weights, the best option is to classify cases qualitatively into different categories and analyze each separately—such as major versus minor decisions, or leading versus following decisions.

A final concern is the appropriate unit of analysis. Rather than each case counting the same, case law can be grouped by separate jurisdiction to assign a legal rule to each location. Doing that enables exploration of how the adoption of particular rules of law relate to other occurrences, including health outcomes.

Conclusion

Content analysis is a valuable research tool for documenting what courts do and what they say. The insights gained from uniform content analysis of large numbers of opinions supplement the deeper understanding of individual opinions that comes from traditional interpretive techniques. The content of judicial opinions can be important in the study of the broader social, economic, and political systems that interact with judicial precedent, but cases are also well worth scientific study in their own right.

The major limitation of content analysis (a limit that applies equally to traditional interpretive methods) is that facts and reasons given in opinions cannot be treated as accurate and complete. Therefore, researchers should be cautious about the meanings they attach to observations made through content analysis. Within these bounds, content analysis is well suited to studying connections between judicial opinions and other parts of the social, political, or economic landscape.

Scientific methods complement conventional legal research methods in three key ways. Content analysis can verify or refute descriptions of case law that are based on more anecdotal or subjective study. Second, content analysis can identify surface patterns (which are sometimes hidden from the naked eye), to be explored more deeply through interpretive, theoretical, or normative legal analysis. Third, systematic numeric content coding of case law opens up major new avenues of research to better understand the many ways in which law affects population health.

Summary

This chapter explored the special considerations in coding text when the relevant legal materials are judicial decisions. The content of case law merits careful study not simply because judicial opinions reflect or respond to the law, but because they *are* the law. But more than this, judicial opinions are detailed repositories that show what kinds of disputes come before courts, how the parties frame their disputes, and how judges reason to their conclusions.

Content analysis of case law boils down to three steps: (1) selecting cases, (2) coding cases, and (3) analyzing (often through statistics) the case coding. Insights gained from content analysis of large numbers of opinions supplement the deeper understanding of individual opinions that comes from traditional interpretive legal research techniques. The content of judicial opinions can be important in the study of the broader social, economic, and political systems that interact with judicial precedent, but cases are also well worth scientific study in their own right. For instance, content analysis can identify previously unnoticed patterns that warrant deeper study, or sometimes correct misimpressions based on ad hoc surveys of atypical cases.

The major limitation of content analysis is that facts and reasons recorded in judicial opinions cannot be treated as accurate and complete. Therefore, researchers should be cautious about the meanings they attach to observations made through content analysis. With this caveat in mind, this chapter described a range of acceptable and best practices for systematically selecting relevant cases, forming coding categories, training coders, and testing for coding reliability.

Further Reading

Friedman, B. (2006). Taking law seriously. *Perspectives on Politics, 4*(2), 261–276.

Hall, M. A. (2003). The scope and limits of public health law. *Perspectives in Biology & Medicine, 46*(Suppl. 3), S199–S209.

Krippendorff, K. (2004). *Content analysis: An introduction to its methodology* (2nd ed.). Thousand Oaks, CA: Sage.

Designing Legal Epidemiology Evaluations

The most important determinant of the quality of a public health law evaluation is the research design. The fundamental objectives of legal epidemiology are to improve knowledge on whether a particular law or regulation *causes* a change in population health and knowledge on the mechanisms of that effect (that is, how the effect was achieved). The level of confidence in a causal interpretation of an observed relationship between law and health is fundamentally related to the quality of the research design. Pollack, Bouris, and Cunningham begin Part Four by describing what is typically deemed the gold standard for research—the randomized controlled trial. Random assignment to treatment versus control group is a very helpful design element to reduce study biases and enhance causal inference. RCTs are feasible and important for two types of studies relevant to legal epidemiology—evaluations of specific causal links or *mechanisms* that might explain effects of existing or potential future laws, and evaluations of interventions in specific study populations that might point the way toward *policy candidates* that could be incorporated into future law. By contrast, randomized trials have been rare for evaluation of existing or newly introduced laws, since researchers usually cannot control passage and implementation of laws and thus cannot randomly assign some persons to get a law and others not. However, the

Legal Epidemiology: Theory and Methods, Second Edition. Edited by Alexander C. Wagenaar, Rosalie Liccardo Pacula, and Scott Burris.

scientific advantages of randomization are huge, and legal epidemiology as a field could do much more to advocate for randomized experiments with new legal and regulatory approaches. Advances in stepped-wedge designs, where everyone eventually receives a similar exposure to the intervention but the timing of that exposure is randomized, are particularly useful for evaluations of actual new laws and regulations. With the creative cooperation of policy makers, public health authorities, and scientists, many more opportunities are possible for randomly timing new legal interventions and randomly rolling out new interventions across persons, organizations, or jurisdictions.

Wagenaar and Komro address the common situation in which laws and regulations are implemented by governments without researcher input and random assignment to treatment or control groups is therefore not possible. The chapter presents many feasible design elements that enhance the plausibility of causal interpretations of observed effects in these "natural experiments" and emphasizes that any particular study should not simply select a workable research design but should creatively incorporate as many of the design elements as possible to maximize the validity of conclusions that a law caused changes in population health.

Two additional chapters follow on other useful approaches to public health law evaluation. Wood describes qualitative research strategies, which enhance quantitative approaches by providing more in-depth or nuanced information on how laws are designed or implemented and how available health outcome measures might not fully encompass the whole of legal effects. Results from such qualitative studies then often feed back into improved measurement and design of quantitative studies, more formally testing the effects suggested in qualitative research. Public health officials and policy makers considering alternative laws and regulations not only want to know how many disease or injury cases are averted, but also want to know whether it is worth it in terms of costs involved. Pacula describes how to conduct cost-effectiveness and cost–benefit studies, attending to the special considerations when estimating the costs and benefits of a law, rather than typical cost–benefit studies involving intervention programs that treat specific individuals.

We conclude the book with a chapter that points to the future of legal epidemiology as an identifiable field of study, highlighting the importance of continual improvement in theoretical integration, strengthening scientific methods, and tighter integration of lawyers, sociolegal scholars, social scientists, and health scientists. The aim should not just be for more and better work in legal epidemiology, but stronger links between research and practice so that healthy policies are more rapidly identified and spread to every place they can help.

Chapter 13

Randomized Trials in Legal Epidemiology

Harold Pollack   Alida Bouris   Scott Cunningham

Learning Objectives

- Recognize the distinct uses of randomized trials in devising, implementing, and evaluating laws to improve public health.
- Understand the different types of randomized trials, and different units of randomization.
- Articulate challenges to internal validity and generalizability of experimental methods.
- Articulate distinctions between randomized trials of specific interventions or policy candidates and experimental law evaluations.
- Articulate the role of implementation science and hybrid trials to explore barriers, facilitators, and contextual factors.

Randomized controlled trials (RCTs) are regarded by many policymakers and researchers as the gold standard of policy evaluation. Trials such as the Oregon Health Insurance experiment demonstrate that expanded health coverage can significantly improve mental health, increase use of prescription medications for chronic conditions, and reduce unmet dental needs, while also protecting individuals from adverse financial outcomes associated with illness and injury (Baicker, Allen, Wright, & Finkelstein, 2017; Baicker, Allen, Wright, Taubman, & Finkelstein, 2018). Conversely, the same trials provided disappointing findings regarding the power of expanded health insurance coverage to substantially affect key health outcomes such as blood pressure

Legal Epidemiology: Theory and Methods, Second Edition. Edited by Alexander C. Wagenaar, Rosalie Liccardo Pacula, and Scott Burris.
© 2023 John Wiley & Sons, Inc. Published 2023 by John Wiley & Sons, Inc.

and debunked assertions that generous health insurance coverage would reduce emergency department use (Finkelstein, Taubman, Allen, Wright, & Baicker, 2016; Taubman, Allen, Wright, Baicker, & Finkelstein, 2014). Other trials have provided important, at-times chastening, results regarding promising models such as health care hotspotting (i.e., reducing costs of health-care "superusers") (Finkelstein, Zhou, Taubman, & Doyle, 2020).

This chapter reviews key issues in randomized trials for public health policy and law. We begin by presenting the need for randomized trials. We describe some different purposes for randomized trials in public health law. We then present basic trial concepts such as intent-to-treat (ITT) and treatment-on-the-treated (TOT) effects in the context of a posited intervention to reduce underage alcohol consumption. We then apply the same concepts in the context of another public health challenge—interventions to reduce the incidence of low infant birthweight by reducing smoking by pregnant patients. We show strengths and limitations of a successful randomized trial of contingency management interventions, and we compare trial results to those obtained through econometric analyses of state tobacco tax policies that also prevent prenatal smoking. We note the different levels of aggregation susceptible to experimental designs with a summary discussion of two cluster-randomized trials. We discuss the connection between cluster-randomized designs, stepped-wedge, and quasi-experimental designs, and discuss the importance of specifying mediating mechanisms and causal pathways in the proper interpretation of these study designs. We then present common critiques of randomized trials, and the use of mechanism experiments, before closing the chapter with a discussion of implementation science designs to address limitations of atheoretical "black-box" randomized trials.

Purposes of Randomized Trials

Randomized trials in legal epidemiology are useful tools for three distinct purposes. *Mechanism experiments* focus on one or a few specific causal links in a broader theory or longer causal chain hypothesized to be the reason a particular law has health effects. Such experiments can provide convincing evidence that a particular policy approach appears sufficiently likely to be effective to be worth trying. Second, well-designed randomized trials are often feasible for specific *policy candidates*—programs and interventions that could be delivered, supported, or facilitated through laws, rules, and regulations. We describe two such policy candidates here: A hypothesized intervention to prevent underage drinking, and contingency management interventions whereby pregnant patients might receive immediate financial rewards as behavioral incentives to reduce tobacco use. An RCT of such interventions could clarify for policymakers whether insurers should be legally required to support such interventions, what might be expected (and what remains unknown) regarding the likely public health benefits if policymakers succeed in supporting the proliferation of such interventions.

There is an important distinction between RCTs on mechanisms and policy candidates, versus RCTs of actual laws and regulations. *Randomized trials of actual laws* to date are rare, but are an important third purpose where randomization as a study design element can be fruitfully used to advance the state of knowledge. Consider, we already know that increased safety belt use reduces automobile fatalities. We already know that driving under the influence of intoxicating substances increases road fatalities, and that underage drinking is associated with many public health harms. We already know that smoking by pregnant patients increases the risk of low infant birthweight and infant mortality. We might want to know more about effects of specific programs and other interventions that address these harms, but that knowledge alone is insufficient to improve use of law to scale those interventions.

Even if we know that a particular intervention is effective, we still need to know whether concrete legislation or regulations based on that intervention will meaningfully improve public health: If state Medicaid programs require insurers to cover prenatal smoking cessation services, will such policies actually improve population infant health? If states or counties intensify traffic enforcement or increase penalties for driving under the influence, does this actually reduce related automobile crashes and road fatalities? That is a question for true policy RCTs, which are informed by—but extend far beyond—rigorous evaluations of specific interventions in specific settings.

The Need for Randomized Trials: Concepts and Examples

Public health laws frequently seek to support, generalize or scale specific interventions that proved efficacious or effective in smaller scale randomized trials. In the absence of these prior trials, the benefits of promising program models often prove illusory or overstated, because initial studies faced methodological limitations that limited causal inference, that failed to illuminate plausible causal mechanisms for observed apparent benefits, or that prevented researchers from ruling out alternative explanations for observed effects. And, randomized intervention trials provide only one scientifically sound path through which one identifies candidates for public health policy. For example, regulatory policies to control particulate pollution may emerge from laboratory or engineering studies that shed light on potential health harms.

To gauge the basic risks of relying on observational studies to infer that an intervention caused a result, consider interventions designed to address underage alcohol consumption—a key public health concern. Suppose policymakers are intrigued by motivational interview (MI)-based interventions to reduce underage drinking and are contemplating changes to Medicaid reimbursement policies to cover such specific interventions, and changes to state curricular standards to encourage or require such interventions. Poignant testimonials by program participants and program staff suggest that participation in this intervention reduces underage drinking. Psychologists and social workers provide a strong conceptual explanation of why such programs might be effective, perhaps drawing on research showing the approach worked for other similar problems.

One might try to test these claims by comparing underage drinking patterns of youth who participated in the intervention to those of youth who didn't participate. This comparison is clearly vulnerable to selection bias. Most obviously, this approach may reflect *favorable selection*, whereby students who care more about health harms of alcohol use (or students whose parents care more about these issues) may seek out the intervention. Of course, many of these youth would have avoided underage drinking absent the intervention. Straightforward comparisons between participants and nonparticipants would thus overstate the intervention's causal impact. Controlling for observed student and family characteristics such as income and parental education might reduce such biases, but would not reliably eliminate them.

Alternatively, the program may exhibit *unfavorable selection*. This can happen if program implementors specifically recruit students they believe have greatest alcohol-related difficulties. Some of these factors might be observed and statistically addressed by researchers. For example, recruited students might have more school absences or lower test scores. Other relevant factors often cannot be fully observed by the researcher: recent social challenges in school, perhaps confidential contacts with school counselors whose records are not shared with the researchers. If this were the underlying dynamic, many intervention participants might still engage in underage drinking, but might have consumed even greater amounts without the intervention. Thus, straightforward comparisons of drinking patterns between participants and nonparticipants would likely understate the value of the intervention.

Controlling for observed student and family characteristics might reduce both kinds of biases. It will not eliminate them. An impressively complex nonexperimental design might even make things worse, by making researchers or policymakers overconfident in the accompanying results. Robert LaLonde's (1986) famous reanalysis of experimental job-training data using nonexperimental methods provides one chastening example. Common nonexperimental econometric approaches yield results far from the experimental results. Even worse, these methods yielded tight confidence intervals that (incorrectly) excluded the experimental results.

A randomized trial may address these concerns, particularly in the evaluation of a specific policy candidate intervention. Suppose one performs an *encouragement-design* randomized trial of our intervention to reduce underage drinking. Here, researchers offer $10 video game gift cards to every high school senior assigned to the treatment group who actually attends the Saturday session. Students assigned to the control group can still attend the session, but would not get the gift card. Researchers keep track of the treatment "dose" each student receives, and track an adolescent drinking measure, say ounces of alcohol consumed in the past month.

In particular, let Z be a dummy variable signifying group assignment. Suppose that 55% of students assigned to the treatment group ($Z = 1$) attend the prevention session, compared with 45% of those assigned to control ($Z = 0$). Let's further suppose that mean monthly alcohol consumption is 61 ounces in the treatment group, and 63 ounces in the control group.

Table 13.1. Hypothetical Encouragement Trial to Reduce Underage Alcohol Consumption.

	Total Study Population (n = 1,000)	Offered Gamecards (n = 500) (Z = 1)	Not Offered Gamecards (n = 500) (Z = 0)
Proportion attending Saturday session	500	275	225
Proportion not attending Saturday session	500	225	275
Mean monthly alcohol consumption (ounces)	62 Ounces	61 Ounces	63 Ounces

These deceptively simple results, shown in Table 13.1, help us to interpret and describe the effect of the posited Saturday intervention, and to present basic concepts of randomized trials.

Intent-to-Treat (ITT) vs. Effect of Treatment-on-the-Treated (TOT)

As we frame this question, it becomes apparent that the "program effectiveness" has two complementary interpretations. Policymakers might ask one bottom-line question: How much, overall, might we reduce underage drinking by offering this voluntary Saturday intervention to everyone who is willing to participate? This is the *intent-to-treat* (ITT) effect. The ITT takes into account that not every patient or study subject actually takes-up the treatment. Perhaps the Saturday intervention is boring or unpleasant, is only offered in English within a multilingual student population, or is offered at a time that many students cannot attend due to work, school, or family obligations. Perhaps some students are simply uninterested in reducing their alcohol use, and thus see little value in participating.

Of course, we might also ask a different question: How much do we reduce underage drinking *among the students who actually attend?* This question is often labeled *the effect of treatment on the treated*, or TOT. This speaks to the specific value and effectiveness of the treatment for people who actually receive it.

Take-Up and Compliance as Central to Effectiveness

ITT and TOT estimates often diverge in real-world trials. A new cancer drug might be powerfully effective for patients who actually take it. This is a critical accomplishment that speaks to the biological effect of the medication on this particular cancer. Yet the medication might have unpleasant or toxic side-effects, and thus low patient acceptability and correspondingly disappointing treatment benefits for the population of cancer patients one seeks to help.

The contrast between ITT and TOT also underscores a critical issue in many public health policies—the importance of exposure, awareness, engagement, and compliance in shaping the magnitude of effects of health laws or interventions. Take-up, compliance, and recruitment are central to program effectiveness. A particular preventive intervention can exhibit a strong TOT effect in a randomized trial. Yet that effect often does not hold up when implemented universally through legal incentives or mandates.

A recent intervention to provide supports for male pre-trial detainees leaving jail provides an illustrative case. The program aimed to prevent homelessness, reduce rearrests, and improve health outcomes among returning citizens who live with serious mental illness, substance use disorders, and related challenges. The intervention sought to improve these outcomes by creating immediate linkages to services and by offering participants a safe place to spend the night. The program significantly reduced risks of immediate rearrest among program participants. Yet program take-up was twice as high among released detainees aged 55 and older as among those aged 18–35. Given these patterns, it is plausible that the program can reduce homelessness, which is quite prevalent among older detainees. But it is much less likely to reduce violent re-offending, given low program take-up among younger offenders in the peak age-group associated with violent crime. Anecdotal evidence from program staff indicated that young men offered the intervention found that the central sales pitch—a place to stay for the night for those who might otherwise be homeless—to be a specifically stigmatizing message, and thus chose not to participate.

COVID-19 vaccination poses analogous take-up challenges, with more dramatic effects for population health and health disparities. An overwhelming body of evidence indicates that vaccination reduces infection risk while dramatically reducing risks of serious illness, hospitalization, and death. Given this body of evidence, differential vaccination rates by political party, race-ethnicity, and other characteristics poses a substantial challenge to population health. The emergence of rural residents and political conservatives as key disparity groups poses a particular challenge to the public health community (Kirzinger et al., 2021). Existing RCTs suggest that culturally competent messages delivered by trusted messengers is likely important to promote protective measures within affected communities (Breza et al., 2021a, 2021b; Torres et al., 2021). Randomized trials might explore the effects of different culturally competent public health messaging strategies in eliciting compliance with work- or school-based vaccine mandates.

Our simplified underage drinking example provides a useful framework to present basic distinctions and nomenclature of the ITT and TOT effects. Under proper assumptions, within this simple framework of a binary intervention, the ITT effect estimate is the difference in drinking between the group assigned to treatment (offered gamecards) vs. the group assigned to the control (not offered gamecards), as in Equation (13.1):

$$\beta_{ITT} = E[\text{Ounces} \mid Z = 1] - E[\text{Ounces} \mid Z = 0] \qquad (13.1)$$

Here Ounces$_i$ is monthly alcohol consumption for participant i measured after random assignment, Z is an indicator for having been offered gamecards. Under these assumptions, the intent-to-treat estimate (ITT) is (63–61) = 2 ounces. That represents the effect of *inviting* students to the intervention. This provides one valuable metric of the likely population impact of this intervention—if the intervention could be scaled at the same level of effectiveness.

What about the TOT effect—that is, the causal effect of the intervention for students who actually attended? Under conventional assumptions, the observed two percentage point difference in alcohol consumption entirely arises from the 10 percentage point increase in attendance between the treatment and control groups. For this binary treatment framework, the classic Wald estimate provides a simple but intuitive approximation to the TOT given binary group assignment, by taking into account differences in intervention dose (i.e., attendance) across groups—how many people in each group actually received the intervention:

$$\beta_{\text{Wald}} = \frac{\overline{\text{Ounces}}_{Z=1} - \overline{\text{Ounces}}_{Z=0}}{\overline{\text{Dose}}_{Z=1} - \overline{\text{Dose}}_{Z=0}} = \frac{63 - 61}{0.55 - 0.45} = 20 \text{ ounces.} \qquad (13.2)$$

Despite the modest 2-point ITT effect, considering attendance across groups suggests that the intervention exerts a surprisingly powerful influence—nearly one-third reduction in underage drinking—specifically for those students who actually attend. Efforts to improve program take-up—e.g., through provision of attractive incentives or even mandates if the intervention were fully imbedded in regular school curricula—might magnify the public health impact of this intervention, assuming that the program can be similarly effective among the new students one attracts as reach expands.

Notice that we *assume* that the entire reduction in alcohol consumption arises from the additional intervention provided to youth in the treatment group. There is no other benefit to being assigned to the treatment group, and there is no benefit to assignment to the control group. A moment's thought calls to mind how these assumptions might be violated. Intervention participants might share program materials with their friends. Sharing materials with friends in the treatment group who prefer not to attend would complicate our interpretation of what this intervention was and how it actually worked. Treatment group participants or intervention implementors might also share materials with students in the control group. Alternatively, some control-group youth could have heard that this intervention seems to help. They and their parents might seek other, similar resources outside the school that the researcher never measured. If such crossover efforts were common, researchers would *understate* the benefits of the Saturday intervention, because some control group participants received benefits similar to the intervention.

Peer effects can also arise in more subtle ways. Suppose the intervention raises school-wide awareness about harms associated with underage drinking—and underscores to students that adults are concerned about the issue. One could imagine that many students in both the treatment and control groups—and others not in the study at all—might be more wary about holding parties where alcohol is served. That could reduce total underage drinking throughout the school.

Other challenges might lead us to overstate or understate the value of the intervention, or may limit generalizability of our results. Students in the treatment group develop personal relationships with program staff. They might conceal some drinking behaviors out of embarrassment or out of a desire not to disappoint program implementors. Researchers might have implicitly or explicitly excluded students from the initial randomization whom they believe might be disruptive or are unlikely to benefit from the intervention. As long as students are properly randomized, this would not undermine internal validity— the causal attribution. It would, however, plausibly undermine generalizability—the population to which the results apply. Another threat to generalizability stems from the virtues of the trial itself. An innovative intervention site might in any number of ways have greater resources or provide higher-quality services than are readily replicated at-scale within representative educational settings. Staff might have higher morale or superior management and training. The research intervention might be implemented within a setting with unusually strong supports to help it succeed, as a showcase intervention strongly supported by the high school principal and teaching staff.

Heterogeneous treatment effects pose additional challenges. We must consider *who* took up the program, and why that might matter if the treatment were more effective for some students than for others. This trial is particularly dependent on the effect of the intervention for students who enjoy video game coupons and thus are disproportionately induced to participate through this specific incentive. Our study design captures the *local average treatment effect*— the benefit accruing to students willing to participate in this intervention who are assigned to the treatment as opposed to the control group.

Similar issues arise in other settings and with other study designs. Suppose a state public health department seeks to reduce the incidence of fatal overdoses caused by the opioid epidemic. It intervenes by distributing free naloxone kits to anyone who requests them, by passing a Good Samaritan law, and by taking other steps to facilitate harm reduction interventions. We might ask an ITT question: If we make naloxone legally available to everyone, how much does this reduce the state's overall opioid mortality? Alternatively, we might want to know what happens to fatal overdoses among those who actually accept the free naloxone. That is a question about the TOT.

There may be divergent answers to these questions. We know from myriad studies and long clinical experience that naloxone, when properly administered, sharply reduces opioid overdose mortality. There's no need for new information there. We have less information regarding the impact of laws and policies designed to expand naloxone use. Suppose few people who use drugs take up the offer for free naloxone. Maybe people accept the kits, but are not able to engage peers, friends, or loved ones to be present and to properly administer naloxone when overdose occurs. Maybe promotion materials are only available in English. Maybe the state does poor outreach. If take-up is low, the population health effect of offering free naloxone will be small, even though naloxone is powerfully effective when used correctly.

Experiments to explore the effectiveness of naloxone *laws* are quite different from experiments to examine effects of naloxone itself. There will be questions ranging from drug users' awareness of legal changes to whether or not pharmacists or physicians take advantage of expanded authority to dispense or prescribe the medication. As discussed below, a state might support an experimental test of the policy by implementing it through a *stepped-wedge* randomized design, whereby an initial group of randomly selected counties are first to roll it out, with other counties randomly selected to roll out the policy 6 months later, 1 year later, and so on.

However the evaluation is designed, the ultimate impact of the naloxone policy will be shaped by the size and behavior of the group of service providers and people who use drugs who actually engage the program. If the program is powerfully protective for those who embrace naloxone, yet take-up is low, we will observe a policy effect analogous to the underage drinking intervention described above: An impressive TOT, accompanied by a disappointing population ITT effect because so few people embrace the intervention.

A Real-World Example: Contingency Management for Prenatal Smoking Cessation

Prenatal smoking provides a classic challenge, one at the boundary of clinical care and population health (Nighbor et al., 2020). Measures to address this challenge provide another illustration of the necessity and the limitations of randomized controlled trials to improve population health. Here randomized intervention trials may play an important role in state health insurance coverage mandates and in other regulatory policies.

Epidemiologists have long documented that tobacco use during pregnancy is associated with increased incidence of low birthweight, particularly low birthweight arising from fetal growth restriction. Such low birthweight is associated with infant mortality and other adverse outcomes. Researchers have established clear biological pathways for some of these associations and have documented large observed birthweight differences between infants born to pregnant smokers and those born to nonsmokers (Lewandowska, Wieckowska, Sztorc, & Sajdak, 2020).

It is plausible that initiating smoking cessation interventions for pregnant patients can improve infant health. Yet for many reasons, large observed differences in health outcomes may overstate the direct causal impact of smoking during pregnancy. Some of the birthweight effect of prenatal smoking may arise during the preconception period if patients become pregnant in poor health.

Prenatal smoking is strongly negatively correlated with patient income and education (Higgins et al., 2009), correlated with maternal depression and other risk-factors (Yang & Hall, 2019; Yang et al., 2017) and correlated with other forms of substance use. For example, the majority of pregnant patients with opioid use disorders are also tobacco users (Isaacs et al., 2021).

Many forms of co-occurring substance use are more deeply stigmatized than tobacco use, and are correspondingly less likely to be disclosed to clinicians or to researchers. If such substance use contributes to adverse birth outcomes and are more common among pregnant smokers, direct birthweight comparisons of infants born to pregnant smokers with infants born to nonsmokers may overstate the causal role of prenatal smoking (Noble et al., 1997; Vega, Kolody, Hwang, & Noble, 1993) and may correspondingly overstate potential health benefits of laws, policies, and clinical interventions designed to reduce prenatal smoking.

A randomized trial of a feasible smoking cessation intervention may help unpack some of these questions. Higgins et al. (2010) reported on the combined outcomes of three pertinent controlled trials. One hundred sixty-six pregnant patients were randomly assigned to either a contingency-management intervention arm (wherein patients earned vouchers exchangeable for retail items by abstaining from smoking) or a control arm (wherein patients earned vouchers independent of smoking status).

This RCT is well-suited to examine the specific effect of reduced smoking, because participants provided urine samples that allowed biometric verification of seven-day smoking status through cotinine tests. On this metric, researchers reported final-trimester smoking abstinence to be markedly higher in the intervention vs. the control group (34.1% vs. 7.1%) (Table 13.2). Compared with other smoking cessation interventions, this contingency-management intervention proved quite powerful to reduce smoking in this patient population. Such a trial may influence public policy through several routes, including state regulatory policies requiring insurance coverage for smoking cessation interventions and state requirements imposed on cigarette manufacturers regarding package warning labels.

As previously, let Z represent a binary indicator for group assignment, whereby $Z = 1$ represent assignment to the contingency management intervention, and $Z = 0$ represents assignment to controls. The incidence of low birthweight was significantly lower in the intervention vs. controls (5.9% vs. 18.5%).

Table 13.2. Infant Birth Outcomes.

	Contingency Management Group ($n = 85$)	Noncontingent Group ($n = 81$)
Percent low birthweight	5.9%	18.5%
Percent preterm birth	5.9%	13.6%
Percent NICU admissions	4.7%	13.8%
Final trimester smoking abstinence	34.1%	7.1%

Source: Adapted from Higgins et al. (2010, table 2).

The *intent-to-treat* (ITT) effect of the contingency-management intervention on low birth weight was thus

$$\beta_{\text{ITT}} = E[\text{LBW} \mid Z = 1] - E[\text{LBW} \mid Z = 0] = 5.9\% - 18.5\% = -12.6\%. \quad (13.3)$$

That's arguably the most important bottom-line measure of the public health impact of this intervention. If we offered this same intervention to 1,000 pregnant smokers similar to the patients offered this intervention, we can anticipate that we would prevent 126 low-birthweight deliveries. Given the modest costs of contingency management interventions and the immediate benefit to both pregnant patients and to infants, prenatal smoking cessation ranks among the most cost-effective interventions in clinical care, with estimated costs of approximately $3,000 per pregnant patient who actually quits smoking due to the intervention (Mundt et al., 2021). Such findings provide a strong policy argument for states to require insurers to cover this service for pregnant smokers, and thus is a good example of *policy candidate* randomized trials.

Because this intervention specifically focused on cotinine-verified smoking cessation, it is plausible to believe that the reduction in low-birthweight incidence was entirely due to reduced smoking. However, we should also be open to the possibility that the intervention influenced birthweight through other channels. For example, the intervention may strengthen the therapeutic alliance between patients and providers. If so, this may lead patients to seek medical help more aggressively for other health concerns, or to reduce other risk behaviors. If so, the ITT would still provide an unbiased estimate of the intervention's treatment benefit. The policy arguments to cover this service would not be undermined or weakened. Yet our causal interpretation of the findings would be misplaced.

This intervention also shows the potential weaknesses of available strategies to estimate TOT effects, even within an excellent trial. In this case, the TOT corresponds to the estimated effect of smoking cessation on the probability of a low-birthweight outcome. If we posit that last-trimester smoking is the key behavioral parameter, we would be tempted to apply the standard Wald estimator to the available published data, to take into account actual smoking cessation:

$$\beta_{\text{Wald}} = \frac{\overline{Y}_{Z=1} - \overline{Y}_{Z=0}}{\text{Dose}_{Z=1} - \text{Dose}_{Z=0}} = \frac{0.185 - 0.059}{0.341 - 0.071} = \frac{0.126}{0.27} = 0.467 \quad (13.4)$$

Taken at face value, these estimates would imply that for every 1,000 pregnant smokers who actually participate in this intervention, we prevent 467 low birthweight deliveries. Note, however, that this interpretation lacks face validity. After all, low birthweight prevalence within the *control group* of pregnant smokers is only 185 per 1,000. One possible explanation would be that prenatal smoking cessation interventions induce valuable reductions in smoking intensity among the 65.9% of the treatment group who *do not* achieve third-trimester complete abstinence from smoking. A second possibility is that smoking cessation interventions solidify the treatment group's connection to prenatal care, thus allowing clinicians to address other health challenges associated with greater risk of low birthweight.

Trials such as this could also face threats to generalizability and external validity. The intervention might be performed at an excellent medical center. The particular approach may be designed for rural non-Hispanic whites and may be less culturally-competent, and thus less effective (due to reduced take-up or reduced patient engagement) when offered to other patients. Policymakers would want to complement this study with other study designs, perhaps including a true policy experiment that includes random assignment when a policy is first implemented, to understand how best to design legal requirements for these services in the entire population.

Randomization at Different Units of Observation

Many randomized trials seek to evaluate specific interventions provided for individual students, patients or service recipients. These include familiar randomized trials in clinical care. The posited causal pathway resides in changing medical care, social services, or other treatments provided to individual participants, with corresponding changes in behaviors and circumstances at the individual level. Evidence from such trials can thus inform legal and regulatory policies that require or facilitate delivery of services and interventions found to be effective.

Even when a trial randomizes individual patients, contextual and institutional factors play fundamental roles, but are often not analyzed in the study. An intervention that proves attractive and accessible in one population may prove less so in another. As discussed below, the burgeoning field of implementation science has brought systematic attention and rigor to the effects of implementation facilitators and barriers as policymakers seek to generalize findings from a trial that serves a specific study population in a particular setting to other different populations in different settings (Eccles & Mittman, 2006; Hirschhorn, Smith, Frisch, & Binagwaho, 2020; Hoagwood, Purtle, Spandorfer, Peth-Pierce, & Horwitz, 2020; Proctor et al., 2011; Shelton, Cooper, & Stirman, 2018).

Cluster Randomization

Randomized trials to improve population outcomes are often most useful when applied at higher units of aggregation. A recent cluster-randomized trial by Abaluck et al. (2021) exemplifies the importance and global reach of such methods. Within a year of the first documented COVID-19 case, these authors conceived and executed a cluster-randomized trial of measures to increase mask wearing within 600 villages in rural Bangladesh, involving more than 342,000 adult participants. The authors demonstrated that public health measures could increase the prevalence of proper mask wearing from 13.3% in the control group to 42.3% in the intervention group. The authors demonstrated accompanying reductions in symptomatic COVID-19 prevalence, particularly among older adults in villages where surgical masks were distributed.

In similar fashion, Victor et al. (2011) performed a cluster-randomized trial of Black barbershops as intervention sites for pharmacy interventions to reduce systolic blood pressure among Black men with high systolic blood pressure (exceeding 140 mm Hg). Barber shops within the treatment group promoted follow-up with a specialty-trained pharmacist. Pharmacists met regularly with customers who frequented barber shops in the treatment group, prescribed anti-hypertensive medications, and sent progress notes to customers' primary care providers. Barber shops within the control encouraged patrons with high blood pressure to pursue healthier lifestyles and to attend medical appointments. Black male patrons with high systolic blood pressure in both treatment and control arms experienced improved systolic blood pressure relative to baseline (6-month reductions of 27.0 mm and 9.3 mm, respectively). Patrons who frequented barber shops in the treatment group were substantially more likely to reduce their systolic blood pressure (63.6% of participants below 130 mm Hg, compared with 11.7% among participants in the control). These group differences appear to reflect greater use of anti-hypertensive prescription medication among treatment-group participants. Benefits provided to the control group are also noteworthy. These underscore the public health benefit of even modest measures (within the control group) by trusted community members. These findings also provide a useful reminder that RCTs can be properly designed to provide important health benefits to all participants.

Saltz et al. (2021) provide another valuable example, examining community-level interventions on alcohol-related crashes. This study examined effects of a bundle of actually deployed public policy enforcement practices on important population health outcomes. Through a cluster-randomized trial of 24 small cities in California, these authors found that enforcement measures to reduce underage drinking, drunk driving, and other behaviors associated with harmful alcohol use induced a 17% reduction in single-vehicle nighttime crashes among drivers 15–30 years of age.

Stepped-Wedge Designs for Policy Experiments

Using cluster randomization in *stepped-wedge* designs as a way to evaluate health effects of actually implemented laws provides strong causal inferences. A stepped-wedge design is a cluster-randomized trial in which the clusters are randomly divided into groups (Copas et al., 2015). All clusters initially receive status quo/usual care intervention for a given roll-out period. Then each group receives the evaluated intervention (crossing over from status quo/control to treatment) at a group-specific later time.

A very large literature now establishes the effectiveness of state laws requiring automobile safety belt use. However, decades ago when such laws were first being enacted, legislators might have designed the rollout of such laws to expeditiously provide a rigorous policy evaluation using a stepped-wedge design. For example, Illinois policymakers might randomly assign each of the state's 102 counties to one of three cluster-groups (Figure 13.1). Residents of

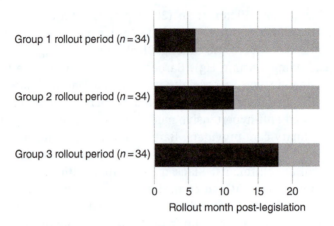

Figure 13.1. Stepped-Wedge Implementation Across 102 Illinois Counties.

Group 1 counties would be required to use safety belts 6 months after the legislation is passed. Residents of Group 2 counties would be required to do so 1 year later. Finally, residents of Group 3 counties would be required to do so 18 months after the legislation passed.

Because counties are randomly assigned to the three groups, researchers can verify similar baseline prevalence and pre-intervention trends in road injuries and fatalities. They can then examine whether one can observe a break in these trends that match the new law's implementation. Researchers might explore mechanisms, for example by examining the rate of safety-belt-related road citations independent of crashes, and by collecting data on belt usage among individuals involved in crashes. Researchers might also explore contextual facilitators and barriers, for example by comparing effects across urban and rural counties or by comparing across counties with high and low levels of safety belt law enforcement.

In like fashion, a county might employ a stepped-wedge design to evaluate clean indoor air smoking regulations. Here local officials might randomly divide workplaces and restaurants into multiple groups subject to focused enforcement in a staged roll-out, examining facility-specific trends in respiratory complaints, worker sick days, and other outcomes in relation to the implementation of such regulations.

Notice that random assignment of jurisdictions addresses some common threats to the validity of quasi-experimental designs (see Chapter 14). Quasi-experimental evaluations of state policy efforts such as Medicaid expansion face the obvious challenge of policy endogeneity—the law is in part a result of other factors also affecting health outcomes. States with stronger commitment to public health may have been first to embrace such policies. If so, quasi-experimental approaches may overstate the public health benefits of early expansion because early-adopter states already had more favorable public health trends. Alternatively, early-adopter states may have included those facing new and alarming public health challenges such as the opioid epidemic. If so, quasi-experimental approaches may understate the public health benefits of early expansion, because early adopters turned to Medicaid expansion as a tool to address worsening trends. Given sufficiently large numbers of jurisdictions, stepped-wedge cluster-randomized designs help to address both challenges.

Notice in our safety belt example that roadside injuries and deaths are immediately proximate to the behaviors that one seeks to deter, and are readily observed. A stepped-wedge design is thus well-suited to evaluate such legal interventions. Much the same might be said regarding laws to deter driving under the influence of intoxicating substances, policies to facilitate naloxone distribution or jail-based opioid disorder treatment to reduce fatal overdose, and mandatory COVID-19 vaccination policies, all having a proximate effect on related hospitalizations (Bajema et al., 2021; Tenforde et al., 2021). A stepped-wedge design might also be effective in evaluating a law mandating insurance coverage for the contingency-management intervention discussed above to reduce prenatal smoking. State policymakers might require insurers to cover such services on a staggered basis across counties or other defined groups.

Stepped-wedge designs are more challenged to evaluate policies whose mechanisms, outcomes, and effects follow a more complex dynamic process. Suppose, for example, that one seeks to evaluate laws that restrict or discourage more general tobacco use. Such policies may take years to appreciably change chronic smoking behaviors. Moreover, many of the health effects one seeks to influence—for example asthma hospitalizations or smoking-related cardiovascular events—themselves unfold over years and are harder to directly link with the evaluated policies.

The internal validity of stepped-wedge designs is threatened when there are important spillover effects. Consider a county-level stepped-wedge design of interventions designed to reduce smoking through local excise tax increases. The ease with which smokers can purchase across county lines or underground-market sellers can smuggle cigarettes across county lines could undermine the research design.

Mediating Mechanisms and Causal Pathways

Both randomized trials and quasi-experimental studies are identified based on effects of interventions on "treatment compliers," whose circumstances or behaviors change as a result of the intervention. In the case of smoking cessation, the posited mechanisms are plausible and direct. In other cases, the pathways are more complex or diffuse.

Specifying such pathways is increasingly important to stakeholders and policymakers seeking to understand and apply scientific results from experimental trials, especially when generalizing from a trial on a specific problem in a specific situation to other opportunities for legal or regulatory intervention. The emerging discipline of implementation science speaks directly to these concerns.

Suppose that we conduct an RCT evaluating effects of small-group cognitive-behavioral therapies to reduce youth violence (Heller et al., 2017). One might reduce youth offending by imparting strategies young men can deploy to deescalate potentially violent confrontations. If this is the key mechanism, the intervention might generalize to broad health benefit. Properly implemented interventions based on this RCT would need to insure proper manualization based on the initial intervention, and proper training of staff to demonstrate fidelity to this initial model. Alternatively, the key mechanism may be less curriculum-dependent, and more dependent on young men building a strong therapeutic alliance with pro-social adults who operate the groups. If this is the key causal pathway, choosing staff with demonstrated ability to build strong relationships with young men may be the key variable and the appropriate focus of program implementation. Once again, the discipline of implementation science provides valuable attention to scale and sustainment in drawing proper policy insights from specific trials.

The National Institutes of Health have imposed increasingly stringent requirements on randomized trials, most obviously in requirements to pre-register trial outcomes and thereby reduce the risks of misleading incidental findings. NIH now also requires investigators to specifically identify and investigate causal mechanisms and pathways. Indeed, beyond exploratory and pilot studies, most NIH institutes will no longer fund or even review fully scaled "black-box" RCTs. As one institute explains:

> NIMH requires an experimental therapeutics approach ... for the development and testing of therapeutic, preventive, and services interventions, in which the studies evaluate not only the clinical effect of the intervention, but also generate information about the mechanisms underlying a disorder or an intervention response. Studies ... must clearly identify a target or mediator of the intervention being tested. A positive result will require that an intervention improves clinical outcomes and has a demonstrable effect on a target, such as a neural pathway, a key cognitive operation, interpersonal or contextual factor that is hypothesized to mediate the intervention's effect (Insel & Gogtay, 2014).

Such requirements have forced researchers to incorporate explicit logic models or explicit theoretical/conceptual frameworks for experimental and quasi-experimental work, in many cases bringing valuable rigor that is sometimes lacking in "black-box" randomized trials. This work is especially important when policymakers wish to draw upon the same mechanisms identified in an RCT, but in support of a different legal or regulatory intervention. For example, an intervention trial might identify additional family resources as a key pathway to reduce criminal offending among affected youth. Such findings could assist policymakers to target child tax credits or other supports to families as a pertinent policy intervention. Another intervention RCT might identify reduced parental alcohol use as a key pathway to improved child outcomes. Such findings could inform state policy debates over alcohol regulatory policies.

This focus on mechanism has attracted criticism, as well. Researchers may identify one plausible clinical target that moves as a result of an intervention, but it may not in fact mediate the intervention's full causal effect. Some black-box

RCTs have great clinical and policy value, even when researchers have poor understanding of multiple accompanying causal pathways.

In like fashion, a policy experiment to expand access to early-childhood education might improve developmental outcomes through multiple pathways that are hard to disentangle through a single study design. Identifying that a feasible public policy actually helps children might be a more important, immediately actionable finding than the findings from a scientifically rigorous study which identified one precise causal mechanism, disconnected from a feasible public policy intervention.

Conversely, a fully informative or generalizable RCT is not always feasible. An RCT may be unethical, too costly, or too complex. For example, the RAND Health Insurance Experiment, the most famous randomized trial in the history of health economics, cost approximately $300 million in 2021 dollars, and took roughly a decade to complete (Frakt, 2010). With occasional exceptions, public health researchers and practitioners rarely have access to such resources for rigorous experimental analysis of public health challenges. Even if an RCT is technically feasible, explicit randomization of a valuable intervention may be socially or politically infeasible. No one was going to randomly assigning millions of seniors to Medicare or to a placebo intervention. Fortunately, randomized trials are not the only path to rigorous policy evaluation. In fact, a much more useful approach is to recognize that randomization is an excellent *design element* to incorporate whenever possible, but is only one of a dozen or more useful design elements enhancing the validity of causal inference. (See Chapter 14 for more on these issues.)

Critiques of Randomized Trials

The rising prominence of randomized control trials and experimental methods has sparked important critiques. Economist Angus Deaton laments that RCTs are wrongly regarded as the top of a hierarchy of research evidence, thus denigrating the importance of other empirical approaches that allow more explicit study of structural factors, and approaches that may bring greater external validity than is possible through an RCT. Deaton (2020) notes

> RCTs are affected by the same problems of inference and estimation that economists have faced using other methods, as well as by some that are peculiarly their own ... RCTs have no special status, they have no exemption from the problems of inference that econometricians have always wrestled with, and there is nothing that they, and only they, can accomplish ...

Deaton and others note several ways RCTs are misinterpreted or overinterpreted: Evidence from one trial conducted in one population is uncritically assumed to apply to very different populations, even when there are strong reasons to expect heterogeneous treatment effects. Deaton notes that data acquired for randomized trials often include "gross outliers," missing data, and data quality challenges that can profoundly influence estimated program effects. Deaton suggests that one very costly pregnancy played an important role in findings from the RAND health insurance experiment (Manning et al., 1987). Such challenges are especially important in violence prevention research, when a single homicide can dominate economic valuations of program effects.

In related fashion, Mosley et al. (2019) express concern that an RCT-based "what works" analytic framework disvalues community-based knowledge, and often fails to develop proper understanding of organizational and community context essential to successful, sustainable interventions that earn legitimacy among service providers, affected communities, and other stakeholders. The rise of implementation science represents one effort to bridge these perspectives (Shelton et al., 2018).

Deaton (2020) also notes an important addition and caveat to critiques of RCTs: "Just as none of the strengths of RCTs are possessed by RCTs alone none of their weaknesses are theirs alone." Many pitfalls commonly associated with RCTs also arise in quasi-experimental studies and other designs. Given heterogeneous treatment effects, the results of a "natural experiment" study design cannot simply be generalized to policy innovations that serve very different populations. More subtle challenges also arise. Suppose one wishes to study the mortality effects of the Affordable Care Act's Medicaid expansion. There is some evidence that states which most eagerly and promptly embraced Medicaid expansion experienced more-favorable prior mortality trends in the years before Medicaid expansion took effect. If so, early quasi-experimental analyses may overstate Medicaid expansion's mortality effects (Kaestner, 2012; Miller, Johnson, & Wherry, 2021).

Heckman and Smith (1995) presented in succinct form many insights now widely presented by scholars worrying about the reification of randomized trials. These authors note the importance of "substitution bias," whereby members of an experimental control group find ways to obtain close substitutes for the studied treatment, and of "randomization bias," whereby individuals willing and able to voluntarily participate in an RCT differ from people likely to participate in a nonexperimental intervention based upon the randomized trial. These authors cite one pediatric drug study (Kramer & Shapiro, 1984) that included an experimental and nonexperimental component. The nonexperimental component experienced a 4% refusal rate, compared with a 34% refusal rate within the randomized sub-trial.

Heckman and Smith (1995) note the widespread belief among social service providers that randomized evaluations are unethical, particularly when an RCT results in denial of services to control group subjects. Such critiques echo criticisms within the public health community, e.g. whether it is ethical to employ site-randomized trials to examine the efficacy of syringe support services (Leary, 1996). At minimum, such debates underscore the importance of ensuring that both intervention trials and policy experiments are conducted with cultural competence and legitimacy with all stakeholders, particularly when such experiments serve vulnerable or stigmatized populations.

Statistical Complexities in Randomized Trials

Researchers and policymakers often hope that an RCT will allow simpler, and thus less-fragile or less-contestable statistical analysis. Such hopes are often dashed.

Differential attrition poses one challenge. Control group participants have less frequent contact and have less of a personal relationship with individuals operating a given study. They may be correspondingly more likely to be lost to follow-up. Such loss to follow-up may be ameliorated if researchers have access to administrative data such as birth and death certificates, arrest records, academic attendance, or grade data. The challenges are more significant if one relies solely on self-reported information or other subject data that requires continued study participation.

Differential attrition can bias the analysis of RCT data, overstating or understating benefits of an intervention. Suppose, for example, one conducts an RCT of a school-based intervention in which members of the treatment group receive valuable counseling to address substance use. The most vulnerable youth in the control group may change schools or leave the school district in an effort to obtain comparable services. Such a pattern might lead researchers to understate the benefits of the studied intervention. Conversely, treatment-group youth who do not benefit from the intervention may leave the school or drop out of the intervention. If researchers only examine data from the remaining students in the treatment group, they might easily overstate the benefits of the studied intervention.

Differences in data quality between treatment and control can create other biases. Individuals exposed to intensive safe-sex or crime prevention counseling may feel greater rapport to candidly describe their sexual practices or criminal behavior than would corresponding individuals not exposed to such messages. Alternatively, treatment group members may be reluctant to reveal information about risk-behaviors they know will disappoint researchers and program implementors. Biases can arise in more subtle ways, as well. For example, the research team may have greater opportunities for data cleaning or to resolve data discrepancies regarding members of the treatment group— particularly if such information is used for operational purposes.

Norms, Long-Term Institutional Changes, and Equilibrium Effects

Randomized trials are implemented in particular institutional and social contexts, serving particular populations with a particular set of implementation resources. Understanding these contexts, populations, and resources is essential to properly interpret trial results and to understand potential challenges as one seeks to bring a particular intervention "to scale." Independent of any question of internal validity, randomized trials are often poorly suited to study effects of institutional changes, changes in social norms, and general equilibrium effects that might be induced if specific interventions were implemented on a broader scale. One can design an RCT to examine the effects of naloxone distribution and syringe support services within a particular population of people who inject drugs. It is harder to design an RCT to understand what drug-use practices would look like if states removed all legal barriers to naloxone distribution and syringe support services. Nor can an RCT explore changes in drug-use practices and peer norms if *all people who inject drugs* had access to these resources, and the ecology of drug use organically included these opportunities.

Burtless provides one provocative example in the context of targeted wage subsidies for disadvantaged workers (Burtless, 1985). In this trial, job seekers were given vouchers identifying them to prospective employers as eligible for a generous wage subsidy. This intervention trial was intended to investigate effects of an enhanced Earned Income Tax Credit (EITC) and related policies.

Contrary to prior hypotheses, workers provided with vouchers were significantly *less* likely to find employment than were job seekers who did not have the vouchers. This experiment was valuable in identifying ways that targeted subsidies can bring unintended and unforeseen harms. Such vouchers apparently carried a stigmatizing effect, leading employers to discriminate against voucher holders. Of course, an intervention that directly affects a small subset of the population is qualitatively different from a universal intervention affecting an entire population. Thus, such an experiment with a small subgroup cannot test the potential effects of broader policies such as an expanded EITC universally applied. A change in law would subsidize an entire population of low-income workers, avoiding potential stigmatizing effects that frequently arise for interventions serving specific small groups of disadvantaged individuals.

At an institutional level, randomized trials cannot fully examine effects of altered organizational practices induced by changes in public policy. This is an important point of dialogue between randomized trials and quasi-experimental designs. A randomized trial of a home visiting intervention, for example, supported by a 2-year private foundation grant, sheds light on the immediate responses and outcomes for specific program beneficiaries within existing structures. This is important information as one seeks to study policy candidates for broader evaluation. Such an RCT can't create or test the kind of structural change that permanent Medicaid reimbursement for this service and other legal-policy changes might facilitate, and thus cannot rigorously address the full range of beneficial or deleterious consequences that might accompany a change in law.

In like fashion, suppose researchers conducted a randomized trial in 1980—just prior to greatly expanded Medicaid benefits for prenatal, labor and delivery, and perinatal medical services—in which a treatment group of 1,000 low-income pregnant patients were provided free prenatal care and other medical services associated with pregnancy and neonatal care. One might have observed greater care utilization within this intervention group. One *would not* have been able to observe the effects of care delivered through the expanded network of prenatal and neonatal intensive care facilities implemented by providers in response to the permanent expansion of Medicaid to millions of pregnant women—an important set of institutional responses, induced by these policy changes, now regarded as critical to declining infant mortality (Chung et al., 2010; Currie & Gruber, 1997; Lorch, Rogowski, Profit, & Phibbs, 2021; Phibbs & Lorch, 2018; Phibbs et al., 2007). Indeed, such an individually-randomized RCT would have provided a misleading—or at-best incomplete—guide for policymakers seeking to understand the likely impact of such policies. A quasi-experimental study design would have provided more rigorous assessment of true policy effects (see Chapter 14).

Scaling interventions may alter economic and institutional contexts in other ways difficult to capture within a single RCT. One important challenge arises when bringing an intervention to scale stresses scarce resources, or in other ways alters pertinent wages and prices. A randomized trial may find that assigning precariously-housed individuals to case workers with one-half the normal caseload reduces homelessness. As such interventions are brought to scale, implementors need to hire less-proficient and less-experienced workers to handle the larger caseload, and may thus achieve less benefit (Jepsen & Rivkin, 2009). Interventions may also prove unexpectedly costly if service providers are required to raise wages to achieve the required staffing, which of course would alter trial-related assessments of cost-effectiveness.

Mechanism Experiments

Mechanism experiments offer one set of tools to address the above challenges (Ludwig, Kling, & Mullainathan, 2011). One might design an RCT with the aim of exploring a specific causal pathway rather than to directly scrutinize a feasible policy as a whole. Such intervention designs might be avowedly ill-suited to expand "at scale" to serve large populations. Their purpose is different: to scrutinize one particular causal mechanism or pathway that might facilitate development of other, more feasible public health policies. For example, many citizens and policymakers believe that the lack of local grocery stores offering affordable, nutritious food promotes obesity in Chicago's far south side and other "food deserts." One might test the hypothesis that food deserts play this important causal role by conducting an RCT in which treatment subjects have subsidized access to a service that makes possible the delivery of fruits and vegetables and other nutritious food items (Ludwig et al., 2011). One can then compare body mass index and other related outcomes between treatment and control subjects. If this rather extreme policy candidate fails to improve health outcomes, policymakers can reasonably conclude that policies that subsidize grocery stores that operate in food-desert areas, or regulations imposed on grocery chains requiring them to open stores in current food deserts might bring other important community benefits, but this "mechanism" RCT indicates such policies are unlikely to improve these specific health outcomes tested.

One might hypothesize that financial factors and legal penalties influence individuals' willingness and ability to obtain COVID-19 vaccinations (Campos-Mercade et al., 2021). One might design an RCT in which study subjects are offered $500 if they agree to receive a vaccine. As an aside, this trial also underscores some significant challenges to mechanism-experimental designs in sensitive arenas. The $500 payment raises significant ethical concerns. Moreover, the large incentive may prove counterproductive, if it heightens concerns among study participants or others that any medical treatment requiring such payment must bring large accompanying risks. A second RCT could test effects of intensive enforcement of vaccine mandates where those unvaccinated are suspended without pay to evaluate effects of such disincentives on vaccine receipt. In short, assessing the role of financial factors and legal penalties in vaccination rates might involve a series of focused RCTs on particular components of the larger question.

Mechanism experiments can also be performed at the organizational level. Suppose one believes that outcomes among homeless individuals with substance use disorders are worsened because caseworkers, overwhelmed with large caseloads, cannot provide the individual attention required to effectively serve their most vulnerable clients. One might implement policies requiring social service agencies to maintain lower client-caseworker ratios to receive Medicaid reimbursement. As noted (and dismissed) above, one might also design a mechanism experiment in which 500 homeless individuals are assigned to caseworkers with half of the standard caseload, and 500 homeless individuals are assigned to a usual-care arm in which caseworkers have standard caseloads. This RCT might be operationally unrealistic or unscalable itself, but nevertheless may still provide valuable insights into the potential benefits of such regulatory policies.

The Burgeoning Role of Implementation Science

A traditional view of policy randomized trials draws heavily on the "pipeline" paradigm of randomized trials of new drugs and procedures in medical care. That is, one first establishes the efficacy of a new intervention under ideal (or at least accommodating) conditions. One then brings the intervention "to scale" in a broader population (Landes, McBain, & Curran, 2019). The burgeoning field of implementation science draws attention to the distinctive gaps between research and practice through the use of scientific methods to promote the uptake, implementation and sustainability of evidence-based practices, programs, and policies, with an ultimate goal of improving population health (Eccles & Mittman, 2006; Hirschhorn et al., 2020; Hoagwood et al., 2020). While a full discussion of the discipline is outside the scope of this chapter, we briefly review how greater engagement with implementation science approaches may improve the adoption, implementation, and sustainment of interventions within the field of legal epidemiology.

Hybrid Effectiveness-Implementation Study Designs

Whereas traditional RCTs focus on intervention effectiveness, implementation science has developed hybrid trial designs that focus on both implementation and effectiveness (Curran, Bauer, Mittman, Pyne, & Stetler, 2012; Johnson et al., 2020; Landes et al., 2019). Such trials are increasingly influential within public health, with Curran and colleagues delineating three categories of hybrid study designs:

- *Hybrid type 1* designs primarily focus on testing clinical interventions and outcomes, but pay explicit attention to implementation processes, contextual barriers and facilitators, and needed program adaptations to local context (Landes et al., 2019; Pho et al., 2021). As Landes and colleagues describe, a hybrid type 1 trial often resembles a conventional RCT paired with a complementary process evaluation.

- *Hybrid type 2* designs give equal weight to clinical intervention and implementation related factors, including explicit measures of implementation outcomes. For example, one may have good reason to believe that smoking cessation counseling reduces smoking and improves health outcomes among patients in a diabetes clinic. A hybrid type 2 trial would scrutinize patient-level smoking status and health outcomes but would give equal weight in studying implementation strategies to understand when and how smoking cessation counseling is actually provided, and how staff might be supported in reliably executing such efforts.

- *Hybrid type 3* designs primarily focus on implementation itself and are secondarily focused on patient outcomes. For example, a state prison system might conduct a site-randomized trial in which staff were provided training materials that encourage and facilitate naloxone distribution for returning citizens who leave these facilities. Researchers might seek to track overdose reversals and related outcomes, but the main focus would be on implementation processes that influence whether naloxone is provided (Landes et al., 2019).

Kemp, Wagenaar, and Haroz (2019) recently expanded on this original typology, with an additional 12 hybrid designs. Although not yet widely used, they offer helpful additional perspectives for evaluating the relative weight of the intervention, implementation context, and the implementation strategies used to support implementation.

Implementation Science Theories, Strategies and Outcomes

Implementation science theories. Core to implementation science research is the use of different theories, models, and frameworks (TMFs) to guide, understand, and evaluate the implementation of a new program, practice, or policy. In a seminal review, Nilsen (2015) identified five categories of TMFs: (1) process models: describing how to translate research to practice, (2) determinant frameworks: understanding the contextual barriers and facilitators that shape implementation outcomes, (3) classic theories: from disciplines outside implementation science, e.g., psychology, sociology, or organizational theory, used to evaluate different domains of implementation, (4) implementation theories: developed by implementation scientists to understand or explain different domains of implementation; and (5) evaluation frameworks: specifying the relevant measures and metrics to assess implementation outcomes. Designed to be used before, during and after implementation, TMFs can be assessed with both qualitative (Hamilton & Finley, 2019) and quantitative methods (Smith & Hasan, 2020), and are essential for understanding the implementation context, selecting implementation strategies, and examining implementation outcomes.

Although Fulmer et al. (2020) argue that process models can strengthen the application of legal epidemiology in public health research, implementation science TMFs have not been widely used in legal epidemiology research. This does not mean that legal epidemiology scholars are not exploring knowledge translation processes or the contextual factors that shape the implementation of public health laws; rather, the discipline does not appear to have widely engaged with extant TMFs. One exception has been the use of Rogers' Diffusion of Innovations Theory (2010)—a classic TMF—and related concepts on the diffusion of innovations in the policy surveillance realm (Bae, Anderson, Silver, & Macinko, 2014; Burris, Hitchcock, Ibrahim, Penn, & Ramanathan, 2016; Komro et al., 2020; Politis, Halligan, Keen, & Kerner, 2014). More explicit engagement with TMFs in legal epidemiology not only will strengthen the field's ability to document the multiple factors that shape the implementation of public health laws, but also can strengthen the role of implementation science in improving population health (Damschroder et al., 2009; Feldstein & Glasgow, 2008; Nilsen, 2015).

Implementation strategies are the specific activities used to support the implementation, enforcement or delivery of an evidence-based intervention. Recent scholarship has provided greater conceptual clarity on the definition (Powell et al., 2015), selection (Powell et al., 2017) and reporting (Proctor, Powell, & McMillen, 2013) of such strategies. Because most of this scholarship has been developed within the context of health services research, additional work is necessary to fully specify implementation strategies for legal interventions.

Implementation scientists are also actively engaged in understanding *implementation pathways of influence*—the mechanisms of action through which an implementation strategy operates to achieve desired implementation outcomes (Boyd, Powell, Endicott, & Lewis, 2018; Lewis, Klasnja et al., 2018; Lewis, Scott, & Marriott, 2018). Relatively little is known about the actual pathways through which implementation strategies affect change on implementation actors and organizational actors, especially within the context of legal interventions. Dual work on identifying and testing implementation strategies in the context of legal interventions would be welcome.

Finally, implementation outcomes are the "effects of deliberate and purposive actions to implement new practices, programs, and policies" (Proctor et al., 2011, p. 65). Two evaluation frameworks commonly used in implementation science are the Multilevel Implementation Outcomes Framework (Proctor et al., 2011) and the RE-AIM Framework (Glasgow, Vogt, & Boles, 1999). Although both frameworks are widely used within the field of implementation science, they have had limited application to date within legal epidemiology.

Table 13.3 lists the outcomes from each framework, their definitions and an example of how to operationalize each one in the context of a legal policy

Table 13.3. Implementation Outcomes.

Implementation Outcomes Framework (Proctor et al., 2011)

Outcomes	Definition	Research Questions
Acceptability	"perception among implementation stakeholders that a given treatment, service, practice, or innovation is agreeable, palatable, or satisfactory" (p. 67)	How do key stakeholders view a state law permitting over the counter (OTC) access to naloxone? Do perceptions of acceptability differ among stakeholders who bear a disproportionately high burden of overdose deaths?
Adoption	"intention, initial decision, or action to try or employ an innovation or evidence-based practice" (p. 69)	To what extent do owners of local businesses, e.g., pharmacies, drug stores, community-based organizations (CBOs), other permitted settings, agree to provide OTC access to naloxone?
Appropriateness	"perceived fit, relevance, or compatibility of the innovation or evidence based practice for a given practice setting, provider, or consumer; and/or perceived fit of the innovation to address a particular issue or problem" (p. 69)	To what extent do key stakeholders perceive that a state law permitting OTC access to naloxone is appropriate for their community and will help to reduce overdose deaths? Do perceptions of appropriateness differ among stakeholders who bear a disproportionately high burden of overdose deaths?
Feasibility	"extent to which a new treatment, or an innovation, can be successfully used or carried out within a given agency or setting" (p. 69)	To what extent is legislation permitting OTC access to naloxone feasible within different settings (e.g., pharmacies, drug stores, CBOs, etc.) in a state? To what extent is feasibility different in low and high resourced settings?
Fidelity	"degree to which an intervention was implemented as it was prescribed in the original protocol or as it was intended by the program developers" (p. 69)	To what extent are pharmacists or other permitted actors providing OTC naloxone as specified by the law?

(Continued)

Table 13.3. (Continued)

Implementation Outcomes Framework (Proctor et al., 2011)

Outcomes	Definition	Research Questions
Penetration	"integration of a practice within a service setting and its subsystems;" it also "can be calculated in terms of the number of providers who deliver a given service or treatment, divided by the total number of providers trained in or expected to deliver the service" (p. 70)	How many pharmacies in a given geographic area provide OTC access to naloxone?
Sustainability	"extent to which a newly implemented treatment is maintained or institutionalized within a service setting's ongoing, stable operations" (p. 70)	How many businesses continue to offer OTC access to naloxone within 1 year of the law coming into effect?
Equity	Extent to which access to the program is equitably distributed across the population. Extent to which the policy does not worsen outcomes, especially for marginalized populations.	How do we ensure that communities disproportionately impacted by overdose deaths have equitable OTC access to naloxone?

RE-AIM Framework (Glasgow, Vogt, & Boles, 1999; Glasgow et al., 2019; Shelton, Chambers, & Glasgow, 2020)

Outcomes	Definition	Research Questions
Reach	At the individual level, the number, proportion, representativeness of individuals who participate in the intervention under study (Shelton et al., 2020)	How many people can access OTC naloxone? To what extent are the populations disproportionately impacted by overdose deaths able to access OTC naloxone?
Effectiveness	At the individual level, "the impact of an intervention on important health behaviors or outcomes, including quality of life (QOL) and unintended negative consequences; consider heterogeneity of effects" (Shelton et al., 2020, p. 4)	Does offering naloxone OTC reduce overdose deaths and affect other QOL outcomes? What are the unintended consequences of OTC naloxone? Which groups bear a higher burden of unintended negative consequences?
Adoption	At multiple levels, "the number, proportion, and representativeness of: (a) settings; and (b) staff/interventionists who deliver the program, including reasons for adoption or non-adoption across settings and interventionists" (Shelton et al., 2020, p. 4)	Two of four pharmacies in a rural county offer naloxone OTC. How do the adopting pharmacies/staff differ from those that do not offer naloxone? Did lower-resourced pharmacies adopt OTC naloxone to the same extent as higher-resourced pharmacies?

Table 13.3. (Continued)

RE-AIM Framework (Glasgow, Vogt, & Boles, 1999; Glasgow et al., 2019; Shelton, Chambers, & Glasgow, 2020)

Outcomes	Definition	Research Questions
Implementation	"At multiple setting and staff levels, continued and consistent delivery of the EBI (and implementation strategies) as intended (fidelity), as well as adaptions made and costs of implementation" (Shelton et al., 2020, p. 4)	To what extent did each adopting pharmacy implement OTC access to naloxone as described in the law? What adaptations did pharmacies make and why? Did all pharmacies have access to the resources necessary to successfully offer naloxone? What was the cost of offering naloxone OTC? What social-contextual factors shaped the implementation, including the social determinants of health?
Maintenance	"At the setting level, the extent to which a program or policy becomes institutionalized or part of the routine organizational practices and policies. At the individual level, maintenance has been defined as the long-term effects of a program on outcomes after a program is completed" (Holtrop et al., 2021, p. 3). Typically 6 months and 1 year after implementation, and an ongoing basis	Which settings continued to offer OTC naloxone over time and why or why not? Which populations continue to be reached; do they continue to benefit or experience negative outcomes; why or why not? What factors shape sustainability low-and high-resource settings?

intervention on over-the-counter access to naloxone. For each framework, we also include a focus on equity, which has drawn significant attention in recent implementation science research (Baumann & Cabassa, 2020; Brownson, Kumanyika, Kreuter, & Haire-Joshu, 2021; Shelton, Adsul, & Oh, 2021; Snell-Rood et al., 2021).

Conclusion

Randomized trials are more common and more influential than ever before in legal epidemiology and public health policy. Such research often produces more rigorous outcome evaluations than has ever been possible in public health, particularly when evaluated in terms of internal validity—the plausibility of inferring a causal effect. The growth of RCTs has produced other benefits as well. Not least of these benefits is an increase the proportion of social scientists who step out of the seminar and computer lab into the field, gaining tactile familiarity with public health challenges while performing intervention research (Blattman, 2016). Federal, state, and local policymakers are also more aware of the importance of strong research designs, and are increasingly willing to partner with researchers to perform experimental research.

Also critical have been more disciplined and systematic efforts to move beyond atheoretical "black-box" randomized trials. These include measures to rigorously establish specific causal mechanisms and pathways that underlay important public health interventions. Such innovations move the field beyond black box randomized trials that prove incapable of replication. More subtly, such innovations move the field beyond an arrogant "pipeline" model, in which researchers and practitioners regard policy innovation as the search for best-practice models that yield excellent results with strong internal validity with minimal attention paid to whether and how such interventions could truly be implemented, at-quality, on a broad scale, in diverse contexts and diverse populations. The rise of implementation science underscores new awareness of the importance of contextual factors and the need for well-designed experiments to better understand implementation processes and outcomes.

Newfound respect for experimental approaches brings new risks. One challenge arises from complex mutual dependencies between researchers and policymakers or organizational leaders, who control data and access to intervention sites. The realities of intervention research require long-term relationships. The spoken and unspoken exigencies of data use agreements within long-term relationships raise conflicting incentives for researchers and for policymakers alike. As researchers note the value of experimental methods, they must also guard against the loss of broader analytic and policy reflection than is typically engaged in experimental research. Experimental methods cannot directly explore changes in social norms, or large-scale institutional changes, such as broad long-term changes in medical practice associated with changes in Medicare policy. No experimental study could have documented the full health benefits of Medicaid expansion; nor could any randomized trial capture the downstream health harms associated with the Tuskegee experiment by reinforcing earned distrust of the American medical system among African-American men (Alsan & Wanamaker, 2018; Alsan, Wanamaker, & Hardeman, 2020). Nevertheless, randomized trials have significantly improved the quality of public health research.

No one methodological approach provides the gold standard, and RCTs are no exception. Many of the limitations of RCTs can be addressed by carefully designed quasi-experimental studies, to which we turn in the next chapter. As discussed there, quasi-experimental designs often face surprisingly similar challenges, yet often have available tools to address questions that cannot currently be addressed through randomized trial designs.

Summary

This chapter reviews the utility of randomized trials to study *policy candidates*, establish specific causal links and *mechanisms* of action, and *evaluate effects of actual laws* implemented in the real world. It begins by presenting the need for randomized trials to address selection bias and related challenges that arise in policy evaluation. It presents basic trial concepts such as intent-to-treat and treatment-on-the-treated effects using the example of a simplified intervention to reduce underage alcohol consumption. It explores strengths and limitations of randomized trials by discussing a successful experimental evaluation of a contingency management intervention to prevent prenatal smoking. We describe cluster-randomized trials, and discuss the importance of specifying mediating mechanisms and causal pathways in the proper interpretation of randomized trials. Finally, we present common critiques of randomized trials, and the use of mechanism experiments and hybrid implementation science designs to address limitations of "black-box" randomized trials, which do not address causal mechanisms of observed effects.

Further Reading

Cunningham, S. (2021). *Causal inference*. New Haven, CT: Yale University Press.

Kemp, C. G., Wagenaar, B. H., & Haroz, E. E. (2019). Expanding hybrid studies for implementation research: Intervention, implementation strategy, and context. *Frontiers in Public Health, 7*, 325.

Proctor, E. K., Powell, B. J., & McMillen, J. C. (2013). Implementation strategies: Recommendations for specifying and reporting. *Implementation Science, 8*, 139. doi:10.1186/1748-5908-8-139

Chapter 14

Natural Experiments

Research Design Elements for Optimal Causal Inference Without Randomization

Alexander C. Wagenaar   Kelli A. Komro

Learning Objectives

- Understand advantages of time-series data, with many repeated observations before and after a change in law, for evaluating the law's effects.
- Create a nested multiple comparison group study design for evaluating health effects of a law.
- Combine several design elements in a single study to strengthen causal inference.
- Identify resources for further study of legal epidemiology methods

Evaluating the health effects of a law or regulation, or any treatment or intervention, most fundamentally requires a comparison of the experience *with* the law to the experience when everything is the same but *without* the law. Imagine the pure counterfactual, which involves the same people at the same time in the same place experiencing a law, compared to the same people at the same time and same place not experiencing the law (Rubin, 1974). The counterfactual requires the same people at the same time and place in the two conditions—with and without a specific law—to ensure that everything is identical between the two conditions, except the specific law. If everything but the law is identical, the difference in health outcomes of interest then directly represents the effect of the law. But such a comparison is impossible since the same people at the same time cannot experience both conditions. Thus the

Legal Epidemiology: Theory and Methods, Second Edition. Edited by Alexander C. Wagenaar, Rosalie Liccardo Pacula, and Scott Burris.

fundamental quandary of scientific research—how do we know that the difference in outcomes observed is really caused by the law, since the difference might be due to something else and not be a true effect of the specific law under study?

Random assignment was a major advancement in creating the counterfactual (Fisher, 1935). Relying on the law of large numbers, randomly selecting sets of people from the whole population, randomly selecting times of intervention implementation, and randomly selecting from the set of all places or settings creates groups of people, times, and settings that *on average* are expected to be equivalent in every way but for the law or intervention we exposed one set to but not the other set. Thus, any single experiment might be wrong, because the treated and untreated groups might simply, by chance, differ in some unknown way and that difference might be the true cause of an observed difference in outcome. But, on average, over many replications of the randomized experiment, the two sets of people, times, or settings compared are expected to be the same, and any difference in outcome can be confidently attributed to the effects of the one planned difference between the two conditions—one is exposed to the law under study and the other is not.

Despite its appeal, randomly exposing treatment groups and control groups is rarely possible when evaluating most new laws and regulations. Most laws are implemented at particular times and in particular settings and, obviously, passage and implementation are not under the control of researchers. They are therefore commonly called *natural experiments*. When laws are changed, they almost always of necessity apply to everyone in the given jurisdiction. Characteristically, there are few units in the study—for example, one or a few cities or states pass an innovative law, and the entire population within the unit is exposed to the new law all at once. In short, randomization is rarely available as a strategy or *design element* to improve the likelihood of correctly assessing a law or regulation's effects.

There is an unfortunate tendency by many scientists and others to dichotomize studies into strong "experimental" studies (that use random assignment to treatment and control groups) that are assumed to provide clear evidence regarding the effects of an intervention, and weak "observational" studies (not using random assignment) that are assumed to provide ambiguous and often inaccurate evidence of effects (Benson & Hartz, 2000; Concato, Shah, & Horwitz, 2000; Guyatt, DiCenso, Farewell, Willan, & Griffith, 2000). This is a false dichotomy. Random assignment is only one of a dozen or more design elements that increase confidence in a causal interpretation of an observed difference (Bärnighausen, Røttingen, Rockers, Shemilt, & Tugwell, 2017; Bärnighausen, Tugwell, Røttingen et al., 2017; Leatherdale, 2019; Shadish, Cook, & Campbell, 2002). When evaluating the effects of local, state, or national laws and regulations, under which random assignment is rarely feasible, careful attention to full use of many other design elements is warranted. Moreover, effectively combining many design elements into a single study can produce real-world legal evaluations with higher overall levels of validity and strength of causal inference than randomized trials, which are typically limited to special circumstances or artificial environments. The objective of this chapter is to review design elements of particular importance when evaluating laws and regulations that naturally occur in the field and improve the quality of empirical studies of public health law by illustrating their use. In this chapter, we assume as a prerequisite the data on the laws under study have been carefully collected and coded using reliable and valid methods, as described in Chapters 11 and 12.

Design Elements for Strong Legal Evaluations

There are several design elements for strengthening causal inference of particular importance when random assignment to treatment conditions is not possible.

Many Repeated Measures

A fundamental criterion for inferring whether a given law or regulation caused a change in outcomes is that the cause preceded the effect. For this reason, we measure the outcome before the law is implemented and again after. But having just one observation before and one observation after produces weak inference, because any difference observed might simply reflect the natural variation in the outcome over time. Figure 14.1 illustrates a situation in which a simple before-and-after design shows a major effect of the law, but that effect is no longer considered real when seen in the context of more observations both backward and forward over time further away from the effective date of the law.

Collecting dozens or hundreds of observations in a *time series* before and after a new law takes effect makes it easier to see whether changes in the outcome of interest right around the time of the new law are larger than typical variation over time, and enhances confidence an observed difference occurring just at the time a new policy legally takes effect is due to that law. Any time series of observations can be viewed as a single sample (one window) from a time series that runs infinitely back in time and infinitely forward in time. The larger the time window observed around the time of a change in law, the easier it is to reliably assess that law's effects.

Beyond collecting many repeated measures, one must choose an appropriate *time resolution* for the observations. Are the observations a measure every minute, day, week, month, or year? Selecting the optimal time resolution

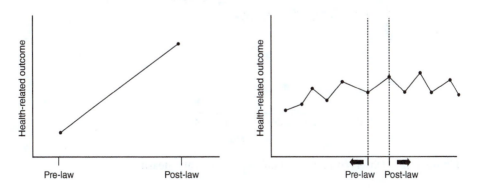

Figure 14.1. Observed Effect: Simple Pre-Post Design Versus Time-Series Design.

is a complex tradeoff of multiple considerations. First is the speed by which a new law is expected to show effects. If the effects are expected to show up within weeks of the law's effective date, using weekly or monthly observations will make that effect easier to discern than using annual observations (Figure 14.2).

A second consideration when selecting the best time resolution to measure is the variation in the outcome over time at each time resolution. If there is little to no variation week by week in an outcome a new state law is meant to improve—say, math ability of teens—then monthly or even annual measures might be more appropriate. Consideration of the variation in the outcome over time interacts with a third important dimension, whether the underlying phenomenon being measured is *continuous*, or a *count*. For example, math ability, air pollution levels, water quality—like the temperature—all are continuous. The outcome is always there, we just choose intervals when we

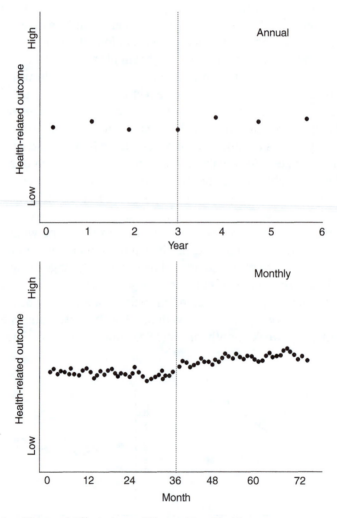

Figure 14.2. Observed Effect: Annual Versus Monthly Measures.

check the level. For continuous outcomes, the most important basis on which to choose the time resolution of the measures is theory regarding the mechanism of a law's effect—when is the law first expected to show a difference in the outcome, and when (that is, at what interval) are further improvements expected?

Many public health outcomes are not continuous, but are counts or frequencies of new infections or disease cases, counts of injuries, or counts of deaths. For count outcomes, the time resolution must roughly match the frequency of the event. If there is only, on average, one or two infections, injuries, or deaths per month in the geographic unit under study, choosing a daily or weekly time resolution is not appropriate since it will not help discern a law's effect on that outcome. Conversely, for example, if there are 50 or a 100 car crash deaths per month, lumping those data up to the yearly level for evaluating a new law's effects impairs the ability to accurately measure the law's effects. At the extreme, the problem of low counts expresses itself as numerous observations that are all zeros. Anything more than a very small fraction of zero-count observations complicates statistical analyses and makes discerning policy effects difficult or impossible. Thus, when the study design is being finalized, one must be aware of the expected outcome frequencies, and if numerous zero counts are expected at the preferred time resolution, the typical practical solution is moving to the next lowest resolution (for example, moving from monthly to quarterly counts).

Selecting the best time resolution for count data presents a tension between the desire for high-time-resolution observations and the resulting time series being "well-behaved," that is, exhibiting smooth regularities, cycles, or trends and not dominated by random unpredictability. In any study, minimizing the random, unpredictable variation from one observation to the next is important for maximizing the ability to detect the underlying "signal" of the law's effects. This is also known as maximizing statistical power (Cohen, 1988).

A fourth factor affecting the best time resolution to measure is exactly when the law took effect—a January 1 effective date works well with annual data, but typical effective dates of public health laws are distributed throughout the year. Using annual data with laws that take effect mid-year requires assumptions that the effect is going to be, say, half the size of effect in the subsequent full-year implementation (if the effective date is July 1), but those annual data will not permit the investigator to evaluate the validity of that assumption. Sometimes anticipatory effects of a new law are seen starting a couple of months before it takes effect, or there are lagged effects that do not start until a few months after it legally takes effect. Perhaps the short-term effects are much larger than long-term effects, a situation common with laws that require public attention and active enforcement. Or the longer-term effects might be larger than the short-term effects, a situation common with laws that require construction of or refinements in an implementation structure before the full effects are seen. All these situations are obscured by selecting outcome data at too coarse a time resolution (for example, annual rather than monthly).

Keep in mind that a date may seem like a straightforward data element, but actually requires careful thought. Several dates are important to consider in evaluating a law's effects. There is the date the law is *introduced for debate;* the date it is *enacted,* passed by a legislative body or signed into law by the executive; the date specified by law that it *legally takes effect*; the date *actual implementation* of the law begins. The specific dates of most interest in the evaluation are based on hypothesized mechanisms of action drawn from theory.

Finally, when designing a study with lower time-resolution measures of continuous outcomes, it is critically important to take the measure at exactly the same time each year. This is because most physical, behavioral, and social phenomenon are characterized by seasonality—a nonrandom cycle within the time unit of observation. Pollution levels, dietary vegetable intake, infection rates, injuries, and most other health-relevant outcomes exhibit cyclic or other systematic differences across hours of the day, days of the week, weeks of the month, or months of the year (Figure 14.3).

So, if one is surveying individuals once per year, or inspecting restaurants or schools once per year to collect an outcome for evaluating a public health law, it is important to do the data collection the exact same month of the year. This applies at all time resolutions of measurement—if one is collecting data once per month, measure the same day each month (for example, first Wednesday of the month). If one is collecting data weekly, measure on the same day and same time of day each time. The further the data collection procedures diverge from measurement at the exact same time within the time unit, the less confident one can be in interpreting observed differences from before to after a new law is implemented as representing the effect of the law—it might be just because the measures were taken at a different point in the cycle.

In summary, a strong public health law evaluation has as many observations as possible before and after the law takes effect—a lengthy time series—and uses the highest time resolution possible, constrained by the nature of the hypothesized effect, the frequency of underlying outcome counts, and feasibility limits due to resources or data available.

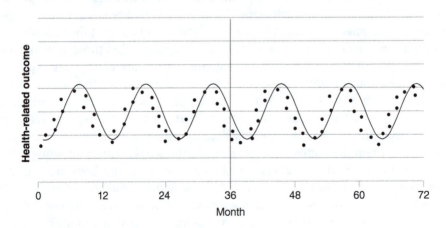

Figure 14.3. Time Series Illustrating Seasonality.

Functional Form of Effects

High-time-resolution data have another important advantage furthering the quality of a policy evaluation. On the basis of theory regarding mechanisms of a law's effects, one has an implicit or (even better) explicit hypothesis on the expected pattern of the effect over time (Figure 14.4).

Imagine one's theory of legal action is based on deterrence. In that case, one may expect a lag before effects are seen due to enforcement taking time to ramp up and news about enforcement actions taking time to spread in the relevant population. Alternatively, if one's theory focuses more on normative compliance, initial timing of expected effects is based on when the relevant population first hears about the new law, suggesting that effects might be

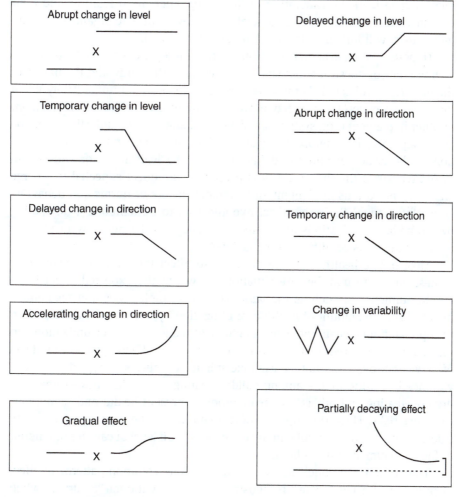

Figure 14.4. Possible Patterns of Policy Effects Over Time.

Note: **X** equals policy change.

Source: Adapted from Glass, Wilson, and Gottman (1975).

observed even before it legally takes effect, due to attention gained by hearings on the proposed law or to publicity surrounding a governor's signing the law. Therefore, one might expect effects to emerge at the enactment date, rather than the more typical expectation of little or no effect until the new law legally takes effect. The amount of time between enactment and the date the law takes effect might affect the magnitude and timing of expected effects. A longer lead time may enhance effects if it allows for better design and ramp up of implementation structures and practices. Some statutes include specific provisions for implementation, but most do not; such provisions might affect the hypothesized timing and size of effects. Implementation is not limited to the public sector. Private organizations and individuals also might require time to put in place what is needed for the law to fully take effect (e.g., train staff, purchase compliance equipment). Furthermore, implementation might vary significantly across sub-units of the jurisdiction (e.g., counties might differentially implement a state law). Consideration of likely implementation features and their timelines, both by public sector officials and relevant private organizations and individuals, will influence facets of the research design.

Hypothesizing particular functional forms for legal effects leads to the following types of questions that shape the design of the study and the nature of the data to be collected. Is the effect expected to show up immediately when the law takes effect? Or is a delay of weeks or months expected, as enforcement or other implementation systems are developed and ramped up? Might there be an anticipatory effect before the legal effective date, due to publicity and attention to the issue surrounding debate on the new legislation, or widespread media reports at the time the law is passed? Is the effect expected to emerge gradually, as various implementation systems change or norms and behaviors gradually change? Or is the effect hypothesized to be temporary, dissipating over time as organizations and individuals adapt to the new law in ways to maintain previous conditions or behaviors?

Most public health laws are designed to affect the *level* of relevant outcomes, but there may be rare situations in which the expected effect is on another dimension, such as the *variance*. For example, laws and regulations might affect the amount of health care utilization by individual citizens, when the optimal public health objective might be to reduce both over-utilization and under-utilization—reducing the variance—while not affecting the overall level of services provided. Another example might be policies designed to reduce variance in caloric intake among children eating school lunches—some children overeating and others undereating both represent health and school performance risks. Thus, the objective of regulations may be to reduce variance in calories consumed at school with no effect on overall level of calories or amount of food consumed at the school.

The bottom two panels in Figure 14.4 illustrate common patterns of effect of public health laws. The first illustrates the conventional "S-curve," when change starts slowly until reaching some "tipping point" at which change accelerates, followed by a leveling off at the (new) long-term level (Granovetter, 1978). The last panel of Figure 14.4 illustrates a sizable, fairly immediate effect that then partially dissipates over time (perhaps due to reduced attention to the issue), resulting in a much smaller, but often still important, long-term effect. One can see this in effects of strengthened driving-while-intoxicated laws, which often receive considerable media attention around the time they are passed or implemented, sometimes magnified by advocacy groups such as Mothers Against Drunk Driving, substantially raising the perceived probability of being detected and punished for driving impaired. As the short-term publicity declines, the magnitude of effect on driving behaviors also declines. But as the strengthened laws are integrated into ongoing enforcement efforts, the real and perceived probabilities of detection and punishment remain higher than baseline before the law, with a more modest but still important long-term effect.

In short, decisions on time resolution of outcome data to collect and their analyses should be informed by expected patterns of effect over time. It is important to note that if the observed pattern of effect closely matches the hypothesized pattern that is based on a particular theory regarding the operating legal mechanism, the level of confidence in causally attributing the observed effect to the change in law or regulation is substantially strengthened.

Comparison Jurisdictions

With many repeated observations correctly measured and analyzed, it is possible to determine with a high degree of accuracy whether a change in the outcome coincides with the time of implementation of a new law or regulation—a change that is larger than expected from normal variation over time, and a change that matches the theoretically expected pattern. However, we still have the problem of the counterfactual—what if the same change in outcome would have occurred regardless of whether the new law was implemented or not? The observed change might have been caused by something else happening at the same time. A fundamental way to further improve causal inference—to assess whether the law caused the change in outcome or whether something else caused it—is to use comparison jurisdictions that did not implement the law under study. One collects the same outcome data for another city or state that did not change their law, and examines whether the observed change in the "experimental" jurisdiction is also seen in the comparison jurisdiction. If no similar change is seen in the comparison, one is more confident that the observed change at the time of the law is in fact due to the law, and not to some other factor occurring in common across jurisdictions. On the other hand, if a similar change is seen in the comparison, the observed change in outcome in the experimental site cannot be attributed to the change in law.

A key design consideration is selecting an appropriate comparison site. This is most commonly described as a site that is similar to the experimental site in terms of observable factors correlated with the outcome if not the outcome itself (in terms of level, trend line or variance). Typically, evaluators select a site with broadly similar sociodemographic profiles of the population, or similar counts or rates on the key outcome variables. There are many dimensions on which one might assess degree of similarity, so it is important to consider the underlying reason why one seeks similar jurisdictions. Choosing a site with similar counts or rates on the outcome is a helpful but relatively minor consideration—it makes it easier to determine whether the comparison site experienced a change in outcome that is similar to the change observed in the experimental site. In other words, it helps ensure approximately equal statistical power to estimate change in the outcome in both the experimental and comparison sites.

The fundamental criterion for comparison site selection has much deeper significance, since it is directly connected to achieving the best possible counterfactual. The fundamental criterion for selection of a comparison site is that all the *causes* of the outcome variable are similar across the two sites. Thus, the conventional approach to choose sites of similar demographics might be appropriate *if* demographics are a key influence on the outcome under study. But in many cases, other factors are more important in any particular study. For example, if car crashes are the outcome, similar urbanization and climate are likely more important than demographics, with the exception perhaps of proportion of young drivers, since they are at such elevated risk.

Stratification before selection of comparison sites optimally is based on multiple characteristics. For example, in policy research focused on promoting healthy food environments, it may be important to find comparison sites based on urbanity, sociodemographic factors, and the overall food environment, all of which are generally associated with outcomes of interest. The goal is to achieve two groups as similar as possible in an attempt to mimic the counterfactual— what a particular outcome would look like with or without a particular policy among the same group of people at the same time in history. Selecting an optimal comparison group is an attempt to rule out competing alternative explanations for the outcomes observed post-intervention. The goal is to be able to attribute any difference between the jurisdictions to the legal intervention of interest and rule out any other plausible explanations as best as possible. For example, if the goal was to evaluate effects of a new food policy, it would be critical to select comparison sites with similar socioeconomic and food environments prior to the new policy to help rule out alternative explanations for change in outcomes. If data for a longer baseline period with many observations are available (as is recommended), a useful tactic is to examine the correlation of the outcome variables between the experimental site and candidate comparison sites during the baseline period only; then select comparison sites with the highest correlations.

Of course, a perfect comparison jurisdiction is unachievable, because no two jurisdictions are identical in every way but for the law under study. For this reason, it helps improve inference by including multiple comparison jurisdictions. If a clear change in outcome is observed in the one with the law change, but no such change is seen in several other similar jurisdictions that did not change their law, inference that the law caused the change in the first site is enhanced.

Synthetic Comparisons

The discussion of comparisons thus far has focused on finding the best available comparison jurisdiction(s), selected from the set of all available comparison jurisdictions. But none of those jurisdictions is likely to be the perfect comparison—exactly the same as the focal jurisdiction in every way but for the specific law being evaluated. This has led to the development of synthetic control methods (Abadie, 2021) that build on ideas from propensity score methods (Holmes, 2014). Synthetic controls are a creative and important advance, but the idea is simple: instead of selecting one (or a few) comparison jurisdictions, a single weighted average of the units in the pool of comparisons is constructed and used as the comparison. This weighted average is constructed in such a way as to maximize the correlation between the experimental jurisdiction (the one that changed a law) and the synthetic control over the baseline time period. Thus, a long baseline with many repeated measures is essential for valid construction of a good synthetic control.

Depending on the structure of available data, there are additional ways to improve the construction of synthetic controls. Many applications of synthetic controls remain at one level of aggregation. For example, imagine a US state changes a law, perhaps making mask use compulsory, and the study design is using the pool of other states that have never implemented compulsory mask use as candidate comparisons to assess effects on state-level COVID-19 test positivity rates. When constructing the synthetic control, we have, at most, measures on $n = 49$ other states in the comparison pool to use as the "raw material" to construct the optimum synthetic control. However, there are also many times when we have data available measured at a sub-unit of the research design unit—data on individual state residents, for example, while the research design is evaluating a state-wide law by comparing to other states. In such a case, we have outcome measures on thousands or millions of people, and individuals can be differentially weighted to create the optimum synthetic comparison group.

Synthetic controls are a great design element to minimize the risk of some types of selection bias—differences between the treatment and comparison groups (other than the law being evaluated) that may confound a causal interpretation of observed effects. However, they do not eliminate the risk of history confounds. To take our example further, imagine many of the states that did not make masks compulsory made vaccines mandatory at about the same time the focal states were making masks mandatory. Despite the synthetic control closely matching the treatment states in outcome rates during the baseline period, it nevertheless is not a good comparison because of the contemporary history confound. It is always best to layer in multiple design elements to strengthen causal inference.

Comparison Groups

The notion of incorporating comparisons not expected to be affected by the law under study can be fruitfully extended in other directions beyond comparison jurisdictions. If a law or regulation is targeted to particular groups of people or organizations within a jurisdiction, effects on that focal group targeted should be compared with other similar groups within the same jurisdiction that are not likely to be affected. The benefit of within-jurisdiction comparisons is the equal exposure of treatment and comparison groups to the totality of all other laws and conditions present in the state, except for the specific law under evaluation. For example, consider a new state regulation intended to reduce worker injuries in auto-repair shops. The injury rate can be tracked before and after the new regulation, and an observed reduction in injuries among auto-repair shop personnel is suggestive of an effect of the law. But inference of a causal effect would be strengthened by tracking similar measures of injuries among workers in the state that work in types of workplaces other than auto-repair shops. If similar declines in injuries were observed, then the observed auto-repair injury reductions are likely due to some other broader factor and are not an effect of the new regulation specific to auto-repair shops. On the other hand, an observed reduction in injuries *only* for the specific group covered by the new law, with no reduction for workers in other similar settings not covered by the law, substantially strengthens the inference that the new law caused the reductions in auto-repair injuries. Most laws and regulations are inherently targeted in some way, opening important opportunities for enhancing causal inference regarding the law's effects by incorporating relevant within-jurisdiction comparison groups. For example, zoning rules that prohibit elementary schools from being sited adjacent to major highways (as a means to reduce air pollution exposure and asthma) can be evaluated by incorporating comparisons consisting of preschool, or middle- and high-school students not covered by the law.

Comparison Outcomes

Additional options for comparisons are provided by outcome variables. Appropriate comparison outcomes are related to the primary outcome, but, of importance, are not affected by the law or policy under study. For example, to evaluate the effect of New York City's regulation to post calorie information in chain restaurants, one might compare sale receipts for food purchased at chain restaurants to receipts from non-chain restaurants. To evaluate effects of motorcycle helmet laws, comparisons of car to motorcycle fatality and injury rates have been conducted (Sosin & Sacks, 1992). To evaluate effects of a graduated driver's license for teen drivers that forbids night-time driving, comparisons have been made between daytime and nighttime teen driver fatalities (Morrisey, Grabowski, Dee, & Campbell, 2006). The difference between labeling a comparison a "group" or an "outcome" is sometimes just a matter of convention. The central importance of the notion of comparison outcomes is to expand one's thinking and highlight the many comparisons, even within the jurisdiction enacting a new law or regulation that can be effectively used to create strong research designs for evaluating the law's effects.

Replications

A fundamental way to strengthen causal inference regarding a law's effects is to replicate the evaluation across jurisdictions. Naturally, the larger the number of sites in the treatment and control groups, the more (statistical) power one has to measure potential effects. And, if similar effects are observed in each place a similar law is implemented, confidence in causal inference is clearly enhanced. If multiple jurisdictions implementing the policy are included in an initial study, observed effect sizes can be directly compared across sites. If statistical power remains too low to reliably compare site-by-site effects, incremental removal of one site at a time from the analysis model can help determine whether the observed effect is driven by a subset of sites, rather than consistently across sites. But often, replications happen later and are separately studied, perhaps by other investigators. If the initial observed effect is not seen in subsequent replications, suspicion increases that some other idiosyncratic or uncontrolled factor accounts for the observed effect in the first jurisdiction, and the law under study may have had no effect.

It is often better to evaluate each instance of a law, rather than the all-too-common practice of lumping all similar laws together into a single group and estimating the average effect across all specific instances. Consider the situation in which such a pooled analysis hints that a law might have small effects, but the effect is too small to be reliably measured (that is, is not statistically significant), leading to the conclusion that the regulatory approach is ineffective. Now imagine that in that pooled analysis lurk five states with large clear beneficial effects but 10 other states with no effects. The pooled analysis might prematurely discredit the regulatory approach and miss the opportunity for more in-depth analyses of the individual states to better understand why the law works in some cases and not in others, leading to improvements in implementation and further replication of effective approaches.

Replications occur not only across sites but also over time. As jurisdictions change the law on a particular subject in different years or decades, evaluation designs incorporating those replications ensure that observed effects are not due to other factors specific to a given era, again increasing confidence the observed effects are caused by the law under study. A whole area of research design in general involves manipulating the timing of a treatment or intervention. As expected, random assignment of a treatment to a particular time of implementation is a great strategy, just like randomly assigning a treatment to groups or jurisdictions, but it is rarely feasible. However, even without random assignment, naturally occurring (that is, induced by legislatures, courts, or administrators) variation over time in law in a single jurisdiction can be used effectively to dramatically strengthen the evaluation.

Psychologists call these "ABAB" designs, in which a treatment is applied, then removed, then later reapplied, and they can support strong causal inference (Kratochwill et al., 2010). Thus, we know with little doubt the causal effects of compulsory motorcycle helmet laws, since some states implemented such laws, later rescinded them, then still later reinstated them, creating an

ABAB design (an "A" period without compulsory helmet law, then a "B" period with, then an "A" period without, followed by another "B" period with the law, all within one jurisdiction). The match between the legal changes and morbidity or mortality outcomes in both directions supports strong causal inference (deaths decline abruptly when helmets become compulsory and abruptly return to the higher levels again when the law is rescinded [Mertz & Weiss, 2008; Ulmer & Preusser, 2003]).

Dose Response

The notion of replications, when a similar law is implemented in multiple jurisdictions, and reversals, when a law is implemented and then removed, can be straightforwardly extended to replications in which the dose of a particular regulatory approach varies by jurisdiction or within jurisdiction over time. Dose can represent many different dimensions, tied to theory on the mechanism of the law's effects. All good legal evaluation studies should be based on a clear understanding of the underlying theory regarding legal mechanisms. This is especially true for designing a good dose–response study, because what constitutes different "doses" of the law is inherently tied to how one thinks the particular law works. It could be the size and speed of application of a penalty in a deterrence-based statute, for example, or many other dimensions of breadth, strength, or reach of a law. After effects of the law are assessed within each jurisdiction, jurisdictions are arrayed in order of low to high "dose" of the law. If the magnitude of observed effect tracks the dose—low-dose jurisdictions have small effects and high-dose jurisdictions have large effects—the causal attribution of the observed effects to the laws is substantially strengthened.

Dose–response studies substantially strengthen causal inference, but can have complications. Because the dosages are not randomly assigned to different jurisdictions and different times, it is possible the dose applied in a particular situation is correlated with some other characteristic of that situation or that time period. For example, if all high-dose locations are highly urbanized areas, and all low-dose locations are rural, perhaps dose does not truly affect the magnitude of legal effect and the observed dose–response relationship is really due to urbanism. The risk of such misattribution of effect is lowered by examining the pool of jurisdictions with differing doses for other differences that plausibly might explain the pattern of effects observed.

Multiple Design Elements

Evaluating effects of laws on public health outcomes should be guided by optimum use of multiple design elements for constructing experiments and quasi-experiments. For most cases, when randomization is not feasible, the use of matched comparisons (jurisdictions, groups, and outcomes) in combination with many repeated measures is recommended. Keep in mind that comparisons need not be matched one for one. One jurisdiction implementing a new law is typically compared with a similar jurisdiction that has not. Causal inference is often enhanced by using several jurisdictions in comparison with the one implementing a new law rather than just one. And comparisons of different kinds nested in a hierarchical fashion substantially strengthen the design. Finally, when multiple sites pass new laws, replications can be built directly into the design.

An illustration of such a combination of design elements that produced strong causal inferences about a law's effects can be seen in studies of the legal drinking age (Figure 14.5).

Two states that changed the legal age for possession and consumption of alcoholic beverages (Maine and Michigan) were compared to two states with, at that time, an unchanged drinking age (New York, with a consistent legal age of 18 since Prohibition ended, and Pennsylvania, with a consistent legal age of 21). Experimental states versus comparison states constituted the first level of comparison. Second, nested within each state, the focal age group affected by the change in law (18- to 20-year-olds) was compared to younger and older age groups. Third, nested within each age group, frequencies and rates of alcohol-related car crashes were compared to frequencies and rates of non-alcohol-related crashes. Fourth, to avoid the possibility that the law changed reporting of alcohol

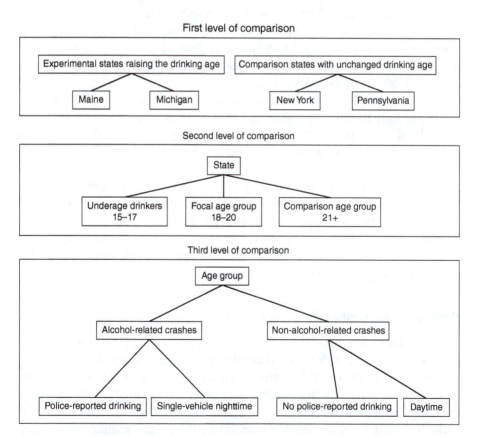

Figure 14.5. Hierarchical Multilevel Time-Series Design: Legal Drinking Age Example.

Source: Wagenaar (1983a)/U.S. Department of Justice.

involvement perhaps more than the actual incidence of such crashes, two measures of alcohol-related crashes were observed—one based on normal crash reports by police officers regarding drivers' drinking, and an alternative that did not rely on officer reports of drinking (single-vehicle nighttime crashes, which are well-known from other research to have a high probability of involving a drinking driver). These two measures were compared with crashes with no police report of drinking and crashes occurring during the day—providing two measures of non-alcohol-related crashes.

For each cell in this hierarchical design, outcomes were measured monthly for many years before and after the legal changes. The pattern of observed effects—reductions in crashes beginning the first month after the new law, only in the "experimental" states that raised their legal drinking age (and not in the comparison states), only among teenagers (not among drivers 21 and over who were not affected by the change in legal age from 18 to 21), only among alcohol-related crashes (and not among non-alcohol-related crashes, and confirmed with two alternative measures of alcohol-related crashes)—together produced an inference with high levels of confidence that this particular law caused a change in car crashes. Replications in other states that raised the legal age confirmed this pattern of effects. Moreover, a look back to reports and studies from a decade earlier in the 1970s, when 29 states lowered their legal age for drinking, produced an implicit ABAB or intervention reversal design. After many states lowered the legal age for drinking in the early 1970s, teen car crashes increased; when a decade later the legal age was returned to 21, crashes decreased, reversing the earlier increase.

Despite periodic renewed attention to the legal age issue, with various individuals and organizations occasionally arguing in favor of returning again to a lower legal drinking age, the fundamental findings from the decades-earlier research have not been seriously challenged by scientists or most evidence-based review panels. In fact, the US National Highway Traffic Safety Administration (2010) estimates the age-21 law continues to prevent about 900 teen crash fatalities per year, saving more than 25,000 lives since the 1970s (Fell, Fisher, Voas, Blackman, & Tippetts, 2009; Voas, Tippetts, & Fell, 2003). Empirical legal evaluations that creatively took advantage of numerous design elements for strong causal inference produced important empirical results that have continuing policy relevance decades later.

Regression-Discontinuity Design

All of the discussion thus far has assumed a time-series design, where the treatment assignment cut-point (i.e., discontinuity) is a particular point in time—no treatment before the law takes effect vs. treatment implementation after a law takes effect. The regression-discontinuity design is conceptually similar, except the cut-point being analyzed for a possible treatment effect is along *some other* variable, not time (Cattaneo & Escanciano, 2017). For example, rather than applying universally, some laws might apply only to persons in a jurisdiction below or above some specified criterion. Common examples are income limits—a law applies to anyone below a specified income level and to nobody above that income level. In that case, the income cut-off can be used in a regression-discontinuity design to evaluate the law's effects. The people just a couple dollars above the limit are, on average as a group, plausibly identical to those just a couple dollars under the limit. Another example: consider a state law that makes masks mandatory in any county when the COVID-19 ICU occupancy rate exceeds a specified level. The ICU rate cut-point is then used to evaluate a potential discontinuity in the outcome, such as rate of new infections.

Conclusion

Given the number of design elements available to strengthen empirical evaluations of public health laws and regulations, opportunities for continued improvement in the science on public health laws is clear. Awareness and understanding of available research designs for use in the real world outside the laboratory, where random assignment to both treatment and control conditions is often difficult, is important not only for scientists and legal scholars but also for policy makers, public health professionals, and advocates as well. Advancing the effectiveness of heath policy requires differential weighting of the evidence coming from various studies based on the quality of the research design—how well a given study incorporates multiple design elements and thus produces high-confidence causal conclusions. A simple before-and-after design should get little weight in policy deliberations compared to a high-time-resolution, time-series study that includes a hundred or more repeated observations. A single-state study with no comparisons should get less weight than one that incorporates multiple comparison states and multiple comparison outcomes within each state.

High-quality and consistently implemented monitoring systems of relevant population-level health outcomes is critical for increasing the number of well-designed time-series evaluations. These ongoing data-collection efforts are the "management information systems" for population health, facilitating the monitoring of health status, evaluation of changes in laws, regulations and implementation procedures, and achievement of expected standards of health and safety for the population as a whole. Continuing outcome-monitoring systems are necessary for "continuous quality improvement" in the health and well-being of the population. A great example of the role of such information systems is the Fatality Analysis Reporting System, which collects hundreds of detailed data elements on every fatal car crash in the entire United States. The system was carefully designed and tested by a large community of scientists and engineers inside and outside the federal government in the 1960s and early 1970s. Then, full implementation began in 1975, and has continued ever since. The complete data in analysis-ready formats are publicly and easily available. This data system resulted in an explosion of research on the causes and prevention of car crash deaths, and each year as additional longitudinal data are added, more high-quality time-series evaluations are possible. Because of the knowledge gained from thousands of studies using these data over the past few decades, we have saved hundreds of thousands of lives and millions of injuries. This is a truly phenomenal public health achievement (Hemenway, 2009). For decades, each time a state innovates with laws and regulations designed to further reduce crash injuries, investigators can simply access the data system and build well-designed multistate time-series studies evaluating the effect of the change.

There are many other examples of emerging data systems that will facilitate the use of strong time-series research designs to evaluate the effects of laws and regulations. The dissemination of electronic medical records (Hillestad, Bigelow, Bower et al., 2005), including records on health risk behaviors recorded routinely in primary care practices (Hung, Rundall, Tallia et al., 2007), will provide population-level daily, weekly, or monthly indicators of health-relevant behaviors and outcomes. New technologies implemented at scale, such as the Apple watch, which monitors and records numerous health indicators continuously for millions of users, will open up new opportunities for evaluating laws using high frequency and high-density data in long time series. All these continuing improvements in the breadth, quality, consistency, and availability of continuous monitoring data systems will facilitate further well-designed evaluations of the effects of laws and regulations.

Combining many design elements in a hierarchical multiple time-series research design represents the best approach for evaluating the effects of public health laws and regulations, in many ways providing better knowledge of effect than that gained from randomized controlled trials (RCTs). Randomization to treatment condition is a useful design strategy in many fields (for example, testing specific treatments such as new pharmaceuticals), but has more limited utility in legal epidemiology studies. RCTs can be used productively to study the effects of specific "micro" mechanisms found in many theories of legal effect, and those results help design better laws and regulations. But RCTs, of necessity, are almost always conducted in small, localized, and unnatural laboratory-type settings, with small samples of people. Natural experiments with public health relevant laws, in contrast, are implemented in real-world settings, use the actual legal tools and implementation processes widely available in society, and apply to very broad or universal populations. And results from actual field implementations of laws and regulations are more persuasive to policy makers, public health practitioners, and citizens, facilitating diffusion of successful approaches to other jurisdictions, resulting in major improvements in population health.

Summary

Most changes in laws and regulations affecting population health represent natural experiments, in which scientists do not control when and where these changes are implemented and thus cannot randomly assign the legal "treatments" to some and not to others. Many research design elements can be incorporated in evaluations of public health laws to produce accurate estimates of the size of a law's effect with high levels of confidence that an observed effect is caused by the law:

- Incorporate hundreds of repeated observations before and after a law takes effect, creating a time series.

- Measure outcomes at an appropriate time resolution to enable examination of the expected pattern of effects over time that is based on a theory of the mechanisms of legal effect.

- Include comparisons in the design, such as multiple jurisdictions with and without the law under study, constructed synthetic comparison groups, comparison groups within a jurisdiction of those exposed and not exposed to the law, and comparison outcomes expected to be affected by the law and similar outcomes not expected to be affected by the law.

- Replicate the study in additional jurisdictions implementing similar laws.

- Examine whether the "dose" of the law across jurisdictions or across time is systematically related to the size of the effect.

Combining design elements produces the strongest possible evidence on whether a law caused the hypothesized effect and magnitude of that effect. Well-designed studies of public health laws in natural real-world settings facilitate diffusion of effective regulatory strategies, producing significant reductions in population burdens of disease, injury, and death.

Further Reading

Abadie, A., & Cattaneo, M. D. (2018). Econometric methods for program evaluation. *Annual Review of Economics, 10*, 465–503.

Bernal, J. L., Cummins, S., & Gasparrini, A. (2017). Interrupted time series regression for the evaluation of public health interventions: A tutorial. *International Journal of Epidemiology, 46*(1), 348–355.

Box, G. E. P., Jenkins, G. M., Reinsel, G. C., & Ljung, G. M. (2016). *Time series analysis: Forecasting and control.* Hoboken, NJ: John Wiley & Sons.

Cunningham, S. (2021). *Causal inference: The mixtape.* New Haven, CT: Yale University Press.

McCleary, R., McDowell, D., & Bartos, B. J. (2017). *Design and analysis of time series experiments.* New York, NY: Oxford University Press.

Shadish, W. R. (2010). Campbell and Rubin: A primer and comparison of their approaches to causal inference in field settings. *Psychological Methods, 15*, 3–17.

Shadish, W. R., Cook, T. D., & Campbell, D. T. (2002). *Experimental and quasi-experimental designs for generalized causal inference.* Boston, MA: Houghton-Mifflin.

Shadish, W. R., & Sullivan, K. (2012). Theories of causation in psychological science. In H. Cooper (Ed.), *APA handbook of research methods in psychology* (Vol. 1, pp. 23–52). Washington, DC: American Psychological Association.

Chapter 15

Qualitative Research Strategies for Public Health Law Evaluation

Jennifer Wood

Learning Objectives

- Identify and distinguish the key qualitative methods of public health law research.
- Compare and contrast standards of research quality for quantitative and qualitative research.
- Describe the role of qualitative research in a causal pathway from law-making to population health.

The field of legal epidemiology occupies a rich space where interdisciplinary theoretical perspectives meet rigorous empirical methods to examine law as an independent variable and population health as the ultimate outcome of concern (Burris, Wagenaar, Swanson et al., 2010). Systematic qualitative research strategies can help form our understanding of relationships between and mechanisms influencing law, legal practices, and public health. Qualitative research can shed light on the nuanced ways law works; how human decision makers, organizations, and whole environments may act or behave differently as a direct or indirect response to legal constraints; and how these changes, in turn, can reshape the physical and social landscape of health risk and well-being for populations.

Because of its inductive nature, qualitative research can generate insight into previously unstudied (or understudied) mechanisms of legal effect (see Chapter 9). It can explore new theoretical ideas, identifying previously uncharted terrain that may not be found through deductive hypothesis testing.

Legal Epidemiology: Theory and Methods, Second Edition. Edited by Alexander C. Wagenaar, Rosalie Liccardo Pacula, and Scott Burris.

Qualitative research often dominates the initial phase of research on a new topic, building a foundation of understanding for later quantitative studies. Qualitative methods help uncover ways in which laws have effects that lie outside existing theories and models, and for which standardized quantitative measures do not exist. It can also inform the study of law's implementation, peering into the gap between "law on the books" and law in action. Those charged with the administration or enforcement of law can be vital sources of empirical data, as can populations and subgroups that are targeted by law. Understanding how law is applied, and in some cases contested in various real-life situations, is an integral piece of the puzzle that seeks to explore law's effects on public health, including unintended consequences. Understanding the factors that drive and shape lawmaking is also an important aspect of legal epidemiology, and the texts capturing legislative debates, including testimonies and committee reports, provide the empirical material for qualitative analysis.

The purpose of this chapter is to situate qualitative research on the wider stage of legal epidemiology and describe ways in which it can be rigorously and effectively used. It outlines examples of broad research strategies and data-collection methods they employ, both alone and in combination. The utility and appropriateness of each method will be discussed in relation to examples of research questions or studies. The chapter closes with a discussion of core criteria for guiding high-quality empirical research.

Qualitative Research in Context

Qualitative research is centrally concerned with the study of *meaning*, including people's understandings of and beliefs about aspects of their experiences. The focus of qualitative studies can range from a few people to small social networks to large groups that are defined by a shared characteristic, experience, or institutional membership. Based on the definition of *empirical* as "relying on direct experience and observation" (Janesick, 2004, p. 18), the task of qualitative research is to provide an authentic account of how people think about the world and act within it. Human thought and action are shaped by social, cultural, organizational, political, and geographic conditions or contexts. Such contexts can be seen, or rendered visible, through various representations including written text (such as laws, policies, or procedures), oral texts (including personal narratives or stories), researcher field notes, and video or audio recordings (Denzin & Lincoln, 2005, p. 3).

Qualitative research is vital to empirical legal studies of "law in the real world" (Genn, Partington, Wheeler, & Nuffield Foundation, 2006, p. iii), including the realities of enforcement and compliance behaviors (McBarnet, Voiculescu, & Campbell, 2007). Sociolegal or "law and society" scholars care about the effects or consequences that law in action may have on populations and social institutions (McBarnet et al., 2007; see Fitzpatrick & Hunt, 1987; Unger, 1983, on the field of "critical legal studies"). In bridging law and social science, law and society scholarship treats law not as neutral or purely technical, but rather as "meaning-making" in the way that Stryker describes (see Chapter 4). As such, qualitative inquiry has long been integral to the study of law (Jabbari, 1998).

Many theoretical frameworks and methodological approaches are being advanced and refined as the field of legal epidemiology advances. Taken together, these frameworks and approaches provide a comprehensive toolkit for answering questions of *whether* and *how* law influences population health. Beyond revealing the patterns, nature, and distribution of laws, qualitative tools can produce evidence to support causal inference, enhancing what we know about the theoretical mechanisms of law. Robust causal inference obviously is vital to evaluations of law's effectiveness, and qualitative tools can help assess both the intended *and* unintended effects of a law, including such effects on particular groups, by exploring the causal mechanisms and identifying potentially important but previously undetected effects.

Data Collection Methods and Sources

Qualitative research typically involves analyses of written texts and the collection of data from, and in conjunction with, human subjects. At the outset, one must determine the nature of one's data sources and their accessibility. Documents capturing processes of lawmaking or law's implementation may be searchable on the Internet or made available by public agencies. Access to human subjects can in some cases be challenging, particularly in studies of a law's effects on vulnerable or protected groups, such as people affected by mental illnesses, or prisoners. Of course, access is only the first consideration. Depending on the characteristics of interview respondents (are they members of an elite professional group, or do they have language or literacy challenges?), the content of interviews and the manner in which interviews are performed affect the ethics and difficulty of the research.

Interviews

The purpose of an interview is to elicit peoples' knowledge and perspectives that might otherwise remain unknown, simply because they weren't asked before. Such individuals might include those involved in lawmaking or in the implementation of the law, or those who experience law's enforcement. Interviews are a useful vehicle for tapping into people's experiences, assuming such individuals are comfortable sharing information with researchers and through two-way verbal communication.

Researchers must decide how much structure to impose on interviews, and whether interviews should be with one individual at a time (one on one) or with groups. Semi-structured interviewing is most useful because it is both systematic and flexible, allowing for the generation of rich qualitative data. A researcher directs an interview by following an interview guide containing general questions to which interviewees can respond with as much detail as is relevant. The researcher strives for depth in responses, using general, open-ended questions that make sure to avoid "yes" or "no" answers. As the interviewee replies, the researcher actively listens for insights. This may prompt the interviewer to ask new questions to gain a deeper understanding of the initial response (see Miller & Crabtree, 2004).

The semi-structured approach therefore aims to strike a balance between guiding the interview to cover preplanned topics while asking unplanned questions that cover new, previously unexplored ground. Therefore, it is an approach that is appropriate when a topic is partially understood and some key research questions are known in advance. Yet "the best probing is that which is responsive, in the moment, to what the interviewee is saying" and having an interview guide allows for comparison of answers to key questions across interviews, therefore ensuring that data gathering is systematic (Cohen & Crabtree, 2006). This semi-structured approach stands in contrast to highly structured interviewing, or survey research, in which respondents must choose from a list of answer options provided in a set of preordered questions (Willis, 2007), and the data generated are numerical and subject to quantitative analyses.

When law is a topic of exploration, care must always be taken not to bias responses through questions that assume law is important. Sociolegal research has shown that law often influences behavior and attitudes at a deep or unconscious level, defining options and setting bounds of possibility. It may be at work defining norms that are not recognized as coming from law, or people may have folk beliefs about what the law is that are not factual. So, when an interview is designed to explore how the law influences behavior, it may be useful to allow law to emerge in a semi-structured interview rather than prompting people to define their legal knowledge or explain how law influences them. An example of this more patient but revealing process is Engel and Munger's (1996) work on how disability rights law has changed the lives of people with disabilities. In their "autobiographical" approach, they asked interviewees to tell their life stories, waiting for the law to emerge, or not, in the narratives of their subjects.

A semi-structured approach was used by Dodson et al. (2009) to better understand the various conditions influencing the development and passage of childhood obesity laws and regulations. The researchers argued that knowledge was lacking on the complex dynamics of the policy-making process, and that those involved directly in this process would be best placed to help deepen and extend existing knowledge. To this end, the team conducted semi-structured interviews with legislators and staffers from various states with different political climates. The researchers used interview guides that contained questions on basic demographic information (for example, respondents' educational backgrounds) as well as open-ended questions designed to probe respondents on their perceptions and experiences of the legislative process. The interviews elicited information that served to validate existing knowledge about lawmaking dynamics in general while illuminating factors specific to the area of childhood obesity prevention. For example, the research affirmed that concerns with the costs of legislation can serve as a barrier to enacting law, while having wide stakeholder support is an enabling condition. At the same time, interviewees illuminated factors specific to the childhood obesity debate, namely the influence of lobbyists representing companies in the production of obesogenic foods, as well as the problem of misinformation among constituents, such as the assumption that school districts would lose money with the passage of legislation.

The Dodson study used one-on-one interviews with people involved in law-making. Interviews are also useful for tapping into the knowledge and experiences of people targeted by law. For instance, a study carried out by Cooper et al. (2005) set out to examine whether and how a police drug crackdown shaped the health-risk behaviors of injection drug users in New York City. Drug users themselves are obviously the most direct source of information on this topic because they can express how policing tactics influence their thought and actions, and, in particular, whether such tactics serve to alter their daily health risk habits and routines. Although previous research revealed that police crackdowns can undermine healthy behaviors (by, for example, discouraging users from obtaining or using sterile syringes), Cooper and colleagues wanted to generate an in-depth understanding of users' thoughts and habits in relation to crackdowns. As part of this, they wanted to see whether specific police tactics had differential impacts on the health risk behaviors of individuals with different demographic and social characteristics (race or ethnicity, gender, age, socioeconomic status, enrollment in a syringe exchange program). To this end, the lead researcher recruited a diverse sample of individuals who lived in and around a police precinct that was the site of a police crackdown.

In addition to a brief survey (highly structured interview), the researcher undertook an open-ended, semi-structured interview that addressed core issues such as community-police relations, contributions of police to public safety, the ways in which the sociodemographic characteristics of users influenced police interactions, and drug use behaviors. These individual interviews provided an opportunity for respondents to describe their thoughts and actions—as they were shaped by police crackdown tactics—through stories of daily struggles and rituals. The research revealed both commonalities and differences in experiences and practices of drug users across different subgroups of the sample. For instance, poorer users—particularly those without homes or access to private spaces—were more likely than users with more resources to resort to high-risk drug use practices, such as injecting hastily (to avoid being caught) without proper regard for safe injecting practices (for example, failing to clean their injection site, not heating up the drug adequately). In this research, semi-structured interviews were essential to drawing out details and nuances of these struggles and rituals as shaped by users' individual life circumstances. Interviews were carried out on an individual or one-on-one basis, but in some cases a semi-structured approach with groups—commonly referred to as focus groups—can be used as well.

Focus Groups

A focus group is a type of group interview designed to facilitate a social process in which interaction and sharing of views among people produce valuable information. Sometimes this information emerges through a new awareness of shared understandings that no single individual group member could provide alone if interviewed separately. In simple terms, "participants relate their experiences and reactions among presumed peers with whom they likely share some common frame of reference" (Kidd & Parshall, 2000, p. 294). One common frame of reference could be an occupational position. For example, Eman et al. (2011) conducted focus groups with family doctors in Canada—as well as administering a short questionnaire—to better understand the nature of doctors' concerns about disclosing patient health information in the interests of public health. Previous research had identified privacy issues as a critical barrier, but the researchers wanted to learn more about the legal and extra-legal factors shaping doctors' perception and application of privacy principles, in specific relation to the 2009 pandemic H1N1 influenza outbreak.

With groups of people sharing the same occupation position, the focus group method was able to draw from a common pool of knowledge, eliciting the experiences of people facing similar challenges as medical practitioners, such as protecting patient-physician relationships and maintaining confidentiality, while dealing with larger public health obligations. Focus groups can also serve as an efficient means of gathering information from people who might otherwise be difficult to access on a one-on-one basis. In the case of this study, research participants were recruited from a sample of doctors who were going to attend a family medicine conference, and thus the focus groups were held in private meeting rooms at the conference venue.

Focus groups have other advantages by virtue of bringing together people who have circumstances, characteristics, or experiences in common. Focus groups create opportunities for participants to build on others' insights, contradict them, or refine them (Kitzinger, 1994). Participants may have to explain or justify what they mean by a given statement when prompted by their peers. This may then cause them to explicate or refine their statements; doing so may cause others to do the same. This iterative engagement does not serve to falsify previous statements, but rather helps add nuance and precision to the researcher's understandings of a group's norms or shared experiences, especially in cases when the researcher is working with a group for the first time (Kitzinger, 1994; Morgan, 2004).

Focus groups also help give a voice to participants who otherwise may have little opportunity to offer their knowledge, helping them to have greater control over the research conversation than they would otherwise have in an interview situation (Morgan, 2004). That being said, it is important for researchers, as focus group facilitators, to steer the focus group and ensure that it addresses the key issues of the study. Otherwise, the objectives of the study might get lost. Similar to those conducting individual semi-structured interviews, focus group facilitators follow a general question guide while giving participants the opportunity to provide detailed answers and to draw from relevant personal stories. In a group dynamic though, different strands or insights may emerge in quick order, and it is up to the researcher to keep track of these insights and to follow up with them as is relevant to the study's questions of interest. As in the case of individual stories in interviews, law in focus group discussions may hide in the background, shaping how members understand a notion such as privacy without becoming explicit in the discussion.

Some suggest that focus groups could potentially inhibit participants from speaking fully about their experience, because doing so can involve acts of highly personal self-disclosure in front of others. However, a group setting can create a safe environment for people who share a common life experience or set of risk factors and who might otherwise be less likely to discuss "taboo" subjects in a one-on-one interview (Kitzinger, 1994; Morgan, 2004). Focus groups, for example, have long been an important tool in HIV research (Joseph, Emmons, Kessler et al., 1984). As part of a larger study on the effects of using criminal law as a tool to reduce HIV transmission, a recent Canadian study used focus groups with people with HIV to elicit information on how they perceived and responded to the legal obligation to disclose their HIV status prior to engaging in sexual activity that posed "significant risk" (Mykhalovskiy, 2011, p. 669). The researcher wanted to better understand how people with HIV interpreted and applied the specific provisions of the law, and in particular the law's rather ambiguous legal conception of "significant risk" (which didn't necessarily align with public health-based understandings of risk). Focus groups in this case brought together people with a common characteristic (HIV-positive status) who—through active participation, listening to others, refining and explicating views—generated a multifaceted understanding of a shared phenomenon.

While focus groups are useful for discussing sensitive topics, it is nonetheless important to consider factors that might serve to silence certain participants in a group setting. In studies of occupational groups, such as law enforcement personnel, for example, it is important to ensure there are no power dynamics that allow certain participants to dominate. Holding focus groups with officers that share the same rank (or gender or both) can avoid this, especially if the topic centers on the informal decision-making norms that guide officers' arrest decisions in sensitive areas of concern to legal epidemiology (for example, management of people with mental illnesses, or arrests of drug users).

Researchers may choose to use focus groups in conjunction with interviews. Doing so can combine the depth achieved in interviews with the breadth achieved in focus groups. Focus groups can be used to validate previous findings from interviews while expanding the sample of people involved in a study. Alternatively, focus groups can generate ideas that can be explored in more depth through one-on-one follow-up interviews.

Field Observations

Sometimes direct observations of people's behavior and informal conversations *in situ* are the most appropriate method to address a special topic in legal epidemiology. When people are asked—in the case of interviews and focus groups—to "talk" about what they do, there's a good chance that their narratives mask aspects of what they actually do. It is human nature to want to be perceived as a good person making sensible choices. People may not always be consciously aware of what they do; they may not reveal some of the minutia of their daily lives that for them is not worth mentioning, but for a researcher may be profoundly insightful. Direct observations provide the opportunity for researchers to judge for themselves what is significant.

Levels of participation in an observation setting can vary, and may change over time (Bailey, 2007). Unobtrusive observations may be most appropriate, in a relatively public setting, such as fast food restaurants or a school cafeteria, if one is interested in observing how healthy foods are explained on menus or displayed on buffet tables, or whether people ask questions about calories or nutritional content. It may, though, be preferable to join a group or to become an honorary member of it. Doing so helps build trust between the researcher and the group, which is important when the behavior of interest is largely hidden from public view, and one needs to be physically close to the actors under study to observe what they are doing. Becoming a semi-participant, or even a full participant, has been used in research on the police, where the focus is on the "practical reasoning" of front-line workers in bureaucratic organizations (Brewer, 2004). Without placing oneself in the group, and building rapport, the researcher may have the figurative door closed to them by organizational gatekeepers, or have the observed behaviors "stage managed" when the outsider is present.

Observations can be used for different purposes. Researchers may be interested, for example, in understanding how something is done, such as the implementation of an intervention. Observations were used by Frattaroli and Teret (2006) as part of a case study on the implementation of the Maryland Gun Violence Act of 1996, which authorizes judges to issue protective orders requiring batterers to surrender their firearms. To see how judges were making use of this authority the researchers observed protective order hearings in a court that specialized in domestic violence cases. The researchers took detailed notes of these hearings and subsequently categorized the judicial activity they observed. These observations revealed that some judges were stricter than others in making sure that the surrender of firearms—as one "relief" option for protective orders—was reviewed with the petitioner. These direct observations of judicial behavior therefore helped the researchers to gauge the degree to which the law was being implemented in practice.

Observations can be used as a tool for understanding the meanings, rules, and norms that guide the behaviors and everyday routines of groups. Such observations can be useful when one is concerned with understanding the norms guiding health risk behaviors, or the norms guiding the practices of those implementing or enforcing the law. This use of observations is central to ethnographic research, which seeks to gather data on culture and cultural practices. What people say or how they talk while they are being observed is just as important as what they do, because their everyday talk can reveal a deeper logic or sensibility that explains actions being observed. Depending on the study, what people wear, how they talk, and their body language could all reveal power relationships, or interpersonal dynamics, that illuminate how a culture operates. The ethnographer documents this social world in as much rich detail as possible. All of these observations then form the data for the analysis of the meaning-making practices of a group.

Written Textual Analysis

In addition to peoples' words and actions, written texts are another valuable source of qualitative data. For instance, a researcher may be interested in gathering and analyzing texts that help us understand how and why a particular lawmaking effort was successful or how it was implemented. As part of understanding law-making, it may be important to examine the nature and extent of arguments used either in support of, or against the passage of a particular piece of legislation. Written texts produced as part of legislative debates can provide detailed information on this argumentation, and because they were produced at the time of the legislative process, can be considered accurate and not subject to the failures of human memory. Written texts, such as standard operating procedures or guidance documents, can also help us understand implementation practices.

As an example of textual analysis, Apollonio and Bero (2009) set out to examine which arguments were used in the passage of workplace smoking legislation. They also wanted to weigh this evidence, seeing how much certain arguments were used more than others. The researchers were particularly interested in discovering whether arguments that deployed research evidence, or scientific discourse, ultimately were associated with the passage of workplace smoking legislation that had strong protections for public health. To this end they performed a content analysis of materials including written and oral testimony, the text of proposed and passed bills and amendments, audiotapes of committee hearings, meeting minutes, and public commentary. Content analysis is a common form of textual analysis that involved, in this case, coding text segments according to argument types and counting the number of times certain arguments were used. Content analysis therefore produced both qualitative data (descriptions of different argument types, categorized by reading and analyzing the narratives) and quantitative data (the number of times different arguments were used). The researchers discovered varying types of argument in the texts, such as those centered on science and health effects and those stressing ideological positions. After analyzing and weighing different forms of argumentation, the authors concluded that "an emphasis on scientific discourse, relative to other arguments made in legislative testimony, might help produce political outcomes that favor public health" (Apollonio & Bero, 2009, p. 1).

Texts can serve as an important data source for legal epidemiology because they capture arguments and discourse that are so much a part of legislative and adjudicative processes. They help us understand thoughts and actions of people, both historically and in present times. Written texts provide good clues into how issues are framed and articulated. They can capture forms of reasoning that help in understanding human practices.

Research Strategies

The data collection methods described can be deployed, singularly or in combination, for different purposes depending on one's legal or health topic, research question, and broader research strategy. This section briefly describes some common qualitative research strategies of use for legal epidemiology.

Ethnography

Ethnographic studies are ideal for understanding the behavioral or cultural norms or rules (both formal and informal) that guide practices of groups or organizations. They help describe and explain everyday activities and logics of groups, about which little may be known. Direct observation of behaviors and practices is the tool of choice in ethnographic studies, but it is common to deploy interviews or focus groups as well. Regardless of how one mixes data-collection tools, an ethnographic study focuses on a group or a collective—its norms, traditions, everyday behaviors, and forms of "practical reasoning" (Brewer, 2004)—as its primary unit of analysis. "Ethnographers," writes Herbert, "unearth what the group takes for granted, and thereby reveal the knowledge and meaning structures that provide the blueprint for social action" (2000, p. 551).

One example of ethnographic research comes from India, where researchers set out to uncover the ways in which an HIV prevention nongovernmental organization (NGO) and female sex worker community-based organizations (CBOs) worked to transform the legal and normative environment in which sex workers were being policed. In a context in which law enforcement practices were arbitrary, corrupt, and a significant threat to the physical and mental health of sex workers, an NGO (with funding from an international donor) worked with CBOs to alter power dynamics. Through extensive community mobilization efforts, sex workers were given tools to identify police abuse and to set new standards of police behavior, thus transforming the "regulatory space" of police work (Biradavolu, Burris, George, Jena, & Blankenship, 2009). An ethnographic approach, involving prolonged engagement in the field, made it possible for researchers to understand this community transformation process, and in particular the sophisticated legal, political, and normative strategies deployed by the various actors to make this transformation happen. The researchers collected data through detailed observations of NGO and other activities, as well as through interviews with sex workers, intimate partners, police, and others. These data were gathered over a 2-year period by four trained observers. The researchers used this extensive time in the field to understand not just what was being done but how all of the activities observed were understood by participants.

Case Study Research

Case studies help illustrate a process, an action, or an event (Creswell, 2007). In legal epidemiology, a case study approach might be best suited for answering questions related to how a law was crafted and passed, or how it was implemented at the administrative level. Methods of data collection include observations; interviews; and analyses of laws, policies, or other guidelines for action. A strong case study uses as many data sources as possible, including individuals involved in the process or event under study and documents that help elucidate what unfolded (for example, media articles, meeting minutes, court decisions). All of these sources shed light on "how things get done" (Cohen, Manion, & Morrison, 2000; Stake, 2005, p. 444).

The case study researcher has to make a choice about parameters of the empirical "case," including a beginning and end time period for an observed process, and size of the subject population or institution involved in the phenomenon (an occupational subgroup, a whole organization, a community). Both of these "time and size" choices determine the scope of the study. Given the need for multiple data sources in a case study, researchers must determine whether they have sufficient time and resources to study multiple sites or whether it is more feasible to focus on a single case. Frattaroli and Teret (2006) focused their research on the single case of Maryland's Gun Violence Act, a law that authorized judges to order batterers to surrender their firearms and police to remove firearms from the scene of an alleged act of domestic violence. Within this case, they studied implementation of these provisions by both judges and police, drawing on three key sources of data: observations of protective order hearings, semi-structured interviews with key informants including judges and law enforcement officers, and documents related to the implementation process, such as training materials. Given the finite resources of the project, the researchers selected four study sites covering urban, suburban, and rural areas within the state and defined an observation period of 1 year.

Grounded Theory

The purpose of a grounded theory approach is to inductively produce a theory of a process, behavior, or interaction through the research, rather than to apply an existing theory at the outset (Glaser & Strauss, 1967). Proponents of grounded theory have provided clear guidelines for using the approach. A central text is *Basics of Qualitative Research*, written by Corbin and Strauss (2008). A grounded theory project starts with a general research question, which guides the start of the data collection. The researcher then moves back and forth between data collection and analysis. Analysis is aided by coding, in which emerging concepts or ideas are linked to segments of the data. Through the coding process, the researcher works to establish tentative relationships between concepts. The researcher then engages in more focused data collection and analysis in a process of "constant comparison," which involves comparing new data with previously collected data in order to discover similarities or differences in their conceptual properties or relationships. The process of constant comparison allows the researcher to refine concepts and identify higher-level concepts (often referred to as categories or themes). Theory emerges through this refinement of concepts and conceptual relationships. The researcher continues this cyclical process of data collection and analysis until no new concepts or conceptual relationships emerge. At this point, described as the stage of "theoretical saturation," the theory developed is determined to be robust enough to explain all of the data gathered, and there are no negative cases (that is, actions or behaviors that cannot be explained by the theory). In other words, the theory is considered to be "grounded" in the data (Corbin & Strauss, 2008; Eriksson & Kovalainen, 2008; Lacey & Luff, 2001).

A grounded theory approach can be used with one or more sources of data, such as narratives from interviews, observations from field notes, written texts such as media clippings or correspondence, or all of the above. Cooper et al. (2005) used the grounded theory approach in analyzing interview data on drug injectors' health risk behaviors in the wake of a New York Police drug crackdown. "Throughout the analysis," they write, "the authors discussed emerging concepts, categories, and their inter-relationships; negative cases were sought to extend and enrich our findings" (p. 677). Using the grounded theory approach, they developed a theory of the relationships between specific policing tactics and drug users' sense of sovereignty over their bodies and the spaces in which they lived, and users' abilities to practice harm reduction. Their theoretical model was general enough to explain experiences of all of the users they interviewed, while providing enough specificity to distinguish between experiences and practices of users with different sociodemographic characteristics or circumstances.

Action Research

In an action research approach, researchers and practitioners (or members of a community of interest) work hand-in-hand in all stages of a research project, from conceptualizing the problem to identifying a needed change to developing ways to improve practice and ultimately human well-being (Brydon-Miller, Greenwood, & Maguire, 2003; Stringer, 2007). Action research involves collapsing traditional boundaries between researchers and subjects. Research teams include members of a targeted group, such as a mental health consumer working with research investigators who are studying a legal intervention to improve community mental health, or HIV-positive individuals providing ideas for a more promising legal intervention that assists in prevention. The assumption is that such participants possess unique insights into the relevant risk behaviors and environments, and how best to study them (Schensul, 1999). Action research therefore centers on "change *with* others," serving as a strong critique of, and alternative to, "ivory tower" research (Reason & Bradbury, 2008, p. 1).

Within legal epidemiology, an action research method called rapid policy assessment and response (RPAR) was developed to bring together researchers and community stakeholders to improve the working of law on the ground. Community-based researchers, together with a Community Action Board, gather and interpret data about the implementation of law in the community and its effect on local health. Researchers and the action board use facilitation techniques such as "power maps" and a "root causes" exercise to analyze who is wielding power in the community, how law relates to practice, and where there might be "pressure points" for healthy change (Temple University, Beasley School of Law, 2004). This approach has been deployed especially in relation to drug and sex-related behaviors, but the method applies to any regulatory problem (Sobeyko, Leszczyszyn-Pynka, Duklas et al., 2006; Vyshemirskaya, Osipenko, Koss et al., 2008).

Models such as RPAR can benefit marginalized populations whose experiences with laws have been unfavorable or whose ability to influence lawmaking has been limited or even nonexistent. While incorporating the knowledge and experience of such groups is key to the research process, participants also benefit by acquiring skills in data collection and analysis. The purpose of action research is precisely to link researchers and the research process to stakeholders in the locale who are in a position to translate knowledge into action.

Mixed Methods

Qualitative research may also form part of a mixed-methods study that integrates numeric and text-based data to offer complementary or a richer set of answers than provided by either quantitative or qualitative research on its own. Mixed-methods researchers adopt the pragmatic view that quantitative and qualitative approaches to research are compatible, with each compensating for limitations of the other (Johnson & Onwuegbuzie, 2004). At the design phase, getting the right mix involves determining the ordering of different research strategies (whether one component should precede the other, or whether data collection should occur simultaneously) (Creswell & Plano Clark, 2007). For example, a focus group study exploring health risk behaviors could assist in refining hypotheses to be tested by a survey of a representative sample of the population. Alternatively, an experimental or quasi-experimental evaluation might produce evidence that a law is connected to a specified public health outcome. Direct observations combined with key informant interviews might then shed light on the mechanisms that "tell us why interconnections . . . occur" (Pawson, 2006, p. 23), as could ethnographies that are nested in randomized controlled trials (Sherman & Strang, 2004).

The term *mixed methods* therefore applies to studies that use both quantitative and qualitative tools and sources, and respective quantitative and qualitative analyses. Various combinations of data sources, tools, and analyses can be used depending on the research questions (see guidance on this by Creswell, Klassen, Plano Clark, Smith, & The Office of Behavioral and Social Sciences Research, 2011). One might choose to conduct two parallel studies of the same thing, such as a random sample survey combined with key informant interviews, comparing or integrating the results. In such a case, qualitative data are interspersed with results from the quantitative analysis as a way to unpack, interpret, or confirm what the numbers are indicating.

Standards of Research Quality

Scholars vary in their views as to whether qualitative research is more of an art (demanding the skills of improvisation) or a science (demanding structure and rigid adherence to procedures).

The former view suggests that researchers need to be flexible, ready to change aspects of their designs as they go along (for example, sampling). Researchers may experience such profound "ah ha" moments that the course of the research must change in order to pursue a potentially groundbreaking finding. Howard Becker, a seminal American sociologist and ethnographer, is a particularly vocal advocate of this improvisational orientation, arguing that "researchers can't know ahead of time all the questions they will want to investigate, what theories they will ultimately find relevant to discoveries made during the research, or what methods will produce the information needed to solve the newly discovered problems" (2009, p. 548). The research process is not linear, nor is the process of designing it. But this does not mean, Becker points out, that it isn't "systematic, rigorous, [and] theoretically informed" (2009, p. 548).

Notwithstanding Becker's view, researchers require guidance as they embark on the most systematic and rigorous study that they can achieve within the scope and resources of their project. From the perspective of funders who support research (quantitative or qualitative), it is important for researchers to justify their financial support by giving careful consideration to every aspect of their research, factoring in the chance that certain design elements may change or expand and ensuring that such changes along the way can strengthen the research and advance its goals. Institutional review boards may also insist on a well-defined research plan and set of objectives.

Undoubtedly, qualitative researchers can't or shouldn't "imitate" guidelines designed for deductive, hypothesis-testing research, but the paradigms of quantitative and qualitative research do share core concerns about quality of data, appropriateness of data collection tools, validity and generalizability of findings, and robustness of the analytical process. Although some prominent qualitative researchers choose not to use such terms (because they align too closely with positivist research) and use others (for example, *confirmability*, *authenticity*), we use the more traditional language here, in a qualified manner, to provide consistency, as well as a source of comparison, with the other chapters in the book. The considerations that follow are particularly complex in the design of mixed-methods research. Fortunately, this complexity is recognized by the National Institutes of Health, which commissioned a guidance document from prominent authorities on mixed methods (Creswell, Klassen, Plano Clark, Smith, & The Office of Behavioral and Social Sciences Research, 2011).

Sampling

Researchers must decide on the particular characteristics of people or texts that make up their sample as well as how large the sample should be. For example, if someone wants to interview injection drug users about their health behaviors, it's important to determine which set of drug-user characteristics should be captured in the sample (for example, people living in certain areas, people of a certain age, males, females, people who are wealthy, or people with few resources). The research question will determine whether a diverse or homogeneous sample is required. Determining how many people to recruit for interviews is equally important, and it is possible that this number can increase or decrease over the course of the research, depending on emergence of new insights or questions. Qualitative researchers aim to reach a point at which additional data collection (increasing the sample) would not generate new insights. The point at which this occurs depends on the research question. There could be little variation in views among a sample of family physicians in terms of their concerns with health information privacy, but there may be huge variation among injection drug users in their experiences of targeted policing, depending on whether users are living in certain parts of a city, or are wealthy or poor, or have access to support networks and social services. Researchers must think carefully about their level of access to the people or to the texts that will allow them to answer their question comprehensively, with depth, and with confidence that there are not parts of the question that have remained unanswered.

Different approaches to sampling in qualitative research can be used alone or in combination. Probability sampling, most commonly found in quantitative research, seeks to make sure that the sample represents the broader target population. This approach can be suitable for large-scale qualitative studies, although higher levels of generalizability can compromise depth, especially in projects with limited resources to collect detailed data (Lamont & White, 2005).

There is a variety of purposeful sampling strategies, and some common ones are highlighted here. Criterion sampling involves selecting participants who meet one criterion or more of interest, such as a legislator working in the area of childhood obesity prevention. Maximum variation sampling consists of choosing sites or participants that differ along various dimensions or criteria, such as injection drug users that differ in terms of levels of wealth, gender, ethnic background, or some combination. Homogenous sampling refers to selecting participants or cases that are similar in some ways, such as judges who work in specialized domestic violence courts in the State of Maryland. Snowball or chain sampling refers to the process of expanding one's sample by asking previous participants to nominate other potential participants (Bailey, 2007). For instance, a police officer involved in a targeted foot patrol intervention in a violent area of a city might refer a researcher to another police officer from a gang unit who has extensive knowledge about drug market dynamics associated with the violent behaviors.

Respondent-driven sampling (RDS) is an innovative approach used in the study of hidden or "hard to reach" populations, such as drug users, sex workers, gay men, or people experiencing homelessness. RDS was developed to help overcome the challenges of achieving probability samples with such groups. Depending on the research question, having a probability sample or random sample is important when the goal is to measure the effect of a law or its enforcement on *all* members of a wider population of interest, not simply those who are most visible or accessible. With hidden populations, however, the sampling frame can be unknown; there is no clear understanding of the extent of such populations or the varying characteristics of their members

(Heckathorn, 1997). The RDS approach uses respondents to recruit their peers (as in snowball sampling), while researchers keep track of peer-to-peer referrals. This snowballing occurs through "waves" (with one wave having been recruited through the previous wave). RDS deploys a mathematical model that helps calculate the non-randomness of the sample, while implementing techniques for reducing bias, including lengthening referral chains and rewarding recruiters (Heckathorn, 2008; see Salganik & Heckathorn, 2004, and Heckathorn, 2007, for further information on the RDS process).

Validity

In qualitative research, the representation of data is very much a product of a researcher's own interpretation of meaning (Creswell, 2007, pp. 206–207). "Qualitative data," write Corbin and Strauss (2008), "are inherently rich in substance and full of possibilities. It is impossible to say that there is only one story that can be constructed from the data" (p. 50). There are, however, several strategies that researchers can employ to make sure that findings are valid, which in the context of qualitative research refers to findings that are credible (capturing the truth of peoples' experiences and perceptions), transferable (applicable to other contexts), and neutral (not distorted by researcher bias) (Cohen & Crabtree, 2006; Lincoln & Guba, 1985).

"Negative case analysis" (Creswell, 2007, p. 208) involves identifying or collecting data that might not be explained by one's existing analysis, and may even contradict it (Cohen et al., 2000). A related form of analytical scrutiny is "communicative validity," a process in which researchers subject their claims to other researchers with relevant content and theoretical expertise. Entering into such a dialogue with one's intellectual community can create an opportunity for one's interpretation to be refuted or refined (Hesse-Biber & Leavy, 2006).

In ethnographic research, the validity of one's findings is strengthened when one commits a sustained period of time in the field and offers a reflective account of the ways in which one gained access to a setting, developed trust with participants, and made sure that one's own cultural predispositions did not distort or skew one's interpretations (Creswell, 2007, pp. 207–208). "Pragmatic validity" is particularly important in action research and is important to legal epidemiology more generally. Pragmatic validity is the ability of a research study to enable participants to better understand and navigate their environment, thus enhancing their ability to effect change, either to the lives of participants or to the contexts in which people live and work (Hesse-Biber & Leavy, 2006; Marks, Wood, Ali, Walsh, & Witbooi, 2010).

Regardless of sampling strategy or size, it is important to be very clear about the ways in which one's findings may have relevance beyond the individuals, cases, or sites studied. Although generalizability to the whole population, in the sense claimed by quantitative researchers, is usually not the goal of qualitative research, it is nonetheless important to discuss whether and why one's findings could be more widely applied to other groups, institutions, or processes (Lamont & White, 2005). Researchers can help readers judge this transferability by providing as much detail as possible on the research setting and characteristics of one's data and sample. With this information, others can compare with the characteristics of other potential research sites or settings.

Reliability

A reliable study is one in which findings would be consistent if the data were to be collected for a second time or if the study were to be repeated. In qualitative research involving observations and interviews, it's not really possible to collect the same data twice (Trochim, 2005). For instance, if a researcher is observing people's behavior, there is no single instance when a behavior will be exactly the same as it was in a previous moment (although there are presumably common and repeated patterns in the behavior). An interview respondent could answer the same questions differently from one day to the next. Nonetheless, it is important to guarantee the reliability of the procedures for data gathering and analysis. This involves providing transparency into how the data were collected and analyzed. This transparency is important not only to the outside world but to members of teams that have different people collecting and analyzing data.

In large projects, it is critical to ensure that data are collected in the same way by different team members, and that the processes of data organization and coding are the same. In ethnographic or other observational studies, for example, observers should be similarly trained and should be producing the same quality of field notes. Being a good note taker is not a trivial skill, and it is a true craft (Emerson, Fretz, & Shaw, 1995). If interviews are being carried out by multiple researchers, it is important for each person to follow the same general guide. Assuming there are open-ended components in such interviews, all researchers should be trained on interviewing techniques that elicit as much relevant information as possible from respondents.

Finally, if there are multiple people coding data, it is important that there be constant dialogue in the development and definitions of codes and emerging themes so that there is a shared overall interpretive framework and process. Team members must discuss their analysis regularly, particularly as new codes and themes emerge. It is also useful in the beginning of an analysis phase for two people to code the same piece of data to ensure that they do not differ fundamentally in technique or in the interpretation of codes. For very large, multisite projects involving teams of qualitative researchers, it is useful to seek guidance on specific techniques for achieving consensus in the coding and analysis process (Guest & MacQueen, 2008).

Analysis: Inductive–Deductive Engagement

Qualitative research requires the researcher to cyclically engage descriptive data and higher levels of abstract understanding (Janesick, 2004). In conducting one's analysis, researchers must engage in a meaningful and iterative dialogue between theory and data. This analysis begins while the researcher is collecting data. Analytical insights gleaned from initial data can drive researchers to collect more or different data as the study progresses, meaning that the qualitative research processes we have described tend to be more fluid than quantitative research. Research findings along the way can inform further sampling procedures, or choices about which elements or phenomenon in the data will become center stage as one works to form a story from the empirical material.

It is common for researchers to take advantage of qualitative analysis software that can assist with the organization and coding of data. Software such as *Atlas.ti* or *NVivo* (see Creswell, 2007) does not, however, serve to replace the analytic work of the researcher. The software helps enhance efficiency of the analysis process and provides useful tools for presenting data, such as charts and visual diagrams, including network views of relationships between concepts. The software also makes it easy for researchers to code text segments as well as to write and organize memos or reflections on those segments. Technology helps analysts become more efficient in an otherwise laborintensive task.

Conclusion

When evaluating the effectiveness of law, it is critical for researchers to design studies that can help support causal inferences (see Chapters 13 and 14). Thinking in causal terms both depends on and contributes to a fundamental understanding of mechanisms, or the ways in which law has effects. In tracing causal pathways beginning with lawmaking and ending with health, qualitative research helps answer questions along the way that are important to practice and essential to theory. Moreover, it can help identify law's unintended consequences on health behaviors and risk environments.

As a complement to quantitative research, qualitative research strategies and methods help answer important questions about what law means to people, how it is experienced, and how law's agents might do a better job in furtherance of public health. Advancing the field of legal epidemiology therefore depends in part on advancing qualitative research that is empirically rich, theoretically innovative, and pragmatically useful. Exactly how this is done in practice requires careful consideration by academics in partnership with agencies and communities intended to benefit from, and ideally contribute to, the design and conduct of research that matters.

Summary

Qualitative research helps form our understanding of relationships between law, legal practices, and public health. Because of its inductive nature, qualitative research generates insight into previously unstudied (or understudied) mechanisms of legal effect. Its various methods and strategies help uncover ways in which laws have effects that lie outside of existing theories and models, and for which standardized quantitative measures do not exist.

Different data collection tools can be used alone or in combination. Semi-structured one-on-one interviews involve open-ended questions that generate detailed narrative data on an individual's unique knowledge and experience. Focus groups create opportunities for participants to build on others' insights, contradict them, or refine them, generating insight that would not emerge through individual interviews. Direct observations help in understanding how an action is carried out and can reveal cultural norms that guide behaviors. Collection and analysis of written texts help us understand how issues are framed and articulated, and capture forms of reasoning that help us understand human practices.

Qualitative tools can be deployed within broader research approaches or strategies. Ethnographic studies are ideal for understanding the behavioral or cultural norms that guide the practices of groups or organizations. Case studies illustrate a process, and are suited to answering questions of how a law was crafted, passed, or implemented. A "grounded theory approach" produces a theory of a process, behavior, or interaction—generating theory inductively from the data. Action research involves researchers and practitioners (or members of a community of interest) working hand-in-hand in all stages of a research project, from conceptualizing the problem to identifying a needed change to developing ways forward to improve practice. Qualitative research is often part of mixed-methods research that integrates quantitative and qualitative data to offer a richer set of answers than either could provide alone.

Regardless of research strategy, studies must be designed with appropriate sampling strategies, and researchers must ensure validity and reliability. Purposeful sampling strategies are common in qualitative research, and their choice depends on the research question, types of data collection methods deployed, availability of participants, and resources of the researcher. There are several strategies that researchers employ to ensure that findings are valid, including use of "negative case analysis" or "communicative validity" processes in which researchers subject their claims to other researchers with relevant content and theoretical expertise. It is important to guarantee the reliability of qualitative research by using consistent and systematic procedures for gathering and analyzing data. Finally, good qualitative research involves a robust cyclical engagement between descriptive data and higher levels of abstract understanding, which is facilitated by a process of coding (assigning concepts to segments of data).

Further Reading

Apollonio, D. E., & Bero, L. A. (2009). Evidence and argument in policymaking: Development of workplace smoking legislation. *BMC Public Health, 9,* 189.

Corbin, J. M., & Strauss, A. L. (2008). *Basics of qualitative research: Techniques and procedures for developing grounded theory* (3rd ed.). Los Angeles, CA: Sage.

Creswell, J. W., & Plano Clark, V. L. (2007). *Designing and conducting mixed methods research.* Thousand Oaks, CA: Sage.

Guest, G., & MacQueen, K. M. (Eds.) (2008). *Handbook for team-based qualitative research.* Lanham, MD: AltaMira Press.

Chapter 16

Using Cost-Effectiveness and Cost–Benefit Analysis to Evaluate Public Health Laws

Rosalie Liccardo Pacula

Learning Objectives

- Understand the value of economic evaluations.
- Identify specific steps involved in conducting a careful economic evaluation.
- Understand the unique complexities and considerations when conducting an economic evaluation of an intervention targeting population health versus an intervention targeting individuals with a health problem or specific disease.
- Identify a strong research design for cost–benefit analysis (CBA) or cost-effectiveness analysis (CEA) focused on evaluating public health law from a societal perspective.

Economics is the study of markets and other mechanisms used to efficiently allocate society's scarce resources to their most valued purpose. Economic evaluation, which is an analytic framework for identifying the most efficient approach to achieving a stated objective, involves the identification, measurement, valuation, and comparison of the true economic costs and consequences of two or more interventions, programs or policies seeking to achieve

Legal Epidemiology: Theory and Methods, Second Edition. Edited by Alexander C. Wagenaar, Rosalie Liccardo Pacula, and Scott Burris.
© 2023 John Wiley & Sons, Inc. Published 2023 by John Wiley & Sons, Inc.

that objective. While methods for conducting economic evaluations of targeted health care interventions (new medical devices, prescription drugs, or therapeutic approaches) have existed for several decades (Drummond & Stoddart, 1985; Gold, Siegel, Russell, & Weinstein, 1996), standards for conducting economic evaluations of more macro interventions targeting population-level objectives have only more recently been the focus of research groups and government agencies (Crowley et al., 2018; Levin, McEwan, Belfield, Bowden, & Shand, 2017; National Academy of Science, Engineering and Medicine [NASEM], 2016; Yates, 2018). This is due in part to the tremendous growth in the scientific tools and applications of cost-effectiveness and cost–benefit analysis, the two most common forms of economic evaluation, applied in the evaluation of population-level interventions.

Unlike evaluations done in the private sector, where the focus is on return on investment to the private firm or individual, economic evaluations of policies and initiatives for a community focus on return to the community as a whole. This population-wide focus fundamentally changes how one measures both the costs incurred and the outcomes or benefits experienced. For example, while many medical and/or health interventions target specific patients with particular acute or chronic diseases, public health laws and interventions target a whole population or community, and often permanently change structures and practices in ways that affect not only the targeted population in the current generation but future generations as well. There are unique challenges to doing these types of evaluations, which have led many public agencies (NASEM, 2016; NICE, 2014), and even classic textbooks on the conduct of economic evaluations (Drummond, Sculpher, Claxton, Stoddart, & Torrance, 2015; Levin et al., 2017), to develop new standards for evaluating "social interventions" and public policies aimed at the population level.

The goal of this chapter is to introduce the reader to current methods used in the conduct of a careful economic evaluation of public health law effects on population health. It outlines specific steps involved in conducting a proper analysis and the different choices made when dealing with issues at each step. I highlight that even when best practices are used, variability in the final calculation of cost effectiveness or net benefit often remain due to different underlying assumptions that an analyst might reasonably make within a given study. I present ways in which this uncertainty can and should be communicated to a decision maker. An educated consumer of these analyses will need to understand the relevance of this uncertainty in terms of implications for the reliability of recommendations based on cost-effectiveness or cost–benefit analyses. While this chapter provides an overview of the recommended steps for cost-effectiveness and cost–benefit analysis, as well as key issues that have to be considered within each, the interested reader is encouraged to dive into the additional resources referenced at the end of this chapter to gain a greater understanding of the many details I can only touch on here.

Steps in Conducting a Proper Economic Evaluation When Assessing a Public Health Law

Public and scientific organizations have only just begun defining their preferred standards for conducting economic evaluations of social interventions and refinements of these have already occurred (Drummond et al., 2015; NICE, 2014; Wilkinson et al., 2016, 2019). Nonetheless, there are certain common principles that have already emerged that are consistently recommended when conducting a scientifically rigorous, high-quality evaluation targeting a population-level outcome. I begin by breaking down the activities involved in conducting an economic evaluation, presenting them as nine basic steps, and highlight current best practices for approaches and methods in each step for evaluating a public health law in particular.

Step 1: Define the Public Health Law Being Evaluated as well as Relevant Alternatives

While this is a seemingly obvious first step, it is in many instances given inadequate attention. While many public health policies involve the same terms, such as "legalization," "payment reform" or "eligibility," the laws referred to by these terms can differ dramatically. For example, the term "medical marijuana law" has been used to describe a wide range of laws that may: (1) prohibit any legal supply system, (2) allow for only home cultivation or private cooperative growing groups, or (3) allow for retail stores that may sell to any patient providing proper verification. Using the same term to describe these very different supply mechanisms is improper as well as confusing and generates conflicting research from analysts who try to evaluate effects of these laws on specific outcomes such as teenage access (Pacula, Powell, Heaton, & Sevigny, 2015). A guide produced by the National Academy of Sciences, Engineering and Medicine (NASEM) (2016) explains that a clear statement of the purpose of the law requires a statement of the law's goals or objectives, the intended target population or recipients of the benefits of the law as well as the intended payers of costs, the intensity and/or duration of the initiative developed by the law, the scale of benefits/costs, and specifics related to its context. While this recommendation is helpful, it misses the subtlety that someone who is not an expert in the policy area may not understand, which is how small deviations in the law (e.g., different supply mechanisms for of medical cannabis) influence the policy's objective or impacts. That's why the Society for Prevention Research takes this recommendation a step farther and recommends that the description of the law be detailed enough that readers who are not experts in the policy area can easily understand the essential elements of what is being considered as part of the policy, particularly elements of the law that describe the mechanisms through which behavioral change is expected to occur (Crowley et al., 2018). In short, economic evaluation research, like any evaluation research on a law, has as a foundation not only the specifics of the legal texts but also a theory-based conceptual model of the purpose of the law, its intended targets, mechanisms and pathways of effect, and expected institutional and behavioral changes resulting from the law.

In addition to a clear description of the policy of interest (in terms of the precise elements of that policy that are believed to be important for affecting population health), it is important to thoroughly describe what the full set of alternative policy options are that the targeted policy is being evaluated against. This full set of alternative policy options might be quite large when CBA or CEA is being used prior to policy adoption (i.e., "ex-ante") because a thorough analysis would consider the full range of possibilities, not just the few most likely candidates. The set of policy options are typically smaller when conducting CEA or CBA post policy adoption (i.e., "ex-post"). At a minimum, and regardless of whether the economic evaluation is being done ex-ante or ex-post, one of the policy alternatives that should be included is the "status quo" (which may mean the absence of a policy or the continuation of an existing policy). The policy alternatives might also include alternative laws or seemingly minor variants of the main policy being proposed. This is the subtlety that I was referencing above in the case of medical cannabis laws, where the policy options considered are those with different supply mechanisms.

Comparing the status quo just to the specific law adopted or of interest is too restrictive if the decision makers have other options available, because economic evaluations will only identify the most efficient allocation of society's scarce resources when all possible options are considered. Clearly articulating what that full set of alternatives actually is can be challenging, so many analysts in practice simply focus on the options that appear to be most feasible given the political and/or social environment.

Step 2: Articulate the Question Being Addressed by the Economic Evaluation

Just as it is important to clearly articulate the specific public health law being considered, as well as its alternatives, so too it is important to clearly articulate the question being considered in the economic evaluation being conducted. The specifics of the question being asked will determine what information is required to answer it.

For example, an economic evaluation considering effects of legalizing cannabis for recreational purposes on adolescent use of cannabis would focus on a very different set of outcomes, costs, and benefits than an economic evaluation that evaluated effects of legalization on adult use. The former would require information on youth initiation, escalation, use of different products and modes of administration, and risks associated with unexpected or long-term exposure given the scientific evidence of harmful effects of cannabis on brain development (Hall, Leung, & Lynskey, 2020). The latter would require information on adult use, intensity and duration, use of different products, and a more nuanced discussion of both the beneficial and harmful effects of occasional, regular, and chronic use of different formulated products, as not all use has been shown to be harmful (Hall & Lynskey, 2020). From a population health and societal perspective, neither of these studies would be adequate to fully consider the effect of cannabis legalization, as adults and youth are just particular subsets of the entire population affected by the change in policy. However, if the question is posed too narrowly, focusing on only one of these two population segments, then a full consideration of costs and benefits will not be undertaken.

Similarly, an economic evaluation that asks about the effects of Medicaid expansion on health care access would involve a different set of outcomes and data than an economic evaluation that asks about the effects of Medicaid expansion on health. The former would focus on the ability to obtain any health care services (e.g., primary care services, mental health services or addiction services), perhaps distinguishing access to clinically appropriate care from any health care service, while the latter would emphasize effects on health outcomes, including possibly mortality (Gruber & Sommers, 2019). From a population health perspective, it is how insurance influences health that is of greatest interest and that might be missed if the focus is just on health care access. Thus, it is important to consider the question being asked in the economic evaluation to understand whether the output from it provides sufficient information to fully evaluate the policy, in terms of outcomes, costs, and benefits at the population level.

Step 3: Clearly Identify the Perspective to be Taken

Common perspectives taken when conducting economic evaluations of health laws include (1) program or agency perspective, (2) recipients' perspective, (3) payer (usually government) perspective, and (4) societal perspective. Depending on the perspective taken in the evaluation, not all stakeholders' costs, benefits, and outcomes are considered. The stated perspective also influences valuation of the resources used to achieve an outcome (a point I will return to in Step 6). When considering health laws, the most appropriate perspective is the societal perspective. Nonetheless, narrower perspectives are still used, often because they are easier or more feasible to conduct given time and resource constraints. These narrower perspectives limit the outcomes, benefits and costs considered and therefore can have important implications for the ultimate recommendation that comes from the study, not unlike the framing of the question. These distinctions in perspectives and how they shrink or expand what is considered in the analysis are perhaps best demonstrated through an example.

Let's consider an analyst conducting an economic evaluation of the effects of the ACA's Medicaid expansion on health care utilization of low-income individuals. An economic evaluation of the impact of the ACA on health care utilization conducted from just a program or agency perspective would consider those costs, benefits and outcomes that are most relevant to the agency/program and its implementation of the policy. These would likely include the administrative cost of expanding and managing new enrollees, the costs of health care utilization of newly covered individuals, and whether enrollees shifted utilization from high cost (emergency) care to lower cost (preventative care) services (Gruber & Sommers, 2019). The agency perspective might also include some effects on the newly insured (i.e., the recipients), such as improved access to a primary care provider and/or management of chronic health conditions, if the question being asked in the evaluation includes effects on access and health. However, an evaluation using only the agency or program perspective would ignore many other beneficial effects experienced by the newly insured, such as lower out-of-pocket expenses, reduced medical debt, reduced travel time to a health care provider, and/or reduced stress associated with medical issues (Finkelstein, Hendren, & Luttmer, 2019; Finkelstein, Taubman, Wright, et al., 2011). These are costs that are solely experienced by the recipient and are frequently not tied to an agency's objective in implementing the policy.

An evaluation that fully considers the recipient perspective (in this case potential Medicaid enrollees) would consider all the financial, physical health, mental health, and time effects associated with this new coverage experienced by those gaining coverage under this policy, but would ignore the potential spillover effects this coverage might have in terms of the cost of insurance and/or healthcare received by the commercially insured, higher taxes paid by taxpayers to cover the agency cost of providing the additional health care services, or the effects of expanded patient loads on health care providers (Gruber & Sommers, 2019). The program recipient perspective, therefore, focuses on the costs, benefits, and outcomes experienced by the population targeted by the program or policy, not necessarily all those affected. It is increasingly common for analysts conducting economic evaluations of health care interventions today to account for both agency and patient perspectives, but accounting for the full range of population-wide societal benefits and costs remains extremely rare.

When considering a policy targeting population-level outcomes, most guidelines suggest an even broader perspective then the health agency + patient/recipient perspective (Boardman and Vining, 2017; Crowley et al., 2018; Drummond et al., 2015; NASEM, 2016). While the taxpayer perspective is at times confused with the agency perspective, it is actually broader in that it considers the allocation of the taxpayer's dollars across different government agencies, not just within a single agency. Any single agency is going to be focused on achieving the goals and objectives of that agency (e.g., health, education or criminal justice), while the taxpayer is ultimately concerned about the objectives and goals of all the government agencies they fund. So, in the example of the ACA Medicaid expansion, consideration of any possible labor market productivity gains associated with insurance coverage, which have the benefit to government of reducing welfare need and/or increasing tax revenue through employment, would be a non-health agency outcome that someone taking the taxpayer perspective would consider if the question is posed generally enough to allow it (Gruber & Sommers, 2019).

The broadest perspective, and generally recommended as the gold standard when conducting economic evaluations involving society's resources, is the societal perspective. The societal perspective considers not just the taxpayers paying for the policy implementation or the direct targets of a public health law (e.g., drunk drivers, smokers, Medicaid recipients, vaccination programs), but all members of a society that might be indirectly affected by a policy's adoption, including children, the elderly, immigrants and refugees. Depending on the policy, the societal perspective might include future generations who are not yet born but affected by a policy because of health gains achieved by policies implemented today (e.g., maternal nutrition programs, Medicaid expansion, clean indoor air laws). Given this much broader orientation, the societal perspective is difficult to fully implement in practice. It requires a complete accounting and measurement of costs and benefits to all members of a society directly and indirectly affected by a policy, as well as full consideration of spillover effects (both positive and negative) caused by these policies, in both the short and long run. Health laws, just like many other social policies, often influence multiple domains of our economy and society, including education and work productivity (Grossman, 1972, 2000). Thus, investments in health have many additional effects on society besides extending life expectancy, reducing disease and disability rates, and improving quality of life, and the gains can be sustained across generations (Robertson & O'Brien, 2018; Thompson, 2014). Trying to quantify all these effects and their net costs and benefits on the current population as well as future populations requires extensive data typically not readily available. In addition to identifying which costs, benefits, and outcomes to consider in an evaluation, the specification of perspective for the economic evaluation identifies *how* those values should be measured, a point that will be discussed in greater detail in Step 6.

Step 4: Identify the Type of Economic Evaluation to Conduct

As noted by Yates (2018), the absence of an established, unified standard for conducting economic evaluations of public health interventions has meant that various methods have been employed in the literature so far, including cost-minimization analysis, cost-consequence analysis, economic-impact analysis, cost–benefit analysis, cost-effectiveness analysis, cost-utility analysis and social return on investment (Drummond, O'Brien, Stoddart, & Torrance, 1998; Drummond et al., 2015; Yates & Marra 2017). Any one of these methods might be used to consider a law's effects from an agency, recipient, government, or societal perspective (Step 3), and all of these require an estimate of the *causal effect* of the intervention on its intended outcome (described in Step 7). The decision regarding which method to use ultimately depends on the question being asked and the available information to answer the question posed. The three primary approaches that have been widely used to evaluate health policies or compare health options to other social policy options are cost-effectiveness analysis, cost-utility analysis (a specific type of cost-effectiveness), and cost–benefit analysis.

Cost-Effectiveness Analysis (CEA) is an analytic framework for evaluating the desirability of a specific intervention over a set of alternative options by assessing and comparing each option's cost and effectiveness from the same stakeholder perspective, but where effectiveness is measured by a singular outcome of interest. In CEA, results are summarized through a cost-effectiveness ratio, where the numerator captures the net costs (total cost minus any cost savings of the intervention) and the denominator is the outcome measured in its natural unit (e.g., lives saved, illness averted, vaccines administered, and so on). An average CEA calculated in this manner can then be compared across a number of interventions of common duration to identify the intervention that has the lowest cost per unit of outcome. When comparing policy options of different duration, it is more common to construct an incremental cost-effectiveness ratio (ICER), which allows one to assess the incremental difference in net present value of costs (C) of two or more interventions per unit of effect (E) on the outcome, and is commonly represented (in the case of two interventions A and B) as:

$$\text{ICER}_{A,B} = \frac{C_A - C_B}{E_A - E_B}$$

Multiple interventions can then be compared in terms of their incremental cost-effectiveness relative *to the same* baseline scenario (e.g., comparing all the options to option B, for example), enabling a more appropriate basis for comparison of a diverse set of interventions that have varying costs and levels of effectiveness over different time periods.

Cost-utility analysis is a special type of CEA where the outcome being examined is a multi-dimensional measure of health or wellbeing such as Quality Adjusted Life Year (QALY) or Disability Adjusted Life Years (DALY) (Drummond et al., 2015). Construction of these multi-dimensional measures involves a description of health/well-being and a valuation of each health state. A variety of preferred methods have been developed to elicit population-based measures of well-being, including the Health Utilities Index, the EuroQol 5-dimensional questionnaire (EQ-5D), and the Quality of Well-Being Index. However, the bulk of this development has focused on evaluations in health, which is why cost-utility analysis has become the dominate and recommended form of CEA employed when evaluating most health interventions. Outside of health, critics of cost utility analysis argue that the complexities and assumptions needed to construct these measures of social well-being are just as numerous and problematic as cost–benefit analysis, which has been broadly applied to evaluate a wide range of policies outside of health.

Most public health laws influence several health outcomes simultaneously, in addition to outcomes beyond health (Payne, McAllister, & Davies, 2013; Weatherly et al., 2009; Kelly, McDaid Ludbrook & Powell, 2005). Cannabis legalization, for example, has been shown to reduce criminal justice expenditures (Caulkins et al., 2015) and have short-run positive effects on employment for some individuals (Ghimire & Maclean, 2020; Nicholas & Maclean, 2019), while also negatively influencing educational attainment (Chu & Gershenson, 2018; Marie & Zölitz, 2017) and health (Hall & Lynskey, 2020). It is very difficult within the CEA framework to develop a composite measure that captures these very disparate, but important, outcomes. Nonetheless, a true societal perspective requires consideration of each of them. This is why cost–benefit analysis remains a common tool for evaluating social policies, particularly when a broader taxpayer or societal perspective is taken in the analysis.

Cost Benefit Analysis (CBA) is an analytic framework for evaluating the social desirability of a program, policy or intervention in terms of its ability to improve efficiency over an alternative set of choices being considered, but mindful of all the alternative uses of those funds. It stems from welfare economics and has at its core the principal of maximizing efficiency, with the recognition that society's resources are scarce (limited) and hence any resources dedicated to the provision of one set of services are no longer available to be used on other valued services (Boadway 1974; Dasgupta & Pearce, 1972; Vining & Weimer, 2006). CBA is a tool that allows one to choose not just whether a particular health policy is the most effective way of achieving a health objective, but whether the use of those funds necessary to achieve the health objective is preferred to alternative non-health objectives the resources might also be used for.

Unlike CEA, where effects of an intervention or law are aggregated to a singular outcome measure (e.g., disease averted, lives saved, QALYs gained), CBA monetizes the value of all effects on outcomes (i.e., converts all effects to dollars gained or lost), which enables one to consider relative effects on outcomes originally measured in different natural units. The monetization occurs through a set of established techniques that include both revealed preference approaches (which base value from observed market behavior) or stated preference approaches (which acquire values through survey responses to hypothetical situations). The focus in CBA is on calculating the net benefit of policy option A over policy option B, where net benefits are calculated as the difference between the present discounted value of benefits of Policy A over Policy B and the present discounted value of their costs. At times, analysts have constructed benefit-cost ratios, which generate a reduced form estimate of the benefit per unit of cost (again using present discounted value of both). The problem with benefit-cost ratios is that the magnitude of the benefits and costs become hidden. For example, a benefit cost ratio of 3:1 regarding Medicaid expansion might reflect a $300 return per $100 cost per Medicaid enrollee, or a $30,000 return per $10,000 cost. Such magnitude order differences are important for policymakers to consider, which is why net benefit calculations are generally preferred.

There are two primary criticisms of CBA. First, many health agencies and organizations are uncomfortable with the monetization of all outcomes, which require assumptions that are generally not agreed upon either among economists or others (Drummond et al., 2015; Marsh, Phillips, Fordham, Bertranou, & Hale, 2012; Vining & Weimer, 2010; Viscusi & Aldy, 2003; Viscusi & Masterman, 2017). Ultimately, attaching a dollar value to outcomes depends on philosophical values—obvious when attaching dollar values to a person's life or years of ill-health. Second, CBA requires a thorough accounting of all potential effects, intended or unintended, beneficial or harmful, which are typically not known with certainty or reliability, especially when the CBA is being conducted prior to policy adoption. Given this difficulty, it is not uncommon for investigators to assess the sensitivity of findings by conducting a primary analysis in terms of a singular outcome using CEA or a subset of outcomes that are easily identifiable in a limited CBA, and then conducting a secondary extended analysis considering some, albeit not all, intended and unintended consequences using a CBA framework (e.g., Caulkins et al., 2002; Karoly, 2012; Kilmer, Burgdorf, D'amico, Miles, & Tucker, 2011; Kilmer, Caulkins, Pacula, MacCoun, & Reuter, 2010; Weimer & Vining, 2009).

Step 5: Determine Time Horizon and Discount Rate

Some public health laws stay in effect for decades (e.g., minimum legal drinking ages, prohibition of drugs, taxes on cigarettes), while others are short-lived. Thus, identifying the proper time horizon for costs, benefits and outcomes is complicated, particularly when the analysis is being done ex-ante and the duration of the policy is uncertain. Moreover, timing of when costs and benefits occur may differ across legal options under consideration. In some instances, cost of implementing a law is paid immediately or in proximity to the adoption of the law, while benefits (or unintended consequences) often accrue for years and even generations later. In other instances, the cost of a law (e.g., to legalize cannabis) is sustained over a long period of time, particularly if the law involves maintaining a new regulatory infrastructure (e.g., regulation of cannabis products and retail outlets). While often not achieved, the goal is a time horizon long enough to encompass all identifiable economic benefits and costs likely to accrue from the intervention (Office of Management and Budget, 2003).

In legal epidemiology, specifying a time horizon for CEA or CBA can be difficult for at three reasons. First, actual implementation of a law may happen immediately or might take years, or both when implementation requires incremental steps and stages. For example, legalization of adult-use cannabis in multiple states has led to the immediate removal of criminal penalties for possession and/or use of cannabis, but the much slower development of regulations on cannabis products and retail outlets. Second, effects of the law on institutions and behaviors may be immediate (e.g., revenue from taxation of cannabis sold) or evolve more slowly (effects on low-birth-weight babies associated with cannabis use during pregnancy, or increased rates of vomiting and psychosis caused by higher potency products coming on the market). Third, short-run effects may not be indicative of longer-term effects, particularly when a law might stay in effect for generations. A careful evaluator selects a time horizon that ensures the public health intervention has sufficient time to (1) be fully implemented, (2) affect the targeted recipients for a sufficient amount of time to reach a steady-state effectiveness rate, and (3) affect the general population for a sufficient amount of time such that spillover effects or unintended consequences are realized.

Importantly, as time horizon grows, so does uncertainty regarding the sustainability of policy implementation and magnitude of effects on the population's health (Basu & Maciejewski, 2019; Vining & Weimer, 2010). This is where simulation modeling, which can test alternative assumptions regarding rates of decay of effects of the policy on behavior over time, can be helpful. Considerable advancements have been made in the development of population-level single disease and multi-disease simulations. Such simulations consider progression of not just a particular disease on health but also their effects on productivity and income.

Discounting is a method for combining costs and benefits that occur at different times. It reflects both personal preferences and financial realities of markets. Goods and services received today are of greater value (when deemed desirable) than goods and services in the future, as most people are impatient and present-oriented and would prefer to consume them today. Moreover, if received today, they could be used and/or sold, with the proceeds earning a rate of return equal to the interest rate in the future. Thus, goods and services received today are of greater value than those in the future. Similarly costs that need to be paid out in the future have lower value today than their face value in the future because of the ability to earn a rate of return between now and then. Thus, discounting reflects these trade-offs of goods, services and income across time, including health (Claxton et al., 2019; Drummond et al., 2015).

There is general agreement that benefits and costs should be discounted at the same rate (Drummond et al., 2005; WHO, 2006), but not on what that rate should be when considering a social investment (Spackman, 2020). Economists usually use the risk-free rate of return on savings, such as the return on US Treasury bills, as a measure of the discount rate. For an intervention generating costs and benefits that displace other investments in the economy, economists tend to rely on a market rate of return, or the opportunity cost of capital (Council of Economic Advisers [CEA], 2017). The precise values of these social discounts can depend on the country considering the policy. In the United States, the US Office of Management and Budget (OMB) has recommended that US agencies apply both a 3% discount rate and a 7% discount rate for a public good that benefits society, and then assess the sensitivity of findings to these rates (OMB, 2003). The US Council of Economic Advisors (CEA) has suggested that these interest rates may be too high because of persistent declines over the past three decades in both the risk-free and long-term interest rates (CEA, 2017). Studies conducted in other, mostly European, nations following their own national guidelines use a lower range of values from 1.5% to 5% for studies with time horizons of at least 3 years (Haacker, Hallett, & Atun, 2020).

Step 6: Identify and Quantify Outcomes, Costs, and Benefits

Costing has two basic elements: (1) measure quantities of the resource used, and (2) assign the cost per unit (Drummond et al., 2015). There are challenges to both of these steps when examining policies at a population level, as not all resources involved in implementing a policy are easily identified or measured and assigning unit costs to those resources can be difficult. Tangible resources, such as personnel, supplies, technology and services, are the easiest to identify but can still create challenges for analysts assigning unit costs when market prices do not reflect the true opportunity cost of those resources. Intangible resources are particularly difficult to measure. The value of physically safe neighborhoods, for example, or the cost of pain and suffering from losing a loved one are difficult to measure. The value of intangible resources (lost life, feeling of safety and security) usually represent the largest share of total costs or benefits in an economic valuation, so their inclusion and method of calculation are important. A variety of methods have emerged to generate proxy prices for them, each with their own strengths and weaknesses (Boardman, Greenberg, Vining, & Weimer, 2011; Drummond et al., 2015).

Suppose we are analysts being asked to evaluate the economic benefit of a state's adoption of a law requiring physicians and pharmacists to access prescription drug records before prescribing or distributing opioids to patients, frequently referred to as must-access prescription drug monitoring programs (PDMPs). The objective is to reduce overprescribing of prescription opioids, thereby reducing overall access to opioid prescriptions, and hence risk of overdose. Must-access PDMPs involve establishment of state-level electronic databases that collect information from pharmacies, hospitals, physician offices, and other dispensers of pharmaceutical drugs on the controlled medications that are being distributed to each individual when they fill their prescriptions. These data are then made available to authorized users, usually doctors and other prescribers, for the purpose of learning about their patients' full history in filling prescriptions of interest before making additional prescriptions. In 43 states, law enforcement agencies also have access to these electronic databases, to monitor patients who may be seeking drugs by pharmacy and/or doctor shopping, as well as identify prescribers who may be improperly prescribing opioids or other controlled substances. Imagine we are told by the state's health department that they want to know what effect this must-access policy has had on opioid prescriptions per capita in the state—they hope to see a reduction—and how many lives it has saved from fatal opioid overdoses. We know the policy was adopted 5 years ago and fully implemented 3 years ago.

The example thus far provides a clear description of the question being asked and the law being evaluated. What is unclear is the perspective that should be taken and the time period for which this should be evaluated. Both affect the costs, benefits, and outcomes. Without such clarity, we start the exercise with a list of resources we can think will be used due to the adoption of the law, based on our knowledge of the scientific literature examining previously adopted PDMP laws. With this list, we can then check back with the state (our client) to make sure we have in fact considered all the costs they think are relevant. Table 16.1 provides a snippet of that list, describing first in broad categories the type of resources that we know the literature has already considered: health care resources, patient/family resources, and some other non-health care community resources. Concrete examples of specific community resources in each of these broad categories are shown in each row. Because the state did not specify what perspective we should take in conducting our analysis (health care agency + patient perspective or societal perspective), and because we

Table 16.1. Identifying and Valuing a Partial List of Costs and Cost-Savings Associated with a State Must-Access Prescription Drug Monitoring Programs.

	Examples of Costs Included in Category	Valuation of Cost from Health Care Agency + Patient (HCA + P) Perspective	Valuation of Costs from Societal Perspective
Health care resources (costs and potential cost savings)			
Technology implementation	Purchase of hardware and software technology enabling the remote access, lookup, and importation of data into PDMP system across different health systems/IT platforms in a manner meeting HIPAA requirements	Market prices associated with the IT hardware, software, and installation services to get the system functioning, storage capacity (server) for the database, and enhanced cyber security. Rent for facility storing database	Same
IT support and maintenance costs	Labor providing software, hardware IT, and network support, as well as technology costs to meet security requirements	Market prices for IT support, software updates, server maintenance, and cyber security	Same
Provider/ pharmacist training	Develop training materials and implement training	Wages for labor and market prices for materials/travel necessary to develop and deliver training either in person or virtually	Same
Provider/pharmacy monitoring	Labor and software materials needed to ensure use by all providers/ pharmacists	Programmer and management time and wages, market prices of resources used to verify utilization by prescribers/distributors	HCA + P cost plus any potential positive/negative spillovers monitoring has for medical malpractice litigation

(Continued)

Table 16.1. (Continued)

	Examples of Costs Included in Category	Valuation of Cost from Health Care Agency + Patient (HCA + P) Perspective	Valuation of Costs from Societal Perspective
Regulating agency responsibilities	Board or health agency responsible for conducting surveillance of over prescribers and implementation of penalties; and coordinate with law enforcement	Programmer and management time and wages, analyst time and wages to identify and report suspicious behavior as indicated by data	HCA + P cost plus potential negative/positive spillover effects this surveillance and monitoring has on prescribers/pharmacies practices
Treatment utilization associated with opioid misuse (cost savings)	Cost of treating patients with an opioid addiction (inpatient/outpatient detox, behavioral therapy, and/or medication assisted therapy)	Therapist and staff time and wages for scheduling, intake, therapeutic plan development, and delivery of therapy, rental rate of space where therapy takes place for time of therapy	HCA + P cost plus spillover effects (positive or negative) this change in treatment utilization has on access to treatment by other patients in need of treatment
Other non-addiction treatment health care services	Averted or new opioid-involved non-overdose ED visits, outpatient visits, complications caused by opioid-using pregnant women; NICU cost of opioid-dependent newborns plus cost (or cost savings) associated with non-opioid treatment of pain	Insurance-negotiated price of labor, diagnostics, therapies, facility fees, and prescriptions averted due to reduction in prescription opioids + saved out of pocket cost of patients	HCA + P cost plus any rise in health care service use caused by shift to other opioids (heroin, fentanyl) or non-opioid therapies outside of the health care system
Cost of responding to overdose (cost savings)	ER, hospital, and ambulance service providers time and capacity costs	Insurance-negotiated prices of labor, diagnostics, therapies for medical and first-responding staff to manage averted Rx opioid overdose	HCA + P cost plus spillover effects due to increased/reduced capacity of ED and first responders on respond quickly and care for other emergency patients

Patient/family resources (cost and potential cost savings)

Extra hassle created for patients to find docs willing to prescribe opioids	Time costs, transportation costs, hassle of finding new provider, family caregiving while time is spent seeking new care	Wages for lost time and caregiving costs, market rates for transportation/parking/tolls, proxy value for stress/hassle	HCA + P cost plus spillover costs on family members or friends who assist patient in these efforts or cover at home/child care to facilitate search
Increased or decreased functionality and productivity associated with change in opioid prescriptions	Ability to do activities of daily living and/or other activities that could be managed either because opioids provided relief from pain or because opioid addiction impaired functionality	Proxy value for functionality of patient	HCA + P cost plus additional cost/cost savings associated with family members/friends who had to assist patient either due to non-treated chronic pain or addiction
Increased or decreased risk of addiction associated with lower access to Rx opioids	Savings/costs from new opioid-dependent patients due to either lower initiation of Rx opioids, or switch to more potent illicit opioids	Proxy value of cost of living with addiction	HCA + P cost plus additional proxy value for emotional cost/cost savings of family members/friends who are affected by patient
Increased or decreased risk in opioid related mortality	Costs or savings associated with rise/fall in opioid-related mortality	Proxy value for lost/saved life from opioid overdose	Proxy value of pain and suffering of those who lost/saved the loved one, foster care placements (caused by overdose of a parent).

Non-health care community costs

(1) Law Enforcement costs

Surveillance of patients seeking meds through doctor shopping/pharmacy shopping	Labor and software materials needed to set up monitoring algorithms in data, investigate potential suspects	Not considered	Market wages and prices of software and supplies related to monitoring plus proxy price for the opportunity cost of law enforcement time spent allocated to this versus other policing activities

(Continued)

Table 16.1. (Continued)

	Examples of Costs Included in Category	Valuation of Cost from Health Care Agency + Patient (HCA + P) Perspective	Valuation of Costs from Societal Perspective
Surveillance of and actions related to over-prescribers	Labor and software materials needed to set up monitoring algorithms in data, investigate potential suspects, coordinate with health agency	Not considered	Market wages and prices of software and supplies related to monitoring plus proxy price for the opportunity cost of law enforcement time spent allocated to this versus other policing activities
Spillover of patients to black market seeking access to medications there (Alpert et al., 2018)	Labor and investigative resources to monitor and intervene strategically in local illicit market, track domestic/international supply chain, deal with rising drug-related arrests	Not considered	Market wages, market cost of surveillance resources for local and federal law enforcement who track and investigate illicit markets, time spent processing new drug arrests, plus proxy value for the opportunity cost of law enforcement time spent allocated to this task versus other policing activities
(2) Neighborhood/ community costs			
Rise in illicit markets related to reduced access through medical sector (Alpert et al., 2018)	Marginal impacts of growth in illicit market on community safety, cohesion, and economic opportunities	Not considered	In addition to law enforcement costs mentioned above, there are impacts on employment choices of community members (legal or illicit job market and implied trajectories), risk of crime generated by drug markets and overall neighborhood safety, which have to be measured using proxy values

Impact on Emergency First responders system (Pike et al., 2019)	Marginal impacts on EMT and ambulance resources associated with change in fatal overdoses	To the extent that these are paid for by the health care system, they are included above. Any community resources (e.g., fire, police, 9-1-1-lines, and community groups) would be added here	HCA + P costs plus any spillover effects on community agencies (fire, police, community volunteers) due to increase/decrease in opioid related 9-1-1 calls
Impact on social welfare related to infants and children of parents misusing opioids (Feder et al., 2019)	Marginal impacts on social services, foster care, and other agencies who manage children who are in the care of an individual struggling with addiction	Not considered	Market value of labor time and resources used in conducting social service activities (monitoring, evaluation, placement) in addition to proxy value on children for loss of parent
Potential impact on disability and labor markets (Maclean, Mallatt, Ruhm, & Simon, 2021)	Marginal impacts on labor market supply, employment, productivity	Not considered	Proxy value for changes in rates of unemployment, lost/gained wages due to reduced productivity of opioid users, lost/gain tax revenue

know that the societal perspective is the recommended perspective when conducting an economic evaluation of a public health law due to its use of society's limited resources (Drummond et al., 2015; Vining & Weimer, 2010), we construct our list of resources using both perspectives so we can share insights using each with our client.

Let's try to describe a bit more carefully what some of the actual resources are that we want to measure and cost for this exercise. Within the health care system, the implementation of a must-access PDMP requires information technology (IT) infrastructure (hardware, software, networking systems allowing for remote access and real-time updates) that can be assessable from both pharmacies and prescribers' offices. Greater use can be achieved by having this integrated into the prescribers' existing health system software, to avoid double entries and/or multiple look ups, but that could require new IT platforms that allow for communication about patient sensitive data in a manner that meets Health Information Portability and Accountability Act of 1996 (HIPAA) requirements. Ongoing IT support of the PDMP database created as well as the software and hardware supporting it will be required. Training may be required for all end users, and for those responsible for monitoring prescriptions and checking compliance. These are the most obvious tangible health care resources involved in implementing the PDMP system. If the system is effective in reducing unnecessary opioid prescribing and deterring misuse of opioids, then there will be additional outcomes that also affect the health care system and agency resources, such as a reduction (or possible increase) in the number of patients needing opioid addiction treatment, the number of opioid-involved emergency department visits, complications caused by opioid-using pregnant women, and neonatal intensive care unit costs associated with fewer opioid-dependent babies. These changes, if realized within the time period being considered in the evaluation study, would represent resources saved within the health care system on account of the law as well as costs incurred responding to an opioid overdose (Table 16.1).

Must-access PDMPs will also influence patients, and possibly their family members. Exactly how depends on the policy's actual impacts (part of what the evaluation is designed to explore) as well as the time period over which they are considered. For example, some individuals who had been using the health care system to obtain prescription opioids for nonmedical use will now find it more difficult to obtain prescriptions from multiple physicians or fill them at multiple pharmacies, as this sort of doctor shopping and pharmacy shopping behavior is exactly what these PDMPs are designed to discourage. However, the oversight created by PDMPs has also caused some prescribers to be less willing to prescribe an opioid either because of the additional hassle of having to check the PDMP system before doing so (affecting new and existing patients) or because they do not want to trigger investigations into their medical practice by continuing to prescribe high doses of opioids to patients with chronic pain conditions. When comparable non-opioid therapies are available to address pain experienced by patients, this behavioral change by prescribers has no negative effect on patients aside from the time spent trying to find an alternative therapy that works. Moreover, it may lead to an overall societal net benefit as fewer people are at risk of becoming dependent on opioids when fewer opioids are being prescribed for pain. However, when comparable non-opioid therapies are not available to patients who have been using high-dose opioids to manage chronic pain, this behavioral change by prescribers places an additional burden on patients who must now either look for a new provider who is willing to prescribe opioids in high doses or, if that is unsuccessful, find a nonmedical (illegal) supply. The time and hassle spent searching for these new therapies and sources of supply represent a real cost to the patient. Additionally, there may be lost functionality and/or productivity that occurs during this time. Those individuals who choose to turn to illegal sources of supply for opioids are now placed at greater risk of both addiction and unexpected overdose due to the unregulated products available through illegal markets.

An analysis of just the health care agency plus patient perspective would stop there. However, we know from the literature that a robust must-access PDMP policy will necessarily involve resources from law enforcement as well, because law enforcement agencies have primary responsibility for investigating and prosecuting individuals inappropriately seeking medications through the health care system. They may also be directed to investigate prescribers who appear to overprescribe medications for financial gain rather than patient welfare. To the extent that patients seek illicit sources for their medications first, and then cheaper opioid alternatives like heroin and fentanyl, the illicit market will grow requiring even more law enforcement resources to squash incoming supply. The presence of, and profits associated with, illicit markets can generate harms to neighborhoods, by making them less safe. Neighborhoods become unsafe due to actions of both the illicit suppliers seeking to protect new territories as well as by the consumers, who due to their opioid use may become less attentive and engage in risky behaviors (leaving children unattended, engaging in fights, impaired driving, sharing needles, and so on). Regular or persistent consumers of high-potency opioids are likely to become addicted, generating effects on the individual's family members (children, spouses, parents) who may rely on that individual for income, care giving, or emotional support. Those children who are no longer able to be cared for by the consumer are sent to relatives or the foster care system. These are just a few examples of non-health effects that research has already identified, but there is now enough variety in resources already mentioned to start thinking about the challenges of assigning unit prices to each.

Having identified various community resources affected by a must-access PDMP, we will need to consider the time period over which to evaluate these effects and costs. Given rates of opioid mortality are still rising exponentially, it would seem as though the targeted recipients (nonmedical users of opioids at risk of opioid fatality) have not yet reached a steady state in response to the law's adoption, so for the purposes of our hypothetical example, I would suggest we use at least a 10-year period, which would allow some of the spillover effects on the community to be felt and measured. Now, we are ready to start thinking about the costs of these resources.

As mentioned already, market-based valuations are frequently considered to be good approximations of the values of resources, particularly when markets are working efficiently on their own. In our example of the must-access PDMP policy, market prices for labor, hardware, software and supplies needed to build, operate and maintain the PDMP platform (hardware, software and network) as well as train people on it are all appropriate as these goods and services are all sold in highly competitive markets. There are other categories of resources shown in Table 16.1, however, for which market prices will not work for at least two reasons: (1) the market list price or price paid by the agency is not reflective of their true opportunity cost of those resources, and (2) the resources are not formally traded in markets (e.g., time spent looking for non-opioid therapies or alternative prescribers, feeling of safety in a neighborhood, value of a life lost due to an overdose).

In the case of health care, there is a pervasive problem that the list prices or charges that hospitals, physicians and even pharmaceutical companies charge for their products and services do not reflect their true opportunity cost. This is due to the fact that health care markets in the United States are not truly competitive; imperfect and asymmetric information coupled with high barriers to entry do not allow competition to drive prices down to the true social value of the inputs being used in production. So, using list charges or fees, which do not reflect the prices that insurance companies or other payers pay, would not appropriately capture their value as they include overhead costs (the cost of maintaining the hospital or ambulatory care building structure, or training residents) and the fixed/sunk costs of specific investments they already made (having extensive medical technology ready to use, or recovering costs from research and development of new pharmaceuticals). So, when estimating the value of fewer (or greater) opioid treatment admissions in response to must-access PDMP adoption, as shown in Table 16.1, we only want to include the marginal cost of providing this treatment. To do this, we want to consider the time spent by an administrator involved in intaking a new patient, the therapist (or team of therapists) developing a therapeutic plan, and then the provider's time engaged in delivering that treatment. This can be constructed by considering the time of the providers and staff involved in these activities and their wages, not actual charges to patients. Similarly, when considering the cost to the health care system of responding to an overdose, we do not want to consider the price of the ambulance or firetruck responding to the overdose. Instead, it is the time and wages of the team responding to the call as well as any medical services used while treating the person in need. Costing these specific units involved in the delivery of care rather than average cost of delivering care to everyone served better captures the incremental cost of the resources being used for this law.

Table 16.1 also provides numerous examples of patient and non-health care system resources that are not actually traded in markets, such as the patient's time spent investigating alternative treatments or providers, the functionality patients gain through the appropriate use of prescription opioids and lose when these medications become unavailable to them, and the value of lives saved through avoided fatal overdoses. For these intangible effects, analysts typically use proxy prices that are obtained using one of three primary approaches: (1) *human capital*, which try to assess the added or lost value of the nonmarket good in terms of productive time; (2) *revealed preference*, which use real information conveyed in markets for related or similar goods and services; and (3) *stated preference*, which are methods that seek to elicit through surveys and hypothetical scenarios how a consumer values various nonmarket goods.

For a long time, economists have used the value of lost earnings in the marketplace, or the *human capital* approach, as the primary method for measuring the opportunity cost of time and nonmarket goods that are related to time, like a lost life. The basic premise for this approach is that the person's wage is a good measure of what the person is giving up by not working, so whenever the person chooses to not work and do something else instead, it clearly must be valued at least as much as the same time they could have spent at work. There are several limitations of this approach that have been discussed in the literature (Boardman et al., 2011; Drummond et al., 2015), but two are particularly important here. First, this approach ignores serious imperfections in labor markets which are known to exist. Look within any society and you will find subpopulations based on gender, race and ethnicity being paid differential amounts for the exact same work due to discrimination. Similarly, looking across jobs there are enormous inconsistencies in pay per value of the job. For example, entertainers and elite athletes get paid wages that far exceed those of school teachers, police and fire fighters, yet few would argue that these highly paid individuals are worth that much more to society. Second, the use of wages as a proxy price for the value of time ignores the consumption value people place on their time. When we take time to make a meal from scratch with healthy ingredients, the value of the time spent cooking itself may be a pleasurable activity. The fact that pain medication enables a patient to work a productive workday is important and valuable, but only using a measure of the wage ignores the value that patient places on the additional pain-free time that medication allows them to have enjoyable activities at home with friends and family. In light of these two serious limitations, human capital methods have moved somewhat out of favor as a means of valuing nonmarket goods, although they are still used to value lost work time or productivity due to being sick or in pain.

Revealed preference approaches are those that attempt to use information revealed through existing markets for proxy goods (increased safety, lower risk of death) to infer the value of a range of nonmarket goods, including time and lost life. Given the range of nonmarket goods we need to price (e.g., stress/hassle of finding new therapies, functionality when experiencing less pain, safe neighborhoods, and value of lost life), it is perhaps not surprising that a wide variety of revealed preference approaches have emerged, including the market analogy method, intermediate good method, hedonic price method, travel cost methods and defensive expenditures method (Boardman et al., 2011). The validity of the estimates produced from any of these methods depends critically on that method's ability to isolate the unique value of the proxy good itself.

For example, some studies have used differential housing values in high crime neighborhoods versus low crime neighborhoods as a way of valuing a safe neighborhood. In theory this would work great, except that those other attributes of homes also influence their pricing across neighborhoods including proximity to a major freeway or jobs, noise, pollution, school districts, and proximity to green space or beaches. So, if the goal is to isolate the value placed on safety alone, the analyst must use methods that allow them to isolate the variation in housing associated with crime alone and not other factors.

The two main revealed preference approaches commonly used to estimate the value of lost life are (1) wage premium approach and (2) defensive expenditure approach. Both approaches assess the value of a lost life by calculating the extra income (expenditure) people receive (pay) to take on incrementally larger (smaller) risks. The wage premium approach uses information about risk premiums people receive for taking on different risks on the job for similar work, such as doing construction on skyscrapers versus working construction on one- or two-story buildings, as an indicator of the payment that must be received for greater risk of death. Because people have different preferences for risk and different abilities to assess risk, the values of a lost life obtained using this method can range widely, from $920,000 to $20 million (Hirth, Chernew, Miller, Fendrick, & Weissert, 2000). The defensive expenditure approach uses information on how much people pay in the marketplace for safety devices that produce small reductions in the risk of fatality to construct estimates of the value of lost life. Given the range of defensive purchases made (from bike helmets to safer cars), the range of estimates of the value of lost life using the defensive purchase methods also vary widely, from $770,000 to $9.9 million (Viscusi & Aldy, 2003). It is unclear to what extent these large variances result because of variation in the quality of studies (i.e., the analyst doing a better/worse job controlling for other attributes that people like about these goods), the inability of the consumer to understand the change in risk associated with these purchases, or because the valuation of life differs based on number of years of life remaining.

Given the limitations and concerns of revealed preference approaches, alternative methods relying on *stated preferences* have emerged. The two most common stated preference methods are (1) contingent valuation (Arrow et al., 1993; Mitchell & Carson, 2013), where individuals are asked through surveys what they would be willing to pay (or be paid to avoid) a particular outcome (e.g., a reduction in risk of illness or death), contingent upon a hypothetical situation, and (2) discrete choice experiments (Green & Gerard, 2009; Ryan, Gerard, & Amaya-Amaya, 2008), where individuals are given a series of hypothetical scenarios that differ along very specific attributes related to the nonmarket good and, based on responses to these scenarios, a valuation can be calculated. There are several advantages of these methods over previous methods mentioned, particularly when trying to construct an estimate of the value of life, as they can be used to value mortality risks for which we have little reliable market analogs (e.g., cancer risk or terrorism attack), and they can be used to obtain estimates of valuations from children and elderly directly (who often have surrogates purchasing goods for them in the market place). However, these methods also have their limitations, in that they assume that people can reliably understand the implicit tradeoffs of the scenarios described, and accurately assess the likelihood of low and high probability events, which is a common error for many (Thaler & Sunstein, 2009). Moreover, there is evidence that people tend to undervalue hypothetical income or risks, a phenomenon known as "hypothetical bias" (Harrison & Rutström, 2008). Given these concerns, guidelines for the proper conduct of both of these approaches have been developed and continue to get refined, as improper implementation can lead to inconsistencies in valuations derived from these methods (Boyle, 2017; de Bekker-Grob, Ryan, & Gerard, 2012; Johnson et al., 2013; Lancsar & Louviere, 2008). Estimates of the value of a life using these methods also tend to be large, ranging from $100,000 to $25.9 million (Hirth et al., 2000).

Due to the tremendous variation in values for a lost life in the academic literature generated from these three approaches (human capital, revealed preference and stated preference), many government agencies use their own preferred proxy value when conducting studies (Viscusi, 2010). For example, the US Environmental Protection Agency uses $7.5 million (in 2006 dollars) as its recommended standard price for the value of a life saved or lost (EPA, 2012), the US Department of Transportation (United States Department of Transportation (DOT), 2016) uses a value of $9.6 million (in 2015 dollars), and until just recently when values were updated for inflation, the Department of Health and Human Services had been using an average value of $9 million (in 2013 dollars) (US HHS, 2021). These are not trivial differences, as few other costs or benefits considered on a per unit basis have variation in value in the millions. Thus, any analyst concerned about which proxy estimate for the value of lost or saved life to use should check the sensitivity of their result to alternative, reasonable values.

Even though we have not assigned actual prices or counted resources affected in our example, it is clear from Table 16.1 that an economic evaluation conducted from a societal perspective requires additional considerations of factors even if we only focus on counting health care system resources. This is because the societal perspective requires the consideration of unintended consequences associated with the must-access PDMP law that may result from its adoption. For example, the development of the must-access PDMP platform may assist plaintiffs (patients, health insurance companies, and other payers) seeking to sue providers or prescription drug companies for overprescribing of opioids, anti-psychotics, or other medications. Alternatively, the system might make certain providers or pharmacies willing to maintain opioid prescribing and dispensing routines targets of thieves seeking medications. Such spillover effects, which clearly affect certain health care actors although not in expected ways, would be considered when using the societal perspective, but not the health care agency and patient perspective. More importantly, the societal perspective considers effects on a wide range of agencies not directly affected by the PDMP law but involved in addressing the harms and implications of opioid misuse and fatalities, namely law enforcement agencies, extended family members, neighborhoods, and social services. The inclusion of these additional community resources that are utilized in response to changes in medical and nonmedical opioid use can dramatically influence the net impact of the PDMP on the state's resources.

Regardless of which perspective is taken, there are resources in Table 16.1 for which fairly reliable market prices are available (e.g., health IT costs, training costs) and then some intangible effects where there is likely to be pretty large ranges for valuations (e.g., proxy value for functionality of the patient, living with addiction or lost/saved lives). Moreover, the exact number of units of each resource to count may be uncertain due to uncertainty associated with actual effects. For example, if more patients choose to seek alternative treatments in lieu of opioids, then the effects (in terms of resources) of must-access PDMPs on first responders would be less than if more patients decide to use illicit opioids. Similarly, if pregnant women or mothers of young children seek treatment rather than an alternative source of pain medications, there is less need for medical and social services. This sort of uncertainty of effects is not uncommon in many evaluations of social policies (Vining & Weimer, 2010) and is what makes cost–benefit and cost-effectiveness analysis particularly challenging. Recommendations on how to deal with these issues are discussed in Steps 7 and 8.

Step 7: Assess Effectiveness of All Policy Alternatives Being Considered

Effectiveness estimates are typically obtained from original research conducted on small pilots, a randomized controlled trial (RCT), a natural experiment, and/or reviews and meta-analyses of existing findings from established literature. The reliability of information on effectiveness from these sources should still be assessed by the analyst in terms of its applicability to the specific evaluation being done. Reliability and applicability of previous effectiveness findings for the economic evaluation will depend on several factors, including representativeness of the sample that was previously studied vis-à-vis the current population, specific effects considered, quality of the data used to estimate effects, and quality of the research designs used.

Studies evaluating policy candidates often rely on sample data that is not fully representative of the larger and more diverse population the law would eventually affect. One of the most prominent RCTs examining the effect of early preschool on poor, at-risk youth was the Perry Preschool experiment, conducted in the late 1960s on a sample of 123 African American children living in Michigan. While the experimental design and implementation of the study were technically strong and appropriate for the question being asked at the time, the generalizability of these findings for other at-risk youth populations in other settings and time periods has been appropriately questioned, leading to subsequent follow up studies using different populations and settings (Lally, Mangoine, & Honig, 1987; Masse & Barnett, 2002). The effectiveness of the policy is also a function of the targeted population's acceptance and responsiveness to the policy, which may differ from those observed in a pilot or RCT due to factors such as demographics, culture, attachment to institutions, and political philosophies. Finally, effects can differ across subpopulations due to differential implementation, enforcement and/or compliance due to cultural or social differences across populations. For more on RCTs in policy candidate and evaluation research, see Chapter 13.

Even if the population from which the effectiveness measure is drawn is similar to the population targeted by the policy being evaluated, the outcomes measured in the prior research might differ from those being considered in the economic evaluation. For example, an RCT might identify effects of a policy on health care utilization while the analyst doing an economic evaluation is concerned about effects of the policy on health outcomes or lost productivity. In such instances analysts connect findings from various studies to link policy effects on utilization to effects on health and productivity, for example. A more difficult problem for analysts is when studies only evaluate effects over a short period of time, say 3, 6 or 12 months, when the analyst needs to incorporate longer term effects 10 or 20 years later. An analyst cannot simply assume that effects observed over short periods will hold for longer periods. There are too many factors that can change over time, including implementation, enforcement, compliance, and norms, that can cause an estimated effect to decay or grow over time. Analysts facing the problem of unmeasured long-term effects often have to make assumptions about the persistence of effects, using either mathematical function approximations or carefully modeled trajectories accounting for plausible shifts in factors that might influence persistence over time. Regardless of technique, recent guidelines related to the conduct of cost benefit analysis of social policies recommend using modeling techniques that consider multiple assumptions about decay or growth, rather than just one, to illustrate sensitivity of findings to the assumptions made (Crowley et al., 2018; Henrichson & Rinaldi, 2014; NASEM, 2016).

Assumptions regarding persistence of a policy effects are important, and often not given sufficient consideration. The current US opioid epidemic is a good reminder of the dangers of presuming a constant policy effect over time in a dynamic world. By all accounts, the opioid epidemic began in the late 1990s and early 2000s by the overpromotion and excess prescribing of opioids, in particular OxyContin (Alpert, Evans, Lieber, & Powell, 2022). But by 2010, when states started implementing supply restrictions and OxyContin got reformulated to reduce the ability of consumers to crush and snort it, the opioid crisis shifted as consumers who had already become dependent on OxyContin moved to a cheaper, more potent substitute, heroin (Powell, Alpert, & Pacula, 2019; Powell & Pacula, 2021). While PDMP laws were generally found to reduce opioid mortality for much of the early 2000s, after 2010 prescription opioids were no longer the primary driver of opioid mortality, heroin was (and then fentanyl). The effectiveness of PDMPs at reducing opioid drug overdoses, therefore, could not be presumed to be the same after 2010 as it was before 2010 (Kim, 2021).

Finally, data quality is important. Factors influencing the quality of data include the data generating process, the suppression of certain jurisdictions due to lack of reporting from them, and the extent to which the available data truly reflect the outcome of interest. Even widely-used, publicly provided data, such as the Centers for Disease Control National Vital Statistics Surveillance (NVSS) system, the Agency for Health Care Quality and Research Hospital Cost Utilization Program (HCUP) data, and the CMS Medicare/Medicaid data have limitations or have undergone significant changes in data collection processes that influence the quality of the data for studying particular phenomena. Not all researchers are fully informed about these limitations and changes, which can cause them to use the data inappropriately.

In the case of the NVSS data, for example, it is now well-understood that systematic differences in the coding of opioid-involvement, overall and by type of opioid, existed on death certificates across states throughout the first decade of the opioid crisis. This systematic difference in coding occurred because some states use medical examiners (trained medical career professionals) to fill out death certificates, while other states use coroners (politically appointed staffers) to do so (Davis & National Association of Medical Examiners and American College of Medical Toxicology Expert Panel on Evaluating and Reporting Opioid Deaths, 2013). The implication is that death certificates from states which use coroners are less likely to identify the specific type of opioid involved in a drug overdose, while states with medical examiners are more likely to record type of opioid involved when such information can be determined. The differential reporting of these data across states complicates analyses evaluating state PDMP policies on opioid-specific mortality rates (e.g., prescription opioid mortality, heroin mortality or synthetic opioid/fentanyl mortality) as some states get dropped entirely from these analyses because of data limitations despite having relevant laws in place. Researchers who are aware of this issue have developed imputation methods and supplemental analyses to verify the magnitude and direction of estimated policy effects (Ruhm, 2016, 2017). But not all studies reflect awareness of data anomalies, which is why analysts need to consider data quality issues before using a study's measure of effectiveness in an economic evaluation.

Step 8: Conduct Sensitivity Analyses, Examine Primary Drivers of Uncertainty

Uncertainty is expected in any economic evaluation. Uncertainty arises from many sources, including uncertainty regarding the degree of implementation, enforcement, or compliance with an adopted policy, uncertainty regarding estimates of effectiveness on outcomes from existing studies, uncertainty with respect to market valuations of benefits and costs (both now and in the future), uncertainty associated with forecast projection period, and uncertainty associated with models (data and parameters) used to determine presumed effectiveness of a policy on outcomes beyond those measured in the literature. A careful economic evaluation does not eliminate uncertainty, but succinctly and clearly articulates the extent to which this uncertainty matters for decision-making by end users of the economic evaluation.

Best practice includes additional supplementary analyses (referred to as "sensitivity analyses") of estimated cost-effectiveness or net benefit for comparison with "base case" estimates. Base case estimates are those that are calculated using the preferred values of all the variables and assumptions: estimate of effectiveness, value of benefits and costs, preferred discount rate, preferred projection of future trends, and so on. Sensitivity analyses are conducted by using alternative plausible values of variables and modeling assumptions (Crowley et al., 2018; Drummond et al., 2015; Briggs, Sculpher, & Buxton, 1994). The alternative values are usually easy to find. Most published studies evaluating effectiveness of a given policy will report not just the average effect of a policy on an outcome but also the 95% confidence interval. Similarly, it is often possible to obtain lower and upper bound estimates of specific valuations of costs and benefits to capture the heterogeneity in values that might be relevant (e.g., if there is population heterogeneity). Model parameter uncertainty can similarly be considered by rerunning the model with alternative values of specific parameters for which a plausible range of values are likely to exist, testing the sensitivity of the model results to these different parameter values (Briggs et al., 1994). Testing the sensitivity of the base case calculation of cost-effectiveness or cost–benefit to alternative sources of uncertainty clarifies how robust the results are.

Two approaches are used when conducting sensitivity analyses: univariate sensitivity analysis and multivariate sensitivity analyses. The approach depends on the analyst's certainty regarding values used in the base case, which is a function of the quality of the work generating those values. When there are relatively few factors for which the analyst is uncertain and those uncertain factors are not interdependent, then the analyst will usually adopt a univariate approach, sometimes referred to as a partial or one-way sensitivity analysis (Drummond et al., 2015; NASEM, 2016). Implementation of this approach is easy in that the analyst simply conducts the same analysis over and over again, each time varying the single parameter of interest within the pre-specified range of values, holding all the other estimates and values at their baseline case values. Univariate sensitivity analysis, when done iteratively for all potentially uncertain values in a calculation, is useful for identifying which parameter or parameters are key in generating uncertainty about the value of the overall calculation. Many economic evaluations will generate what is known as a tornado graph to demonstrate the sensitivity of the final net benefit or cost effectiveness calculation to alternative plausible model assumptions. Figure 16.1 is an illustration of a tornado graph assuming the median net benefit calculation of our hypothetical PDMP policy discussed in Step 6 is $1.5 million. Each row in the tornado graph shows the impact on that positive net benefit calculation of changing a single parameter used in the baseline estimate, holding all other parameter values constant at the baseline value.

Bars to the right of $1.5 million show that the calculation becomes even more positive than the baseline calculation, while bars to the left show that the calculation becomes less positive. It is not until we assume the lowest value for a statistical life that the net benefit calculation is no longer positive. Thus, this

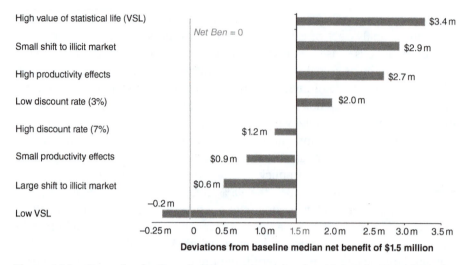

Figure 16.1. Example of a Tornado Diagram Assessing Sensitivity of a Hypothetical Model of Effectiveness of Must-Access PDMPs.

tornado graph conveys to the analyst and decision maker that only one of our uncertain underlying assumptions changes the overall conclusion of the study, although the uncertainty definitely influences the magnitude of that net gain.

The univariate sensitivity approach ignores associations between parameters, that is, their covariance. For example, the size of the shift of consumers to the illicit market is likely to be correlated with lost productivity time in addition to the number of individuals who die from an illicit fentanyl. Monte Carlo methods, which involve repeatedly sampling parameter values from a pre-determined range for all uncertain parameters simultaneously and allowing for joint distributional assumptions across parameter values, allows the analyst to construct an estimate of the variance around the calculated estimate of net benefit or cost-effectiveness in a manner that considers simultaneous changes in multiple parameters. Because multivariate sensitivity analyses comprehensively consider the various types of uncertainty, it is the recommended approach (Crowley et al., 2018; NASEM, 2016; OMB, 2003; Vining & Weimer, 2010). The larger the number of samples drawn through the Monte Carlo methods the more reliable the estimate of the variance; thus, typically simulations are repeated tens of thousands of times. Results of Monte Carlo simulations (e.g., 10,000 trials) can then be plotted using histograms, which show the share of trials for which a particular value of the net benefit or cost-effectiveness ratio emerge, illustrated in Figure 16.2 for our hypothetical assessment of the net benefits of must- access PDMPs.

In CBA, analysts typically summarize uncertainty using the proportion of Monte Carlo trials conducted that yield a positive net benefit calculation, because only policies with a positive net benefit would be recommended (NASEM, 2016; Vining & Weimer, 2010). If the proportion of trials generating a positive net benefit is large, for example 86% in the hypothetical presented in Figure 16.2, then the analyst can be reasonably comfortable that under a range of scenarios the policy will generate a net benefit. However, it is still useful to

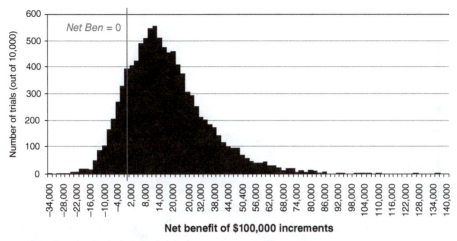

Figure 16.2. CBA Monte Carlo Simulation Results (10,000 Trials).

convey to the decision maker that there are scenarios where the net benefit could be negative. As the proportion of positive net benefit calculations moves further away from 100%, the relative certainty of a societal gain with adoption of the policy decreases.

Similar methods exist for conveying uncertainty around a single incremental cost effectiveness value (Boardman, Greenberg, Vining, & Weimer, 2017; Polsky, Glick, Willke, & Schulman, 1997). However, when conducting CEA, there usually is not always a single target value that analysts are trying to reach. Given the uncertainty in both the underlying assumptions of the CEA construction as well as the threshold values of interest, cost effectiveness acceptability curves have become a common tool for conveying uncertainty when CEA is used. The cost effectiveness acceptability curve summarizes in a single graph the uncertainty associated with any single CEA calculation as well as the threshold value that any particular CEA may be trying to achieve. As shown in Figure 16.3, the cost effectiveness acceptability curve shows the percent of Monte Carlo simulation runs accounting for uncertainty generating cost-effectiveness ratios exceeding different threshold values of willingness to pay (specified in terms of $ per QALY).

One aspect of uncertainty that is often overlooked is the role of benefits/ costs that could not be valued in the exercise, either because they involve nonmarket goods for which valuations are highly contested (e.g., the value of a statistical life, or loss of child during pregnancy) or because evidence on potential spillover effects has not yet been produced, even if such spillover effects are possible (e.g., the extent to which pain patients decide to seek pain medications through illicit markets rather than seek non-opioid therapies within the medical system). Several examples of these were offered in Table 16.1 where the valuation of costs and benefits for a must-access PDMP were considered. In work with my colleagues at RAND, we would refer to these uncertain but potentially important effects as "wild cards"

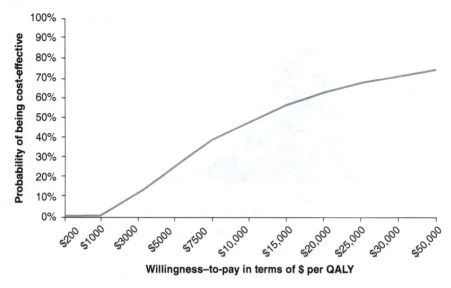

Figure 16.3. Cost Effectiveness Acceptability Curve for Must Access PDMP in Terms of $/QALY.

(Caulkins et al., 2015; Kilmer et al., 2010). While it is not possible to explicitly include them in the economic evaluation, the circumstances under which these unknown factors can switch the final calculation from positive to negative is something that should be conveyed to decision makers if known.

Step 9: Apply Decision Rule Criteria under All Plausible Uncertainty From Step 8 and Clearly Report Results

Depending on the question being asked and the type of economic evaluation undertaken, different summary measures can be generated, and whether a law is a good investment will depend on the summary measure used. For CBA, net benefit and benefit–cost ratios are the most common summary measures employed, but occasionally internal rates of return and return on investment are also used. When using net benefit as the primary decision rule, the reference decision point may be a net benefit > 0, if comparing a policy to the status quo, or it may be a minimal positive value if comparing across policies. As noted previously, benefit–cost ratios might also be used, with any value greater than 1 indicating more benefit to costs (some have also reported cost–benefit ratios, where a ratio < 1 would indicate higher benefit per dollar of cost), but these ratios hide information about the relative magnitude of the benefits and costs vis-à-vis other options that might also be considered, which may also be useful information to the decision makers. For CEA, summary measures include cost-effectiveness ratios or incremental cost-effectiveness ratios for the cost per outcome gained, where the outcome measure can vary from narrow outcomes, such as infection rates, disease rates, or hospitalizations averted, to more comprehensive measures, such as quality- or disability-adjusted life years.

Regardless of the method and measure used, it is critical to clearly communicate the results of the evaluation in a manner that enables understanding of the findings for a broad audience, particularly policy makers (NASEM, 2016). To do this, the study must adhere to a strong principle of transparency, but do so in a manner that does not overwhelm the decision maker with too much information. While several recent guidelines recommend summary tables that provide details of the values of all parameters used in the construction of a base case estimate, the sources used for these effect sizes and valuations, as well as the range of values assessed to address underlying uncertainty (Henrichson & Rinaldi, 2014; ISPOR Task Force, 2013; NASEM, 2016), it is also important to communicate clearly to the reader those parameters and values that create the greatest chance of flipping a decision. When findings of cost-effectiveness or net cost benefit are sensitive to reasonable assumptions others could make, those specific assumptions should be conveyed clearly. Similarly, if there are certain assumptions that can cause the decision to switch from being beneficial to being harmful, those assumptions should be made explicit. While it may be difficult to know with certainty the exact value of parameters that cause these decisions to turn, it may still be possible to convey an understanding of the range of parameters that generate one outcome versus another.

Including measures that summarize the overall uncertainty regarding the metrics used are also recommended. In CBA, analysts typically use the proportion of Monte Carlo trials conducted that yield a positive net benefit calculation as a measure of uncertainty, because only policies with a positive net benefit would be advised (NASEM, 2016; Vining & Weimer, 2010). If the proportion of trials generating a positive net benefit is large, for example 86% in the hypothetical simulation presented in Figure 16.2, then the analyst can be reasonably comfortable that under a range of scenarios the policy will generate a net benefit. However, it is still recommended that the analyst convey to the decision maker what specific scenarios will cause the net benefit calculation to become negative (or fall below a prerequisite value), so they are able to consider for themselves the potential risk of a bad outcome. In CEA, if the government agency or policy maker has a firm perspective of a threshold value of willingness to pay per unit gain, then the analyst can simply report the probability of the policy being cost effective at that specific threshold, but again it is useful to describe what values in the calculation increase the risk of it not being cost effective at that value. More often, in light of uncertainty regarding the preferred threshold value of willingness to pay, analysts are encouraged to present an entire cost effectiveness acceptability curve to enable the decision maker to see the likelihood of an intervention being cost-effective at different presumed levels of willingness to pay.

The purpose of CBA and CEA is to assess efficiency—identifying which laws generate the highest societal value given the resources involved in achieving them. Equity is not a consideration. The ultimate metric of these economic evaluations is still based on the net overall outcome, not an even or fair distribution of benefits and costs. Equity should be a genuine concern for decision makers, so conveying information about the distribution of gains and losses across stakeholders and subpopulations is also useful. Indeed, recent guidelines recommend subpopulation analyses of particularly vulnerable populations, so that the potential inequities generated or exacerbated by a policy might be considered (WHO, 2006; Wilkinson et al., 2016).

Additional Issues for Quality Economic Evaluations of Public Health Law

Basic principles of economic evaluations are much easier to apply in narrow settings where a particular treatment or intervention is applied to a relatively small homogeneous group. A law almost always applies to an entire community or state, creating considerable additional complexities beyond those discussed here (Vining & Weimer, 2010). These include a divergence in valuations caused by differences in status within the community, the limitations of using willingness to pay as a basis for social preference ordering and valuation, and the uncertainty regarding total causal effects of laws, due to interacting causal pathways and feedback loops that exist in our complex society.

A core principle of an economic evaluation is that an average value of a resource, determined by the community through markets or other methods, is a meaningful measure. However, people within a jurisdiction can have substantial differences in these values, particularly when nonmarket goods (time, sense of belonging and security, healthy functioning of the community) are translated into dollar values. The value that someone places on any particular dimension of health reflects not just their individual preferences for that good but also their position in society—where they are in status hierarchies. Most analysts are trained to obtain an average or other measure of central tendency in obtaining values across these different populations, as this is deemed the proper way of capturing value across the full population (e.g., median income, average cost of health care). However, using averages masks important information about equity. Given evidence of growing disparities in health and in the social determinants of health (Chetty, Stepner et al., 2016; National Center for Health Statistics, 2016), analyzing subpopulation valuations of both costs and benefits is important. Moreover, some laws are explicitly designed to achieve distributional goals related to health and wellbeing, not maximize efficiency. The field is far from a consensus on how best to present tradeoffs between efficiency and equity using economic evaluation methods.

A standard neoclassical assumptions underlying economic evaluations is that willingness to pay, as reflected by market demand curves, represent the true social value of the good to society. However, this assumption may not hold in diverse populations, particularly when large segments of the population do not engage in a given market due to disagreement with the use of resources to that purpose (e.g., diesel fuel in cars, plastic bottles containing water, and so on). This assumption only holds when preferences are transitive (Arrow, 1963; Sen, 1969). Preferences are said to be transitive when their ordering is preserved no matter what comparisons are made. If a person prefers option A to option B, and option B to option C, then transitive preferences mean that they will prefer option A to option C. But, even if individual preferences meet the condition of transitivity, in the aggregate as a population the assumption might not hold. While some subpopulations might prefer option A to option B and option B to option C, other segments might prefer option C to option A. In aggregate, depending on the relative sizes of groups with different preference orderings, the transitive preference assumption could easily be violated. This disrupts any agreement on what the "best" policy approach would be for the full population. It also disrupts the assumption that willingness to pay, as reflected by market valuations of the costs, benefits, and outcomes associated with that policy, are indeed an accurate assessment of society's valuation of the resources involved. When segments of society remove themselves from a marketplace, in protest regarding the market, then accurate inferences of willingness to pay cannot be presumed.

A final consideration when conducting economic evaluations of public health laws specifically is the extent to which a study considers all the potentially relevant effects associated with an adoption of a policy, however uncertain. The fact that an outcome is unlikely does not mean it will not come to fruition, as we unfortunately learned with the reformulation of Oxycontin in 2010 (Powell & Pacula, 2021). Regulators presumably understood that the approval and marketing of an opioid formulation labeled as less subject to abuse would lead to much wider medical use, but evidently did not anticipate or discounted the possibility that wider medical use would ultimately lead to such a large-scale change in the illicit market for opioid medications, which brought with it a rise in hepatitis C and fatal overdoses caused by heroin and then fentanyl (Alpert, Powell, & Pacula, 2018; Powell et al., 2019; Powell & Pacula, 2021). Even well intended and well-designed policies can generate negative outcomes in light of the diverse communities and circumstances in which people live, work, and play. An awareness of this potential, particularly in areas beyond health, is important to keep in mind when considering public policies.

Concluding Thoughts

Economic evaluation of a law requires more than just applying a societal perspective when assessing costs and benefits. It requires a serious consideration of all stakeholders, which for public health includes all individuals present in the jurisdiction with the law. The broad range of intended and unintended consequences associated with a law must be included, both in the short term and the longer run. Accounting for multiple beneficial and deleterious population outcomes is difficult, and projecting potential effects into the uncertain future is even more so. Nonetheless, new tools and methods continue to emerge improving economic evaluations and better revealing the uncertainties inherent in them. High quality economic evaluations will keep this broad perspective in mind as it related to outcomes, omitted populations, and valuations, even if the question being asked by decision makers is perhaps too narrowly focused on just the items that can be readily assigned dollar values with current measures and methods.

When conducting analyses of public health laws in particular, it is important to keep in mind that the majority of societies are far from homogeneous in their populations. People within the same jurisdiction live in different circumstances, face different daily stresses, have different cultural or religious values, and start with different baseline levels of health, income, and education. Any population-wide public health policy that is implemented will result in a variety of social outcomes, costs and benefits, given this underlying heterogeneity. While an economic analysis can do a good job of identifying whether a policy on net might be cost effective, it is important to consider the extent to which those who do not benefit from a law, or are possibly harmed by it, might be compensated. Well-intended laws, such as drug prohibitions, have resulted in extremely large costs imposed on particular segments of society. Law frequently addresses actions of institutions and behaviors of persons that are the result of complex social phenomenon, but they address them at times using blunt sticks (mandates or prohibitions). Consideration of the economic, social, and welfare effects beyond health is important and requires the use of outcome measures that captures these dimensions. But consideration of who incurs the outcomes, the costs and benefits, is also important when evaluating the desirability of a law or policy. When economic analyses are comprehensive and done well, they can provide insights into who the winners and losers are, but the decision rule typically does not explicitly consider equity. Equity must still be considered by the analyst in the formulation of the policy analysis in the first place, or by the decision maker after the fact.

Further Reading

Crowley, D. M., Dodge, K. A., Barnett, W. S., Corso, P., Duffy, S., Graham, P., ... Plotnick, R. (2018). Standards of evidence for conducting and reporting economic evaluations in prevention science. *Prevention Science, 19*(3), 366–390.

Drummond, M. F., Sculpher, M. J., Claxton, K., Stoddart, G. L., & Torrance, G. W. (2015). *Methods for the economic evaluation of health care programmes* (4th ed.). Oxford, UK: Oxford University Press.

National academics of Sciences, Engineering, and Medicine (NASEM) (2016). *Advancing the evidence to inform investments in children, youth and power of economic evidence to inform investments in children, youth and families.* Washington, DC: The National Academics Press.

Neumann, P. J., Sanders, G. D., Russell, L. B., Siegel, J. E., & Ganiats, T. G. (2017). *Cost-effectiveness in health and medicine* (2nd ed.). New York, NY: Oxford University Press.

Chapter 17

The Future of Research in Legal Epidemiology

Scott Burris   Rosalie Liccardo Pacula   Alexander C. Wagenaar

Learning Objectives

- Formulate a rationale for the further development of legal epidemiology as a field.
- Recognize how legal epidemiology can contribute to efforts to improve population health.

Legal epidemiology empirically studies the complicated ways that laws and legal practices influence health. Because both *law* and *public health* encompass a vast range of heterogeneous human activities, institutions, and environments, research methods serve as an important mechanism for building unity and coherence in the field. We may study very different laws, environments, behaviors, and outcomes, but all of us in legal epidemiology build on established theory to hypothesize and measure how legal inputs contribute to levels and distributions of health in the population. Individual studies can illuminate particular policy choices; a few studies will be game changers. When those studies lead to very different conclusions of policy effects, as we have seen repeatedly in evaluations of specific laws that get measured differently across studies (Horwitz, Davis, McClelland, Fordon, & Meara, 2021; Pacula, Powell, Heaton, & Sevigny, 2015; Patrick, Fry, Jones, & Buntin, 2016; Powell, Pacula, & Jacobson, 2018; Smart, Pardo, & Davis, 2021), they do neither the science, the policy makers, nor the field any good. We help each other, and strengthen the field, by our efforts to explicitly and transparently define the concepts of interest; use theory to explicate mechanisms of effect and support causal inference; reliably and validly measure the processes under study; incorporate the

Legal Epidemiology: Theory and Methods, Second Edition. Edited by Alexander C. Wagenaar, Rosalie Liccardo Pacula, and Scott Burris.

strongest possible research design features to maximize plausibility of causal interpretations of observed relationships; and analyze the resulting data with the most advanced qualitative and statistical methods available to identify true effects and ensure the robustness of conclusions drawn. Better research makes the field more attractive to new entrants, facilitates transdisciplinary integration, increases the chances the major health research funders will support research on law, and enhances the credibility and utility of research results in scientific and policy-making communities.

A second edition textbook devoted to methods for legal epidemiology is an unmistakable milestone in the development of the field. The chapters in this book have suggested how far the field has come. This closing chapter considers where legal epidemiology might go from here. Although the field has grown (Burris, Cloud, & Penn, 2020) and internationalized (Hoffman, Poirier, Rogers Van Katwyk, Baral, & Sritharan, 2019; Kavanagh, 2016; Kavanagh, Meier, Pillinger, Huffstetler, & Burris, 2020; Phelan & Katz, 2019) since our first volume, we continue to see three priority needs as the field moves forward: further disciplinary integration on several axes; methods improvement through further development of field-specific tools and approaches; and a broad effort to deploy a social determinants framework in legal epidemiology.

Disciplinary Integration

We hope and expect to see more researchers who will identify themselves as primarily focused on legal epidemiology. A core group of dedicated specialists can give the field a clear identity, serving as the stewards of its history and standards. Given the transdisciplinary nature of the field (Burris, Ashe, Levin, Penn, & Larkin, 2016), and the breadth of both law and health, however, the field's boundaries will continue to be fuzzy. We expect that many or even most of the researchers who identify themselves with the field will not be specialists in legal epidemiology. Moreover, we see it as essential to the development of the field that *all* researchers who work on the social and behavioral determinants of health be able and willing to integrate legal questions and legal variables into their research, even if the study is not primarily focused on law. For example, while a primary legal epidemiology researcher might investigate whether laws that require the reporting of HIV test results deter people from being tested (Hecht, Chesney, Lehman et al., 2000), it is equally (or possibly more) valuable for studies examining the behavior of people with HIV to consider including law as one possible influence among many on the decision to test (Myers, Orr, Locker, & Jackson, 1993). Law is rarely the main driver of behavior, but it is very rarely absent from an individual's environment.

An organic connection between legal epidemiology and the field of health policy research is also overdue. Chapter 2 offered concrete ideas for integrating legal epidemiology and public health systems and services research, and legal epidemiologists can draw on well-articulated and tested policy research and translation methods (Eyler, Chriqui, Moreland-Russell, & Brownson, 2015). Although a newer field, legal epidemiology brings from law a commitment to taking seriously the policy instrument—the law, regulation, rule, or other text setting out the behavior or standard constituting the policy—and an explicit understanding that a "policy" is not simply the settled practice of a desirable behavior but a mechanism for deliberately increasing the adoption and enhancing the effects of that practice (Burris, 2017). This attention to the instrument has led to the development of more and better methods and tools for measuring law and sharing legal data. Recognizing that policy is a mechanism for scaling desirable behavior also allows us to better distinguish research that is *relevant* to policy (such as the "policy candidate" experiments described in Chapter 13) and research that actually evaluates whether a policy is succeeding in scaling desirable behaviors or standards.

Two core areas of health policy that are particularly ripe for closer integration with legal epidemiology include policies influencing health care service organization (e.g., the practice of health care by an organization, possibly through the integration of health insurance and/or different health care providers) and health care service delivery (e.g., the appropriate use of telehealth and/or legal limits on opioid prescribing). In the United States, we have seen both with the opioid epidemic and coronavirus pandemic how certain health care delivery laws have influenced the practice of health care through, for example, changes in licensing or scope of practice laws, the legally permitted use of telehealth for delivery of opioid treatment, and changes in allowances regarding home delivery of specific medications (Davis & Samuels, 2021; Pessar, Boustead, Ge, Smart, & Pacula, 2021). While in the United States, we often talk of a market-based health care delivery system, there remain several ways that state and federal laws influence how medical care is delivered, such as by placing limits on location of services (services that can or cannot be delivered by telehealth or in particular settings), types of services that can be provided by particular providers (scope of practice laws), and whether and how particular services are paid (mandated health insurance benefits and the turning on of reimbursement codes by state agencies). Legal interventions are even more common in countries with universal health insurance or nationalized health care.

The need for integration extends as well toward non-health-related empirical legal research (Mello & Zeiler, 2008). The legal epidemiology category of incidental public health law encompasses laws passed, or legal activities conducted, with little or no consideration of possible health consequences. It follows that research on the operation and outputs of such laws can contribute to the legal epidemiology evidence base if data on health outcomes are included in the research scope. For example, many empirical legal scholars have investigated the implementation and effects of the Americans with Disabilities Act. Studies have documented the importance of the ADA and its enforcement processes to people with disabilities, including its effect on their sense of social position and the fairness of the system (Engel & Munger, 2003; Swanson, Burris, Moss, Ullman, & Ranney, 2006). From a legal epidemiology perspective, we would expect that a law protecting basic social and employment rights of people with a wide range of health conditions would have affective effects on people with disabilities, and would regard health outcomes of one kind or another to be important components of its overall impact. Emerging research at the population level supports this view (Montez, Hayward, & Wolf, 2017).

Criminology offers another example. The study of violence and its control by the police is a matter with obvious health implications (Ratcliffe, Taniguchi, Groff, & Wood, 2011). Links between violence, law, and mental health services are well documented (Swanson, Tong, Robertson, & Swartz, 2020), and criminologists themselves have addressed the overlap in proposing a discipline of epidemiological criminology (Akers & Lanier, 2009). The links between policing and public health have driven efforts to harmonize or better integrate work in the two fields (Anderson & Burris, 2017; Wood, 2019). Including actual or self-reported health outcomes associated with crime within the scope of empirical legal studies would enrich both legal and public health research.

Economists, criminologists, epidemiologists, and other empirical scientists evaluating legal and policy effects would be well served by incorporating improved understanding of the sociology of law from sociolegal traditions. Law is much more than a specific statute or regulation, and a more nuanced conceptualization and understanding by health and social scientists of the nature of law and its meanings and diffused operation throughout all of society's major institutions would clearly advance the field of legal epidemiology.

Another form of integration that is important to the future robustness and impact of the field encompasses empirical researchers and lawyers, including legal scholars who do not do empirical research. Lawyers are, we believe, crucial constituents of a multidisciplinary team for a number of reasons. As we discuss in Chapters 11 and 12, lawyers are indispensable to the accurate conceptualization and execution of processes to collect, code, and measure legal variables that meet scientific standards of reliability and validity. Lawyers bring to bear experience and knowledge about how legal systems work, and through training and socialization are professionally suited to identifying issues—including research questions—that other lawyers and legal decision makers are likely to deem important. More importantly, their firm understanding of the public health powers granted to specific jurisdictions (e.g., federal, state, county, and city in the United States) can ensure proper interpretation of laws on the books within a given jurisdiction. This combination of legal mapping skills, proper legal interpretation, and a legal understanding of breadth of impact, when combined with social and health empirical scientists, can produce hybrid legal research and empirical analysis that are both conceptually elegant and highly policy-relevant. Consider, for example, a classic study from the early days of legal epidemiology. Teret et al. (1986) analyzed and categorized state law on child car restraints to determine the population covered. These legal data were then merged with Fatality Analysis Reporting System (FARS) data, which allowed the researchers to estimate the number of child fatalities among children who would have been protected by laws with fewer exemptions or a wider range of covered ages (Teret, Wells, Williams, & Jones, 1986). Integrated cross-disciplinary teams that combine lawyers with empirical social and health scientists are essential for continued advances in the theoretical sophistication and methodological quality of legal epidemiology studies.

The next advance for theory in legal epidemiology is the development and evaluation of transdisciplinary systems theories on how law affects health. Such theories would integrate multiple approaches to law and human behavior in complex systems, sharpening our understanding of policy trade-offs, side effects and feebback loops. It could, for example, draw on the Theory of Triadic Influence (Chapter 8), which integrates numerous micro-theories from sociology and psychology. Or consider the relationship of deterrence (Chapter 5) and procedural justice (Chapter 6) theories of compliance. Procedural justice integrates Weberian legitimacy with experiences of fair treatment as drivers of compliance, but does not heavily engage with deterrence. Integrative theory would advance understanding of the ways these two mechanisms reinforce or mitigate each other and point the way toward proposed laws designed to optimize both types of effects on behalf of population health and well-being. A single grand theory integrating all possible legal effects is neither feasible nor desirable— diversity of perspective is a benefit to research—but seizing opportunities for transdisciplinary theoretical integration will clearly advance the field legal epidemiology.

Theoretical advances will also come from engaging the burgeoning field of implementation science and building on elements it shares with legal epidemiology. Implementation science emerged to fill a knowledge gap in evidence-based policy (Nilsen, Ståhl, Roback, & Cairney, 2013), whereas legal epidemiology started with implementation as a central concern, and drew on a long tradition of policy implementation research (see Chapter 1). Cross fertilization of these traditions and their concerns has already been noted, and more will be better. Studies testing links between law and health outcomes must be expanded to include a greater emphasis on proximal effects of law, including implementation structures and processes, and implementation fidelity across jurisdictions and across time. Such research unpacking the "black box" between law and health will improve theory by expanding the number of causal links considered and improve generalizability of a given evaluation to other areas of law and health.

Finally, legal epidemiology can be part of and promote integration not just across research traditions but across the key domains of professional and social practice in public health. Research findings and researcher knowledge are instrumental at every step of public health law work. Evidence and expertise can instigate and guide the development of policy ideas; they inform the transformation of policy concepts into actual laws; they serve as persuasive tools in the political process to secure enactment; they provide guidance for effective implementation and evidence to support laws against legal challenges (Burris, Ashe, Blanke et al., 2016). Even if legal epidemiology research is funded at a level commensurate with its importance, a professional model in which researchers stand apart waiting for laws to be enacted and implemented long enough to allow credible causal inference studies is inadequate to the challenge of making law a positive force for health. We would better aspire to something more like systematic social experimentation, in which stakeholders and researchers collaborate across all the stages of the policy process to define policy needs, test policy candidates, study implementation, and provide timely feedback beginning with early single-jurisdiction and cross-sectional evaluations (Burris, Korfmacher et al., 2020; Korfmacher, 2019).

Methods Improvement

The section of this volume devoted to elucidating the "mechanisms of law" reflects our belief in the importance of opening the black box that too often fills the causal diagram between law and health effects in legal epidemiology. Theories of how law works to change environments and behaviors can support more robust hypotheses and more confident causal inferences. We hope that the contributions of our authors will support that sort of improvement. As we worked on this volume, however, we identified several topics we expect will require more coverage in a future edition: the need to further develop widely accepted shared standards and protocols for measuring law, and norms of archiving legal data sets for public access; the need for further conceptual and operational clarity regarding indices and scales for measuring theory-based attributes of laws such as stringency; and diffusion of optimal research designs and methods across all topics in legal epidemiology.

Reliable and valid measurement of legal concepts is central for the advancement of scientific evaluation of the many public health effects of law and depends on both good theory and strong methods. The two chapters focused on coding legal variables propose a variety of good practices in conducting, memorializing, and sharing the results of legal research. Anderson and coauthors in Chapter 11 suggest that creators of legal datasets routinely include certain basic attributes (such as exact dates a law takes effect or ceases to be in effect) and use widely accepted geographic tags (such as FIPS codes). Further conventions for consistent citation of statutes and regulations could also be useful. Designing a quality measurement protocol requires conceptual clarity about what dimensions of law one wishes to measure. The design of quality measures is inherently related to the specific research questions at issue in a given study. As new studies accumulate, an improved understanding of the effects of law leads to further specificity about the dimensions of law that need to be measured for the next study. Continued attention to methods focused on the challenges of collecting and coding law across nations for both intra- and cross-national research should be a priority for the field (Kavanagh et al., 2020; Meier et al., 2017).

Many legal epidemiology studies are taking on the challenge of creating an ordered scale of strength or quality of laws in a given area, to permit improved dose–response studies of legal effects (Woodruff, Pichon, Hoerster et al., 2007). In this new edition, Anderson and colleagues make explicit the separation of observation of the apparent features of legal texts and the subsequent phase of transparently building scales, indices, or other composite measures based on those observations. And working through the operational problems and complexity in reliably coding "strength" enhances conceptual clarity about the many meanings of "strength" and which of those meanings are most relevant for the current study.

Increased use of scientific standards and protocols for the measurement of law will provide the opportunity then to create accessible archives of legal data sets across an increasing number of domains relevant to legal epidemiology. Anderson and colleagues also propose a norm of open-source legal data, in which datasets are posted with codebooks and detailed research protocols for replication by other researchers, who in turn post updated and expanded data sets including their own contributions. As open-source legal data becomes more common, it can be harmonized and then integrated into "data dashboards" that aim to aggregate and organize health data for practical action (Politis, Halligan, Keen, & Kerner, 2014; Thorpe & Gourevitch, 2022).

Technology has also proven to be important to leverage the advantages of solid scientific methods. More than one thousand researchers now use the MonQcle software platform to create and publish legal data, and custom platforms have also been effectively used. For example, a team at Oxford University built a platform that allowed more than four hundred volunteers around the world to build and maintain three data sets tracking national COVID-19 policies, accurately capturing more than 1.2 million data points in just its first 6 months (Hale et al., 2021). The deployment of machine learning in research and coding is an exciting possibility on the verge of feasibility.

The importance of high-quality public-use data sets also extends to the dependent variables in legal epidemiology studies—measures of health-relevant exposures, behaviors, and outcomes. These include regularly repeated consistently conducted sample surveys across all states (for example, the Behavioral Risk Factor Surveillance System or National Survey on Drug Use and Health), as well as census records on all adverse events (for example, the Fatality Analysis Reporting System or National Vital Statistics System). Even in these well-used public data systems, there are important data aggregation techniques (the use of sampling or age-adjusted weights, the inclusion of waves of data or jurisdictions in which key populations are defined differently) that the careful researcher must attend when asking particular research questions. Continuing technology and management information system improvements will result in an increasing number of very large longitudinal continuous measures (e.g., uniform electronic medical records, health monitoring devices such as the Apple watch). Such databases will create many opportunities for statistically powerful and precise evaluations of public health law effects once the representation and limits of these data are well understood by the researcher.

The benefits of random assignment as a research design element for social policy research is now widely recognized (Chapter 13). As a result, we have a growing body of high quality randomized controlled trials (RCTs) testing particular preventive or treatment approaches for addressing health outcomes. These trials to date largely do not evaluate actual laws but illustrate potential policy candidates that might be integrated into future law. Such RCTs also advance legal epidemiology by improving understanding of various mechanisms of effect on health-relevant structures, environments, and behaviors. The resulting better theory, in turn, improves the development of legal innovations.

The benefits of randomization as a scientific tool must not be limited to studies of policy candidates or specific legal mechanisms, however. The field must push policy makers to integrate high-quality evaluations of legal effects into new laws. There are many cases where implementation of a new law of necessity is phased, or where resource allocations prevent immediate universal implementation. Recent advances in stepped-wedge randomized trial designs are ideally suited to such situations and substantially improve causal inference regarding a law's effects (see Chapter 13).

Randomization is but one beneficial research design element improving causal inference and often is not feasible when evaluating the health effects of law. Most laws are natural experiments where the scientific team has no influence over implementation (Chapter 14). In that common situation, creative combinations from the many available design elements strengthening causal inference will further establish legal epidemiology as a respected field of scientific and scholarly inquiry. As a collaborative paper between a lawyer and a statistician reminds us (Ho & Rubin, 2011), research *design* always trumps statistical methods. Complex statistical modeling methods imperfectly attempt to make up for poor design. Strong research designs (for example, long time series, multiple comparison groups, and multiple measures) have been used for many years on some topics in legal epidemiology, such as road safety. Such strong designs, which are the studies that produce credible causal inferences, must now be disseminated across all topics in legal epidemiology. The fundamental aim of legal epidemiology is to understand law's effects on health, and it is neither necessary nor proper to shy away from this ambition (Galea, 2013; Hernán, 2018).

Social Determinants

Research to date has made a clear case that social position—particularly income and education—matters for almost all dimensions of mental and physical health. Responding to this evidence is arguably the most important challenge we face in public health, and it is one of particular importance to law. Law clearly acts as a major force structuring our societies, defining our social positions, maintaining or altering existing distributions of resources. It follows that law has the potential to be a major domain of action to address social determinants of health. So far, however, efforts to pursue legal epidemiology aimed at the social determinants of health have been limited.

In a 2002 paper, an interdisciplinary team of authors from legal epidemiology, social epidemiology, and sociolegal research sets out a conceptual framework for research in this area (Burris, Kawachi, & Sarat, 2002); more recent papers have elaborated on the original model (Burris, 2011a, 2011b). The basic idea advanced is that we can study law as a system that creates environments and sorts the people within them to health outcomes based on their positions within those environments. There is now a growing body of research illustrating the effects of laws that affect social position. Studies of natural experiments involving even relatively small changes in social position reflected in changes to mandated minimum wages or tax credits for those with low incomes have shown significant effects on population levels of diverse health outcomes such as suicide, HIV, and infant and child health (Kaufman, Salas-Hernández, Komro, & Livingston, 2020; Komro, Livingston, Markowitz, & Wagenaar, 2016; Markowitz, Komro, Livingston, Lenhart, & Wagenaar, 2017; Spencer et al., 2020; Van Dyke, Komro, Shah, Livingston, & Kramer, 2018). Research examining policy differences have shed important light on the effects of overall policy "dispositions" on state-level differences in key health indicators (Montez et al., 2020; Wolf, Monnat, & Montez, 2021). In work like this, legal epidemiology points to concrete opportunities to changes in core social programs and policy constellations to create environments in which people can be healthy.

Conclusion

Research over time approaches the truth and gains credibility and authority, by accretion. A series of more or less coordinated studies explores a particular phenomenon, producing a body of evidence that in time can be systematically weighed and even reanalyzed to produce a confident statement of the facts. So, with law, the efficacy of interventions ranging from fluoride to safety belts to tobacco and alcohol taxes was established by years of assiduous study. In a field as new and diverse as legal epidemiology, however, this level of sustained attention may be difficult to reach. As individual researchers, we need to keep in mind our place within a larger effort not only to assess the effects of particular laws but to determine the particular mechanisms and mediators of legal effect that are broadly generalizable across public health problems and to illuminate the utility of law generally as a force for better public health. In turn, legal epidemiology will have more visibility, more resources allocated to it from NIH and other health research funders (Ibrahim, Sorensen, Grunwald, & Burris, 2017; Purtle, Peters, & Brownson, 2016), and a larger impact on population health if we have a measure of coherence and identity as a field, and some degree of consensus on major critical opportunities for research advancing the public's health. The field of legal epidemiology asserts and demonstrates the importance of objective inquiry and rational analysis to a policy process that too often seems to undervalue both. Legal epidemiology stands for the propositions that even complicated health problems can be grasped through research and that, sometimes, collective action through social intervention can make us all better off.

Summary

The chapters in this book are points on a long arc of improvement in public health law research methods. Scientific strength is crucial to the field of legal epidemiology in several ways. Better research makes the field more attractive to new entrants, facilitates interdisciplinary collaboration, increases the chances the major health research funders will support investigation of law, and enhances the credibility of research results for informing policy. As the field moves forward, key areas for methodological improvement include disciplinary integration and interdisciplinary collaboration on the theoretical mechanisms and legal components of policy that matter for public health, development of research standards and tools, and better approaches to studying law in a social determinants framework.

As an applied research field, legal epidemiology ultimately will be justified by the extent to which it proves useful to health policy decision makers. To this end, building the field as measured by the quality and quantity of individual studies is only part of the story. We do well, as a field, to think also in terms of our "collective impact." Individual studies can illuminate particular policy choices; a few studies will be game changers. Collectively, the impact of legal epidemiology as a field must exceed the sum of the effects of particular studies. The field asserts and demonstrates the importance of objective inquiry, consistent and rational measurement of laws, and empirically appropriate analysis to better inform science as well as the policy process. Legal epidemiology stands for the propositions that even complicated health problems can be grasped through research and that, sometimes, collective action through social intervention can make us all better off.

Further Reading

Burris, S., Ashe, M., Levin, D., Penn, M., & Larkin, M. (2016). A transdisciplinary approach to public health law: The emerging practice of legal epidemiology. *Annual Review of Public Health, 37*(1), 135–148.

Burris, S., Kawachi, I., & Sarat, A. (2002). Integrating law and social epidemiology. *Journal of Law, Medicine & Ethics, 30*, 510–521.

Epstein, L., & King, G. (2002). The rules of inference. *University of Chicago Law Review, 69*(1), 1.

References

Abadie, A. (2021). Using synthetic controls: Feasibility, data requirements, and methodological aspects. *Journal of Economic Literature, 59*(2), 391–425.

Abadie, A., & Cattaneo, M. D. (2018). Econometric methods for program evaluation. *Annual Review of Economics, 10*(1), 465–503.

Abaluck, J., Kwong, L. H., Styczynski, A., Haque, A., Kabir, M. A., Bates-Jefferys, E., ... Mobarak, A. M. (2021). Impact of community masking on COVID-19: A cluster-randomized trial in Bangladesh. *Science, 375*(6577), eabi9069.

AcademyHealth. (2009). *Advancing research, policy and practice.* Retrieved from www.academyhealth.org/About/content.cfm?ItemNumber=831&navItemNumber=514.

Acevedo-Garcia, D., Osypuk, T. L., McArdle, N., & Williams, D. R. (2008). Toward a policy-relevant analysis of geographic and racial/ethnic disparities in child health. *Health Affairs, 27*(2), 321–333.

Adler, N. E., & Newman, K. (2002). Socioeconomic disparities in health: Pathways and policies. *Health Affairs, 21*(2), 60–76.

Adler, N. E., & Rehkopf, D. H. (2008). U.S. disparities in health: Descriptions, causes, and mechanisms. *Annual Review of Public Health, 29*, 235–252.

Agostino, D., & Arnaboldi, M. (2016). A measurement framework for assessing the contribution of social media to public engagement: An empirical analysis on Facebook. *Public Management Review, 18*(9), 1289–1307.

Agrawal, V., Cantor, J. H., Sood, N., & Whaley, C. M. (2021). *The impact of the COVID-19 pandemic and policy responses on excess mortality* (National Bureau of Economic Research Working Paper Series, No. 28930). doi:10.3386/w28930.

Ahmad, F. B., & Anderson, R. N. (2021). The leading causes of death in the US for 2020. *JAMA, 325*(18), 1829–1830.

Ainsworth, M. D. S., & Bowlby, J. (1991). An ethological approach to personality development. *American Psychologist, 46*(4), 333–341.

Ajzen, I. (1985). From intentions to actions: A theory of planned behavior. In J. Kuhl & J. Beckman (Eds.), *Action-control: From cognition to behavior* (pp. 11–39). Heidelberg, Germany: Springer.

Ajzen, I. (2003). *Constructing a TpB questionnaire: Conceptual and methodological considerations.* Retrieved from people.umass.edu/aizen/pdf/tpb.measurement.pdf.

Akers, R. L. (1977). *Deviant behavior: A social learning approach* (2nd ed.). Belmont, CA: Wadsworth.

Legal Epidemiology: Theory and Methods, Second Edition. Edited by Alexander C. Wagenaar, Rosalie Liccardo Pacula, and Scott Burris.
© 2023 John Wiley & Sons, Inc. Published 2023 by John Wiley & Sons, Inc.

Akers, R. L. (1991). Self-control as a general theory of crime. *Journal of Quantitative Criminology, 7*(2), 201–211.

Akers, R. L. (1998). *Social learning and social structure: A general theory of crime and deviance.* Boston, MA: Northeastern University Press.

Akers, R. L., & Jensen, G. F. (Eds.) (2007). *Social learning theory and the explanation of crime* (Vol. 11). New Brunswick, NJ: Transaction.

Akers, R. L., Sellers, C., & Jennings, W. G. (2020). *Criminological theories: Introduction, evaluation, and application* (8th ed.). Oxford, UK and New York, NY: Oxford University Press.

Akers, T. A., & Lanier, M. M. (2009). "Epidemiological criminology": Coming full circle. *American Journal of Public Health, 99*(3), 397–402.

Albers, A. B., Siegel, M., Cheng, D. M., Biener, L., & Rigotti, N. A. (2004). Relation between local restaurant smoking regulations and attitudes towards the prevalence and social acceptability of smoking: A study of youths and adults who eat out predominantly at restaurants in their town. *Tobacco Control, 13*(4), 347–355.

Aliprantis, D, Fee K, & Schweitzer ME. (2019). *Opioids and the Labor Market (2019)* (Federal Research Bank of Cleveland Working Paper No. 18-07R2) (November 15, 2019).

Allen, E. (2019). Perceived discrimination and health: Paradigms and prospects. *Sociology Compass, 13*(8), e12720.

Allen, S. T., Grieb, S. M., O'Rourke, A., Yoder, R., Planchet, E., White, R. H., & Sherman, S. G. (2019). Understanding the public health consequences of suspending a rural syringe services program: A qualitative study of the experiences of people who inject drugs. *Harm Reduction Journal, 16,* 1–10.

Alpert, A., Evans, W. N., Lieber, E. M., & Powell, D. (2022). Origins of the opioid crisis and its enduring impacts. *The Quarterly Journal of Economics, 137*(2), 1139–1179.

Alpert, A., Powell, D., & Pacula, R. L. (2018). Supply-side drug policy in the presence of substitutes: Evidence from the introduction of abuse-deterrent opioids. *American Economic Journal: Economic Policy, 10*(4), 1–35.

Alsan, M., & Wanamaker, M. (2018). Tuskegee and the health of black men. *Quarterly Journal of Economics, 133*(1), 407–455.

Alsan, M., Wanamaker, M., & Hardeman, R. R. (2020). The Tuskegee study of untreated syphilis: A case study in peripheral trauma with implications for health professionals. *Journal of General Internal Medicine, 35*(1), 322–325.

Al-Tammemi, A. B., & Tarhini, Z. (2021). Beyond equity: Advocating theory-based health promotion in parallel with COVID-19 mass vaccination campaigns. *Public Health in Practice, 2,* 100142.

Altman, D. (1986). *AIDS in the mind of America* (1st ed.). Garden City, NY: Anchor Press/Doubleday.

American College of Pediatricians. (2018). *Marijuana use: Detrimental to youth.* Retrieved from https://www.acpeds.org/the-college-speaks/positionstatements/effect-of-marijuana-legalization-on-risky-behavior/marijuana-use-detrimental-to-youth.

Anderson, E., & Burris, S. (2014). Researchers and research knowledge in evidence-informed policy innovation. In T. Voon, A. D. Mitchelll, & J. Liberman (Eds.),

Regulating tobacco, alcohol and unhealthy foods: The legal issues (pp. 36–63). Abingdon, UK: Routledge.

Anderson, E., & Burris, S. (2017). Policing and public health: Not quite the right analogy. *Policing and Society, 27*(3), 300–313.

Anderson, E., & Burris, S. (Forthcoming, 2022). Imagining a better public health (law) response to COVID-19. *Richmond Law Review*. Retrieved from https://lawreview.richmond.edu/2022/05/12/imagining-a-better-public-health-law-response-to-covid-19/.

Anderson, G., & Horvath, J. (2004). The growing burden of chronic disease in America. *Public Health Reports, 119*(3), 263–270.

Anderson, T. L., Donnelly, E. A., Delcher, C., & Wang, Y. (2021). Data science approaches in criminal justice and public health research: Lessons learned from opioid projects. *Journal of Contemporary Criminal Justice, 37*, 175–191.

Andrews, D. A., Zinger, I., Hoge, R. D., Bonta, J., Gendreau, P., & Cullen, F. (1990). Does correctional treatment work? A clinically relevant and psychologically informed meta-analysis. *Criminology, 28*(3), 369–404.

Apollonio, D. E., & Bero, L. A. (2009). Evidence and argument in policymaking: Development of workplace smoking legislation. *BMC Public Health, 9*, 189.

Ariza, E., & Leatherman, S. P. (2012). No-smoking policies and their outcomes on U.S. beaches. *Journal of Coastal Research, 28*(1A), 143–147.

Arnett, P. K. (2011). Local health department changes over the past twenty years. Unpublished dissertation. University of Kentucky.

Arno, P. S., Sohler, N., Viola, D., & Schecter, C. (2009). Bringing health and social policy together: The case of the earned income tax credit. *Journal of Public Health Policy, 30*(2), 198–207.

Arrow, K., Solow, R., Portney, P. R., Leamer, E. E., Radner, R., & Schuman, H. (1993). Report of the NOAA panel on contingent valuation. *Federal Register, 58*(10), 4601–4614.

Arrow, K. J. (1963). *Social choice and individual values* (2nd ed.). New York, NY: Wiley.

Ashe, M., Jernigan, D., Kline, R., & Galaz, R. (2003). Land use planning and the control of alcohol, tobacco, firearms, and fast food restaurants. *American Journal of Public Health, 93*(9), 1404–1408.

Ashley, M., Northrup, D., & Ferrence, R. (1998). The Ontario ban on smoking on school property: Issues and challenges in enforcement. *Canadian Journal of Public Health, 89*(4), 229–232.

Atwoli, L., Baqui, A. H., Benfield, T., Bosurgi, R., Godlee, F., Hancocks, S., … Vázquez, D. (2021). Call for emergency action to limit global temperature increases, restore biodiversity, and protect health. *New England Journal of Medicine, 385*(12), 1134–1137.

Autor, D. H., Manning, A., & Smith, C. L. (2010). *The contribution of the minimum wage to U.S. wage inequality over three decades: A reassessment*. London, UK: Centre for Economic Performance.

Ayanian, J. Z., Weissman, J. S., Chasan-Taber, S., & Epstein, A. M. (1999). Quality of care by race and gender for congestive heart failure and pneumonia. *Medical Care, 37*(12), 1260–1269.

Ayres, I., & Baker, K. (2004). *A separate crime of reckless sex*. Unpublished manuscript. Yale Law School Public Law & Legal Theory Research Paper Series.

Ayres, I., & Braithwaite, J. (1995). *Responsive regulation: Transcending the deregulation debate*. New York, NY; Oxford, UK: Oxford University Press.

Azagba, S., Shan, L., & Latham, K. (2020). County smoke-free laws and cigarette smoking among U.S. adults, 1995–2015. *American Journal of Preventive Medicine, 58*(1), 97–106.

Backstrom, C., & Robins, L. (1995). State AIDS policy making: Perspectives of legislative health committee chairs. *AIDS & Public Policy Journal, 10*(4), 238–248.

Bae, J. Y., Anderson, E., Silver, D., & Macinko, J. (2014). Child passenger safety laws in the United States, 1978–2010: Policy diffusion in the absence of strong federal intervention. *Social Science & Medicine, 100*, 30–37.

Bagenstos, S. R. (2009). *Law and the contradictions of the disability right movement*. New Haven, CT: Yale University Press.

Baicker, K., Allen, H. L., Wright, B. J., & Finkelstein, A. N. (2017). The effect of medicaid on medication use among poor adults: Evidence from Oregon. *Health Affairs (Millwood), 36*(12), 2110–2114.

Baicker, K., Allen, H. L., Wright, B. J., Taubman, S. L., & Finkelstein, A. N. (2018). The effect of medicaid on dental care of poor adults: Evidence from the Oregon health insurance experiment. *Health Services Research, 53*(4), 2147–2164.

Bailey, C. A. (2007). *A guide to qualitative field research* (2nd ed.). Thousand Oaks, CA: Pine Forge Press.

Bajema, K. L., Dahl, R. M., Evener, S. L., Prill, M. M., Rodriguez-Barradas, M. C., Marconi, V. C., ... Surie, D. (2021). Comparative effectiveness and antibody responses to moderna and Pfizer-BioNTech COVID-19 vaccines among hospitalized veterans—Five Veterans Affairs Medical Centers, United States, February 1-September 30, 2021. *MMWR. Morbidity and Mortality Weekly Report, 70*(49), 1700–1705.

Bandura, A. (1977a). Self-efficacy: Toward a unified theory of behavioral change. *Psychological Review, 84*(2), 191–215.

Bandura, A. (1977b). *Social learning theory*. Englewood Cliffs, NJ: Prentice-Hall.

Bandura, A. (1986a). The explanatory and predictive scope of self-efficacy theory. *Journal of Social and Clinical Psychology, 4*(3), 359–373.

Bandura, A. (1986b). *Social foundations of thought and action: A cognitive theory*. Englewood Cliffs, NJ: Prentice-Hall.

Bandura, A. (2006). Guide for constructing self-efficacy scales. In F. Pajares & T. Urdan (Eds.), *Self-efficacy beliefs of adolescents* (Vol. 5, pp. 307–337). Greenwich, CT: Information Age Publishing.

Bärnighausen, T., Røttingen, J.-A., Rockers, P., Shemilt, I., & Tugwell, P. (2017). Quasi-experimental study designs series—Paper 1: Introduction: Two historical lineages. *Journal of Clinical Epidemiology, 89*, 4–11.

Bärnighausen, T., Tugwell, P., Røttingen, J. A., Shemilt, I., Rockers, P., Geldsetzer, P., ... Atun, R. (2017). Quasi-experimental study designs series—Paper 4: Uses and value. *Journal of Clinical Epidemiology, 89*, 21–29.

Bassett, M. T., Dumanovsky, T., Huang, C., Silver, L. D., Young, C., Nonas, C., ... Frieden, T. R. (2008). Purchasing behavior and calorie information at fast-food chains in New York City, 2007. *American Journal of Public Health, 98*(8), 1457–1459.

Basu, A., & Maciejewski, M. L. (2019). Choosing a time horizon in cost and cost-effectiveness analyses. *JAMA, 321*(11), 1096–1097.

Bauman, K. E., & Fisher, L. A. (1985). Subjective expected utility, locus of control, and behavior. *Journal of Applied Social Psychology, 15*(7), 606–621.

Baumann, A. A., & Cabassa, L. J. (2020). Reframing implementation science to address inequities in healthcare delivery. *BMC Health Services Research, 20*(1), 190.

Bayer, R. (1989). *Private acts, social consequences: AIDS and the politics of public health.* New York, NY: Free Press.

Beccaria, C. (1764). On crimes and punishments. In J. E. Jacoby (Ed.), *Classics of criminology* (2nd ed.). Prospect Heights, IL: Waveland Press.

Beck, A. T., Kovacs, M., & Weissman, A. (1979). Assessment of suicidal intention: The Scale for Suicide Ideation. *Journal of Consulting and Clinical Psychology, 47*(2), 343–352.

Beck, L. F., Shults, R. A., Mack, K. A., & Ryan, G. W. (2007). Associations between sociodemographics and safety belt use in states with and without primary enforcement laws. *American Journal of Public Health, 97*(9), 1619–1624.

Becker, G. S. (1968). Crime and punishment: An economic approach. In N. G. Fielding, A. Clarke, & R. Witt (Eds.), *The economic dimensions of crime* (pp. 13–68). London, UK: Palgrave Macmillan.

Becker, G. S., & Stigler, G. J. (1974). Law enforcement, malfeasance, and compensation of enforcers. *The Journal of Legal Studies, 3*(1), 1–18.

Becker, H. S. (2009). How to find out how to do qualitative research. *International Journal of Communication, 3*, 545–553.

Beitsch, L. M., Brooks, R. G., Grigg, M., & Menachemi, N. (2006). Structure and functions of state public health agencies. *American Journal of Public Health, 96*(1), 167–172.

Beitsch, L. M., Grigg, M., Menachemi, N., & Brooks, R. G. (2006). Roles of local public health agencies within the state public health system. *Journal of Public Health Management and Practice, 12*(3), 232–241.

Benson, K., & Hartz, A. J. (2000). A comparison of observational studies and randomized, controlled trials. *New England Journal of Medicine, 342*(25), 1878–1886.

Bentham, J. (1789). *Theory of legislation.* London, UK: Paul, Trench, Trubner.

Berkman, L. F., & Kawachi, I. (2000). *Social epidemiology.* New York, NY: Oxford University Press.

Bero, L. A., Montini, T., Bryan-Jones, K., & Mangurian, C. (2001). Science in regulatory policy making: Case studies in the development of workplace smoking restrictions. *Tobacco Control, 10*(4), 329–336.

Berwick, D. M., & Brennan, T. A. (1995). *New rules: Regulation, markets, and the quality of American health care.* San Francisco, CA: Jossey-Bass.

Bhandari, M. W., Scutchfield, F. D., Charnigo, R., Riddell, M. C., & Mays, G. P. (2010). New data, same story? Revisiting studies on the relationship of local public health systems characteristics to public health performance. *Journal of Public Health Management and Practice, 16*(2), 110–117.

Bhargava, S., & Loewenstein, G. (2015). Behavioral economics and public policy 102: Beyond nudging. *American Economic Review, 105*(5), 396–401.

Bialous, S. A., Fox, B. J., & Glantz, S. A. (2001). Tobacco industry allegations of "illegal lobbying" and state tobacco control. *American Journal of Public Health, 91*(1), 62–67.

Bicchieri, C., Fatas, E., Aldama, A., Casas, A., Deshpande, I., Lauro, M., ... Wen, R. (2021). In science we (should) trust: Expectations and compliance during the COVID-19 pandemic. *PLoS One, 16*(6), e0252892.

Bilz, K., & Nadler, J. (2009). Law, psychology, and morality. *Psychology of Learning and Motivation, 50*, 101–131.

Biradavolu, M. R., Burris, S., George, A., Jena, A., & Blankenship, K. M. (2009). Can sex workers regulate police? Learning from an HIV prevention project for sex workers in southern India. *Social Science & Medicine, 68*(8), 1541–1547.

Black, J. (2008). Constructing and contesting legitimacy and accountability in polycentric regulatory regimes. *Regulation & Governance, 2*, 137–164.

Blackenship, K. M., Friedman, S. R., Dworkin, S., & Mantell, J. E. (2006). Structural interventions: Concepts, challenges and opportunities for research. *Journal of Urban Health, 83*(1), 59–72.

Blader, S. L., & Tyler, T. R. (2003a). What constitutes fairness in work settings? A four-component model of procedural justice. *Human Resource Management Review, 13*(1), 107–126.

Blader, S. L., & Tyler, T. R. (2003b). A four-component model of procedural justice: Defining the meaning of a "fair" process. *Personality and Social Psychology Bulletin, 29*(6), 747–758.

Blank, R. M. (2002). Can equity and efficiency complement each other? *Labour Economics, 9*(4), 451–468.

Blankenship, K. M., & Koester, S. (2002). Criminal law, policing policy, and HIV risk in female street sex workers and injection drug users. *The Journal of Law, Medicine & Ethics, 30*(4), 548–559.

Blattman, C. (2016). A lot of people think field experiments make scholars ask small questions, but I think they'll push us to answer the big ones. Retrieved from https://chrisblattman.com/2016/01/08/a-lot-of-people-think-field-experiments-make-scholars-ask-small-questions-but-i-think-theyll-push-us-to-answer-the-big-ones/.

Blau, P. (1964). *Exchange and power in social life*. New York, NY: John Wiley & Sons.

Bluthenthal, R. N., Heinzerling, K. G., Anderson, R., Flynn, N. M., & Kral, A. H. (2007). Approval of syringe exchange programs in California: Results from a local approach to HIV prevention. *American Journal of Public Health, 98*(2), 278–283.

Boadway, R. W. (1974). The welfare foundations of cost-benefit analysis. *The Economic Journal, 84*(336), 926–939.

Boardman, A., Greenberg, D., Vining, A., & Weimer, D. (2011). *Cost-benefit analysis: Concepts and practice* (4th ed.). Englewood Cliffs, NJ: Prentice Hall.

Boardman, A. E., Greenberg, D. H., Vining, A. R., & Weimer, D. L. (2017). *Cost-benefit analysis: Concepts and practice*. New York, NY: Cambridge University Press.

Boardman, A. E., & Vining, A. R. (2017). There are many (well, more than one) paths to Nirvana: The economic evaluation of social policies. In *Handbook of social policy evaluation*. Cheltenham, UK: Edward Elgar Publishing.

Boehmer, T. K., Luke, D. A., Haire-Joshu, D. L., Bates, H. S., & Brownson, R. C. (2008). Preventing childhood obesity through state policy: Predictors of bill enactment. *American Journal of Preventive Medicine, 34*(4), 333–340.

Bogenschneider, K., & Corbett, T. J. (2010). Family policy: Becoming a field of inquiry and subfield of social policy. *Journal of Marriage and Family, 72*(3), 783–803.

Bonilla-Silva, E. (1997). Rethinking racism: Toward a structural interpretation. *American Sociological Review, 62*(3), 465–480.

Borgatti, S. P., Mehra, A., Brass, D. J., & Labianca, G. (2009). Network analysis in the social sciences. *Science, 323*(5916), 892–895.

Bouffard, J. A., & Askew, L. N. (2019). Time-series analyses of the impact of sex offender registration and notification law implementation and subsequent modifications on rates of sexual offenses. *Crime & Delinquency, 65*, 1483–1512.

Boyd, M. R., Powell, B. J., Endicott, D., & Lewis, C. C. (2018). A method for tracking implementation strategies: An exemplar implementing measurement-based care in community behavioral health clinics. *Behavior Therapy, 49*(4), 525–537.

Boyle, K. J. (2017). Contingent valuation in practice. In *A primer on nonmarket valuation* (pp. 83–131). Dordrecht, the Netherlands: Springer.

Bradford, B., Murphy, K., & Jackson, J. (2014). Officers as mirrors: Procedural justice and the (re)production of social identity. *British Journal of Criminology, 54*, 527–550.

Braga, A. A., Weisburd, D., & Turchan, B. (2018). Focused deterrence strategies and crime control: An updated systematic review and meta-analysis of the empirical evidence. *Criminology & Public Policy, 17*, 205–250.

Braithwaite, J. (1989). *Crime, shame, and reintegration.* Cambridge, UK: Cambridge University Press.

Braithwaite, J. (2008). *Regulatory capitalism: How it works, ideas for making it work better.* Cheltenham, UK; Northampton, MA: Edward Elgar.

Braithwaite, J. (2020). Regulatory mix, collective efficacy, and crimes of the powerful. *Journal of White Collar and Corporate Crime, 1*, 62–71.

Braithwaite, J., Coglianese, C., & Levi-Faur, D. (2007). Can regulation and governance make a difference? *Regulation and Governance, 1*(1), 1–7.

Braithwaite, J., & Drahos, P. (2000). *Global business regulation.* Cambridge, UK: Cambridge University Press.

Braithwaite, J., Healy, J., & Dwan, K. (2005). *The governance of health safety and quality.* Canberra, Australia: Commonwealth of Australia.

Brand, P. A., & Anastasio, P. A. (2006). Violence-related attitudes and beliefs. *Journal of Interpersonal Violence, 21*(7), 856–868.

Braun, J. M., Kahn, R. S., Froelich, T., Auinger, P., & Lamphear, B. P. (2006). Exposures to environmental toxicants and attention deficit hyperactivity disorder in U.S. children. *Environmental Health Perspectives, 114*(12), 1904–1909.

Brender, J. D., Maantay, J. A., & Chakraborty, J. (2011). Residential proximity to environmental hazards and adverse health outcomes. *American Journal of Public Health, 101*, S37–S52.

Brewer, J. (2004). Ethnography. In C. Cassell & G. Symon (Eds.), *Essential guide to qualitative methods in organizational research* (pp. 312–322). London, UK; Thousand Oaks, CA: Sage.

Brewer, N. T. (2017). Increasing vaccination. *Psychological Science in the Public Interest, 18*, 149–207.

Breza, E., Stanford, F. C., Alsan, M., Alsan, B., Banerjee, A., Chandrasekhar, A. G., ... Duflo, E. (2021a). Doctors' and Nurses' Social Media Ads Reduced Holiday Travel and COVID-19 infections: A cluster randomized controlled trial in 13 States. *medRxiv.* doi:10.1101/2021.06.23.21259402

Breza, E., Stanford, F. C., Alsan, M., Alsan, B., Banerjee, A., Chandrasekhar, A. G., ... Duflo, E. (2021b). Effects of a large-scale social media advertising campaign on holiday travel and COVID-19 infections: A cluster randomized controlled trial. *Nature Medicine, 27*(9), 1622–1628.

Briggs, A., Sculpher, M., & Buxton, M. (1994). Uncertainty in the economic evaluation of health care technologies: The role of sensitivity analysis. *Health Economics, 3*(2), 95–104. doi:10.1002/hec.4730030206

Briss, P. A., Rodewald, L. E., Hinman, A. R., Shefer, A. M., Strikas, R. A., Bernier, R. R., ... Williams, S. M. (2000). Reviews of evidence regarding interventions to improve vaccination coverage in children, adolescents, and adults: The Task Force on Community Preventive Services. *American Journal of Preventive Medicine, 18*(1), 97–140.

Brody, H., Rip, M. R., Vinten-Johansen, P., Paneth, N., & Rachman, S. (2000). Mapmaking and myth-making in Broad Street: The London cholera epidemic, 1854. *Lancet, 356*, 64–68.

Bronfrenbrenner, U. (2005). *Making human beings human: Bioecological perspectives on human development.* Thousand Oaks, CA: Sage.

Brown, A. F., Ma, G. X., Miranda, J., Eng, E., Castille, D., Brockie, T., ... Trinh-Shevrin, C. (2019). Structural interventions to reduce and eliminate health disparities. *American Journal of Public Health, 109*(S1), S72–S78.

Browning, C. R., & Cagney, K. A. (2002). Neighborhood structural disadvantage, collective efficacy, and self-rated physical health in an urban setting. *Journal of Health and Social Behavior, 43*(4), 383–399.

Brownson, R. C., & Bright, F. S. (2004). Chronic disease control in public health practice: Looking back and moving forward. *Public Health Reports, 119*(3), 230–238.

Brownson, R. C., Colditz, G. A., & Proctor, E. K. (2012). *Dissemination and implementation research in health: Translating science to practice.* New York, NY: Oxford University Press.

Brownson, R. C., Eriksen, M. P., Davis, R. M., & Warner, K. E. (1997). Environmental tobacco smoke: Health effects and policies to reduce exposure. *Annual Review of Public Health, 18*, 163–185.

Brownson, R. C., Kumanyika, S. K., Kreuter, M. W., & Haire-Joshu, D. (2021). Implementation science should give higher priority to health equity. *Implementation Science, 16*(1), 28.

Brydon-Miller, M., Greenwood, D., & Maguire, P. (2003). Why action research? *Action Research, 1*(1), 9–28.

Buehler, J. W., Whitney, E. A., & Berkelman, R. L. (2006). Business and public health collaboration for emergency preparedness in Georgia: A case study. *BMC Public Health, 6*, 285.

Bullock, H. L., Lavis, J. N., Wilson, M. G., Mulvale, G., & Miatello, A. (2021). Understanding the implementation of evidence-informed policies and practices from a policy perspective: A critical interpretive synthesis. *Implementation Science, 16*(1), 18.

Burris, S. (1998a). Gay marriage and public health. *Temple Political and Civil Rights Law Review, 7*(2), 417–427.

Burris, S. (1998b). Law and the social risk of health care: Lessons from HIV testing. *Albany Law Review, 61*, 831–895.

Burris, S. (2003). Legal aspects of regulating bathhouses: Cases from 1984 to 1995. *Journal of Homosexuality, 44*(3–4), 131–151.

Burris, S. (2006). From security to health. In J. Woods & B. Dupont (Eds.), *Democracy and the governance of security* (pp. 196–216). Cambridge, UK: Cambridge University Press.

Burris, S. (2008). Regulatory innovation in the governance of human subjects research: A cautionary tale and some modest proposals. *Regulation and Governance, 2*, 1–20.

Burris, S. (2011a). From health care law to the social determinants of health: A public health law research perspective. *University of Pennsylvania Law Review, 159*(6), 1649–1667.

Burris, S. (2011b). Law in a social determinants strategy: A public health law research perspective. *Public Health Reports, 126*(Suppl. 3), 22–27.

Burris, S. (2017). Theory and methods in comparative drug and alcohol policy research: Response to a review of the literature. *International Journal of Drug Policy, 41*, 126–131.

Burris, S., & Anderson, E. (2013). Legal regulation of health-related behavior: A half century of public health law research. *Annual Review of Law and Social Science, 9*(1), 95–117.

Burris, S., Ashe, M., Blanke, D., Ibrahim, J., Levin, D. E., Matthews, G., ... Katz, M. (2016). Better health faster: The 5 essential public health law services. *Public Health Reports, 131*(6), 747–753.

Burris, S., Ashe, M., Levin, D., Penn, M., & Larkin, M. (2016). a transdisciplinary approach to public health law: The emerging practice of legal epidemiology. *Annual Review of Public Health, 37*(1), 135–148.

Burris, S., Blankenship, K. M., Donoghoe, M., Sherman, S., Vernick, J. S., Case, P., ... Koester, S. (2004). Addressing the "risk environment" for injection drug users: The mysterious case of the missing cop. *The Milbank Quarterly, 82*(1), 125–156.

Burris, S., Cloud, L. K., & Penn, M. (2020). The growing field of legal epidemiology. *Journal of Public Health Management and Practice, 26*, S4–S9.

Burris, S., Hitchcock, L., Ibrahim, J. K., Penn, M., & Ramanathan, T. (2016). Policy surveillance: A vital public health practice comes of age. *Journal of Health Politics, Policy and Law, 41*(6), 1151–1167.

Burris, S., Kawachi, I., & Sarat, A. (2002). Integrating law and social epidemiology. *The Journal of Law, Medicine & Ethics, 30*, 510–521.

Burris, S., Kempa, M., & Shearing, C. (2008). Changes in governance: A cross-disciplinary review of current scholarship. *Akron Law Review, 41*(1), 1–66.

Burris, S., Korfmacher, K., Moran-McCabe, K., Prood, N., Blankenship, K., Corbett, A., & Saxon, B. (2020). *Health equity through housing: A blueprint for systematic legal action*. Retrieved from https://phlr.org/sites/default/files/uploaded_images/HousingHealthEquityLaw-Report6-July2020-FINAL.pdf.

Burris, S., Wagenaar, A. C., Swanson, J., Ibrahim, J. K., Wood, J., & Mello, M. M. (2010). Making the case for laws that improve health: A framework for public health law research. *The Milbank Quarterly, 88*(2), 169–210.

Burris, S. C., Beletsky, L., Burleson, J. A., Case, P., & Lazzarini, Z. (2007). Do criminal laws influence HIV risk behavior? An empirical trial. *Arizona State Law Journal, 39*, 467–517.

Burtless, G. (1985). Are targeted wage subsidies harmful? Evidence from a wage voucher experiment. *Industrial and Labor Relations Review, 39*(1), 105–114.

Buse, K., & Lee, K. (2005). *Business and global health governance*. London, UK: London School of Hygiene & Tropical Medicine.

Butler, D. M., & Smith, D. M. (2007). Serosorting can potentially increase HIV transmissions. *AIDS, 21*(9), 1218–1220.

Cabanac, M. (1992). Pleasure: The common currency. *Journal of Theoretical Biology, 155*(2), 173–200.

Call, C. (2018). The community corrections perspective toward sex offender management policies and collateral consequences: Does contact with sex offenders matter? *Criminal Justice Studies, 31*, 1–17.

Cameron, L., Seager, J., & Shah, M. (2021). Crimes against morality: Unintended consequences of criminalizing sex work. *Quarterly Journal of Economics, 136*(1), 427–469.

Campbell Collaboration. (2009). *What helps? What harms? Based on what evidence? Systematic reviews of the effects of interventions in education, crime and justice, and social welfare, to promote evidence-based decision-making*. Retrieved from www.campbellcollaboration.org/artman2/uploads/1/C2_GeneralBrochure_low_May09.pdf.

Campbell, F., Conti, G., Heckman, J. J., Moon, S. H., Pinto, R., Pungello, E., & Pan, Y. (2014). Early childhood investments substantially boost adult health. *Science, 343*(6178), 1478–1485.

Campos-Mercade, P., Meier, A. N., Schneider, F. H., Meier, S., Pope, D., & Wengstrom, E. (2021). Monetary incentives increase COVID-19 vaccinations. *Science, 374*(6569), 879–882.

Cantor, J., Beckman, R., Collins, R. L., Dastidar, M. G., Richardson, A. S., & Dubowitz, T. (2020). SNAP participants improved food security and diet after a full-service supermarket opened in an urban food desert: Study examines impact grocery store opening had on food security and diet of Supplemental Nutrition Assistance Program participants living in an urban food desert. *Health Affairs, 39*(8), 1386–1394.

Carreras, G., Lugo, A., Gallus, S., Cortini, B., Fernández, E., López, M. J., … Perez, P. (2019). Burden of disease attributable to second-hand smoke exposure: A systematic review. *Preventive Medicine, 129*, 105833.

Case, A., & Deaton, A. (2017). Mortality and morbidity in the 21st century. *Brookings Papers on Economic Activity, 2017*, 397.

Case, A., & Deaton, A. (2020). *Deaths of despair and the future of capitalism*. Princeton, NJ: Princeton University Press.

Cast, A. D., & Burke, P. (2002). A theory of self-esteem. *Social Forces, 80*(3), 1041–1068.

Cattaneo, M. D., & Escanciano, J. C. (2017). *Regression discontinuity designs: Theory and applications* (1st ed.). Bingley, UK: Emerald Publishing.

Caulkins, J., Pacula, R., Paddock, S., & Chiesa, J. R. (2002). *School-based drug prevention: What kind of drug use does it prevent? (MR-1459-RWJ)*. Santa Monica, CA: RAND.

Caulkins, J. P. (2007). Price and purity analysis for illicit drug: Data and conceptual issues. *Drug and Alcohol Dependence, 90*, S61–S68.

Caulkins, J. P., Kilmer, B., Kleiman, M., MacCoun, R. J., Midgette, G., Oglesby, P., ... Reuter, P. H. (2015). *Considering marijuana legalization: Insights for Vermont and other jurisdictions*. Santa Monica, CA: RAND.

Cawley, J. (2015). An economy of scales: A selective review of obesity's economic causes, consequences, and solutions. *Journal of Health Economics, 43*, 244–268.

Cawley, J., & Liu, F. (2008). Correlates of state legislative action to prevent childhood obesity. *Obesity, 16*(1), 162–167.

Cawley, J., Sweeney, M. J., Sobal, J., Just, D. R., Kaiser, H. M., Schulze, W. D., ... Wansink, B. (2015). The impact of a supermarket nutrition rating system on purchases of nutritious and less nutritious foods. *Public Health Nutrition, 18*(1), 8–14.

Center for Law and the Public's Health. (2001). *Core legal competencies for public health professionals*. Retrieved from www.publichealthlaw.net/Training/TrainingPDFs/PHLCompetencies.pdf.

Center for Public Health Law Research. (2022). *MonQcle*. Retrieved from http://www.monqcle.com/.

Centers for Disease Control and Prevention (1999a). Achievements in public health, 1900–1999: Decline in deaths from heart disease and stroke—United States, 1900–1999. *Morbidity and Mortality Weekly Report, 48*(30), 649–656.

Centers for Disease Control and Prevention (1999b). Achievements in public health, 1900–1999: Impact of vaccines universally recommended for children—United States, 1990–1998. *Morbidity and Mortality Weekly Report, 48*(12), 243–248.

Centers for Disease Control and Prevention (1999c). Achievements in public health, 1900–1999: Motor-vehicle safety: A 20th century public health achievement. *Morbidity and Mortality Weekly Report, 48*(18), 369–374.

Centers for Disease Control and Prevention (1999d). Achievements in public health, 1900–1999: Tobacco use—United States, 1900–1999. *Morbidity and Mortality Weekly Report, 48*(43), 986–993.

Centers for Disease Control and Prevention (1999e). Ten great public health achievements—United States, 1900–1999. *Morbidity and Mortality Weekly Report, 48*(12), 241–243. Retrieved from www.cdc.gov/about/history/tengpha.htm

Centers for Disease Control and Prevention. (1999f). *Backgrounder: State laws on tobacco Control*. Retrieved from www.cdc.gov/media/pressrel/r990625.htm.

Centers for Disease Control and Prevention (2008). Smoking-attributable mortality, years of potential life lost, and productivity losses—United States, 2000–2004. *Morbidity and Mortality Weekly Report, 57*(45), 1226–1228.

Centers for Disease Control and Prevention (2010). State cigarette minimum price laws—United States, 2009. *Morbidity and Mortality Weekly Report, 59*(13), 389–392.

Centers for Disease Control and Prevention. (2011a). *National Public Health Performance Standards Program (NPHPSP)*. Retrieved from www.cdc.gov/nphpsp/index.html.

Centers for Disease Control and Prevention (2011b). Ten great public health achievements—United States, 2001–2010. *Journal of the American Medical Association, 306*(1), 36–38.

Centers for Disease Control and Prevention (2020a). *Understanding the epidemic*. Retrieved from https://www.cdc.gov/drugoverdose/epidemic/index.html.

Centers for Disease Control and Prevention. (2020b). *An approach for monitoring and evaluating community mitigation strategies for COVID-19*. Retrieved from https://www.cdc.gov/coronavirus/2019-ncov/php/monitoring-evaluating-community-mitigation-strategies.html.

Centers for Disease Control and Prevention. (2021). *HIV and STD criminalization laws*. Retrieved from https://www.cdc.gov/hiv/policies/law/states/exposure.html.

Chalkidou, K., Tunis, S., Lopert, R., Rochaix, L., Sawicki, P. T., Nasser, M., & Xerri, B. (2009). Comparative effectiveness research and evidence-based health policy: Experience from four countries. *The Milbank Quarterly, 87*(2), 339–367.

Chaloupka, F. J. (2004). The effects of price on alcohol use, abuse, and their consequences. In R. J. Bonnie & M. E. O'Connell (Eds.), *Reducing underage drinking: A collective responsibility*. Washington, DC: National Academies Press.

Chaloupka, F. J., Powell, L. M., & Chriqui, J. F. (2011). Sugar-sweetened beverages and obesity: The potential impact of public policies. *Journal of Policy Analysis and Management, 30*(3), 645–655.

Chapman, S. (2006). Butt clean up campaigns: Wolves in sheep's clothing? *Tobacco Control, 15*, 273.

Chatterji, P., Kim, D., & Lahiri, K. (2014). Birth weight and academic achievement in childhood. *Health Economics, 23*(9), 1013–1035.

Chauncey, G. (1994). *Gay New York: Gender, urban culture, and the makings of the gay male world, 1890–1940*. New York, NY: Basic Books.

Chetty, R., & Friedman, J. N. (2011). The long-term effects of early childhood education. *Communities & Banking, Summer*, 6–7.

Chetty, R., Grusky, D., Hell, M., Hendren, N., Manduca, R., & Narang, J. (2017). The fading American dream: Trends in absolute income mobility since 1940. *Science, 356*(6336), 398–406.

Chetty, R., Hendren, N., Jones, M. R., & Porter, S. R. (2020). Race and economic opportunity in the United States: An intergenerational perspective. *The Quarterly Journal of Economics, 135*(2), 711–783.

Chetty, R., Hendren, N., & Katz, L. F. (2016). The effects of exposure to better neighborhoods on children: New evidence from the moving to opportunity experiment. *American Economic Review, 106*(4), 855–902.

Chetty, R., Hendren, N., Kline, P., & Saez, E. (2014). Where is the land of opportunity? The geography of intergenerational mobility in the United States. *The Quarterly Journal of Economics, 129*(4), 1553–1623.

Chetty, R., Hendren, N., Lin, F., Majerovitz, J., & Scuderi, B. (2016). Childhood environment and gender gaps in adulthood. *American Economic Review, 106*(5), 282–288.

Chetty, R., Stepner, M., Abraham, S., Lin, S., Scuderi, B., Turner, N., ... Cutler, D. (2016). The association between income and life expectancy in the United States, 2001–2014. *JAMA, 315*(16), 1750–1766.

Chriqui, J. F., Frosh, M., Brownson, R. C., Shelton, D. M., Sciandra, R. C., Hobart, R., ... Alciati, M. H. (2002). Application of a rating system to state clean indoor air laws. *Tobacco Control, 11*(1), 26–34.

Chriqui, J. F., O'Connor, J. C., & Chaloupka, F. J. (2011). What gets measured, gets changed: Evaluating law and policy for maximum impact. *The Journal of Law, Medicine & Ethics, 39*(Suppl. 1), 21–26.

Chriqui, J. F., Ribisl, K. M., Wallace, R. M., Williams, R. S., O'Connor, J. C., & el Arculli, R. (2008). A comprehensive review of state laws governing Internet and other delivery sales of cigarettes in the United States. *Nicotine & Tobacco Research, 10*(2), 253–265.

Chu, Y. W. L., & Gershenson, S. (2018). High times: The effect of medical marijuana laws on student time use. *Economics of Education Review, 66*, 142–153.

Chung, J. H., Phibbs, C. S., Boscardin, W. J., Kominski, G. F., Ortega, A. N., & Needleman, J. (2010). The effect of neonatal intensive care level and hospital volume on mortality of very low birth weight infants. *Medical Care, 48*(7), 635–644.

Claxton, K., Asaria, M., Chansa, C., Jamison, J., Lomas, J., Ochalek, J., & Paulden, M. (2019). Accounting for timing when assessing health-related policies. *Journal of Benefit-Cost Analysis, 10*(S1), 73–105. doi:10.1017/bca.2018.29

Clay, K., Lewis, J., & Severnini, E. (2016). *Canary in a coal mine: Infant mortality, property values, and tradeoffs associated with mid-20th century air pollution* (No. w22155). National Bureau of Economic Research.

Cloud, D. H., Beane, S., Adimora, A., Friedman, S. R., Jefferson, K., Hall, H. I., ... Cooper, H. L. F. (2019). State minimum wage laws and newly diagnosed cases of HIV among heterosexual black residents of US metropolitan areas. *SSM - Population Health, 7*, 100327.

Cochrane Collaboration. (2009). *An introduction to Cochrane reviews and the Cochrane library*. Retrieved from www.cochrane.org/reviews/clibintro.htm.

Cohen, D., & Crabtree, B. (2006). *Qualitative research guidelines project*. Robert Wood Johnson Foundation. Retrieved from www.qualres.org/index.html.

Cohen, D. A., Scribner, R. A., & Farley, T. A. (2000). A structural model of health behavior: A pragmatic approach to explain and influence health behaviors at the population level. *Preventive Medicine, 30*(2), 146–154.

Cohen, J. (1988). *Statistical power analysis for the behavioral sciences* (2nd ed.). Hillsdale, NJ: Lawrence Erlbaum Associates.

Cohen, L., Manion, L., & Morrison, K. (2000). *Research methods in education* (5th ed.). New York, NY: Routledge.

Cohen, S., Kessler, R. C., & Underwood-Gordon, L. (1995). Strategies for measuring stress in studies of psychiatric and physical disorders. In S. Cohen, R. C. Kessler, & L. Underwood-Gordon (Eds.), *Measuring stress: A guide for health and social scientists* (Vol. 28, pp. 3–26). New York, NY: Oxford University Press.

Collins, J., & Koplan, J. P. (2009). Health impact assessment: A step toward health in all policies. *Journal of the American Medical Association, 302*(3), 315–317.

Commission on Social Determinants of Health (2008). *Closing the gap in a generation: Health equity through action on the social determinants of health.* Geneva, Switzerland: World Health Organization.

Concato, J., Shah, N., & Horwitz, R. I. (2000). Randomized, controlled trials, observational studies, and the hierarchy of research designs. *New England Journal of Medicine, 342*(25), 1887–1892.

Conners, C. K., Sitarenios, G., Parker, J. D. A., & Epstein, J. N. (1998). Revision and restandardization of the Conners Teacher Rating Scale (CTRS-R): Factor structure, reliability, and criterion validity. *Journal of Abnormal Child Psychology, 26*(4), 279–291.

Cook, P. J., Machin, S. J., Marie, O., & Mastrobuoni, G. (2012). Lessons from the economics of crime. In P. J. Cook, S. J. Machin, O. Marie, & G. Mastrobuoni (Eds.), *Lessons from the Economics of Crime'in Lessons from the Economics of Crime.* MIT Press. https://ssrn.com/abstract=2119606

Cook, K. S., Cheshire, C., Rice, E. R. W., & Nakagawa, S. (2013). Social exchange theory. In J. DeLamater & A. Ward (Eds.), *Handbook of Social Psychology* (pp. 61–88). Dordrecht, the Netherlands: Springer.

Cook, P. J. (2007). *Paying the tab: The costs and benefits of alcohol control.* Princeton, NJ: Princeton University Press.

Cooper, D. (1995). Local government legal consciousness in the shadow of juridification. *Journal of Law and Society, 22*(4), 506–526.

Cooper, H., Moore, L., Gruskin, S., & Krieger, N. (2005). The impact of a police drug crackdown on drug injectors' ability to practice harm reduction: A qualitative study. *Social Science & Medicine, 61*(3), 673–684.

Copas, A. J., Lewis, J. J., Thompson, J. A., Davey, C., Baio, G., & Hargreaves, J. R. (2015). Designing a stepped wedge trial: Three main designs, carry-over effects and randomisation approaches. *Trials, 16*(1), 352.

Corbin, J. M., & Strauss, A. L. (2008). *Basics of qualitative research: Techniques and procedures for developing grounded theory* (3rd ed.). Los Angeles, CA: Sage.

Corral-Verdugo, V., & Frías-Armenta, M. (2006). Personal normative beliefs, antisocial behavior, and residential water conservation. *Environment and Behavior, 38*(3), 406–421.

Corrigan, P. W., Watson, A. C., Heyrman, M. L., Warpinski, A., Gracia, G., Slopen, N., & Hall, L. L. (2005). Structural stigma in state legislation. *Psychiatric Services, 56*(5), 557–563.

Coryn, C. L. S., & Scriven, M. (2008). The logic of research evaluation. In C. L. S. Coryn & M. M. Scriven (Eds.), *Reforming the evaluation of research (New directions for evaluation)* (Vol. 118, pp. 89–105). San Francisco, CA: Jossey-Bass and American Evaluation Association.

Council of Economic Advisers. (2017). *Discounting for public policy: Theory and recent evidence on the merits of updating the discount rate.* Retrieved from https://obamawhitehouse.archives.gov/sites/default/files/page/files/201701_cea_discounting_issue_brief.pdf.

Council on Linkages Between Academia and Public Health Practice. (2021). *Core competencies for public health professionals.* Retrieved from http://www.phf.org/corecompetencies.

Creswell, J. W. (2007). *Qualitative inquiry & research design: Choosing among five approaches* (2nd ed.). Thousand Oaks, CA: Sage.

Creswell, J. W., Klassen, A. C., Plano Clark, V. L., Smith, K. C., & The Office of Behavioral and Social Sciences Research. (2011). *Best practices for mixed methods research in the health sciences.* Retrieved from obssr.od.nih.gov/scientific_areas/methodology/mixed_methods_research/index.aspx.

Creswell, J. W., & Plano Clark, V. L. (2007). *Designing and conducting mixed methods research.* Thousand Oaks, CA: Sage.

Croley, S. (2008). *Regulation and public interests: The possibility of good regulatory government.* Princeton, NJ: Princeton University Press.

Crowder, K., & Downey, L. (2010). Inter-neighborhood migration, race, and environmental hazards: Modeling micro-level processes of environmental inequality. *American Journal of Sociology, 115*(4), 1110–1149.

Crowley, D. M., Connell, C. M., Jones, D., & Donovan, M. W. (2019). Considering the child welfare system burden from opioid misuse: Research priorities for estimating public costs. *The American Journal of Managed Care, 25*(13 Suppl), S256.

Crowley, D. M., Dodge, K. A., Barnett, W. S., Corso, P., Duffy, S., Graham, P., … Plotnick, R. (2018). Standards of evidence for conducting and reporting economic evaluations in prevention science. *Prevention Science, 19*(3), 366–390.

Cullen, F. T., Pratt, T. C., Miceli, S. L., & Moon, M. M. (2002). Dangerous liason? Rational choice theory as the basis for correctional intervention. In A. R. Piquero & S. Tibbetts (Eds.), *Rational choice and criminal behavior: Recent research and future challenges* (pp. 279–298). New York, NY: Routledge.

Cullen, F. T., Wright, J. P., & Applegate, B. K. (1996). Control in the community: The limits of reform? In A. T. Harland (Ed.), *Choosing correctional options that work: Defining the demand and evaluating the supply* (pp. 69–116). Thousand Oaks, CA: Sage.

Curran, G. M., Bauer, M., Mittman, B., Pyne, J. M., & Stetler, C. (2012). Effectiveness-implementation hybrid designs: Combining elements of clinical effectiveness and implementation research to enhance public health impact. *Medical Care, 50*(3), 217–226.

Currie, J., & Gruber, J. (1997). *The technology of birth: Health insurance, medical interventions, and infant health.* Cambridge, MA: National Bureau of Economic Research.

Cutler, D. M., & Miller, G. (2004). *The role of public health improvements in health advances: The 20th century United States.* Cambridge, MA: National Bureau of Economic Research.

Cutler, D. M., Lleras-Muney, A., & Vogl, T. (2011). Socioeconomic status and health: Dimensions and mechanisms. In S. Glied & P. C. Smith (Eds.), *Oxford handbook of health economics* (pp. 124–163). Oxford, UK: Oxford University Press.

Dahl, R. A. (1956). *A preface to democratic theory.* Chicago, IL: University of Chicago Press.

Damschroder, L. J., Aron, D. C., Keith, R. E., Kirsh, S. R., Alexander, J. A., & Lowery, J. C. (2009). Fostering implementation of health services research findings into practice:

A consolidated framework for advancing implementation science. *Implementation Science, 4,* 50.

Danila, R. N., Laine, E. S., Livingston, F., Como-Sabetti, K., Lamers, L., Johnson, K., & Barry, A. M. (2015). Legal authority for infectious disease reporting in the united states: Case study of the 2009 h1n1 influenza pandemic. *American Journal of Public Health, 105*(1), 13–18.

Dansereau, D. F., & Simpson, D. D. (2009). A picture is worth a thousand words: The case for graphic representations. *Professional Psychology: Research and Practice, 40*(1), 104–110.

Darley, J. M., Tyler, T. R., & Bilz, K. (2003). The Sage handbook of social psychology. In M. A. Hogg & J. Cooper (Eds.), *Enacting justice: The interplay of individual and institutional perspectives.* Thousand Oaks, CA: Sage.

Dasgupta, A. K., & Pearce, D. W. (1972). *Cost-benefit analysis: Theory and practice.* London, UK: Macmillan International Higher Education.

Daudel, P., & Daudel, R. (1948). The molecular diagram method. *The Journal of Chemical Physics, 16*(7), 639–643.

Dausey, D. J., Buehler, J. W., & Lurie, N. (2007). Designing and conducting tabletop exercises to assess public health preparedness for manmade and naturally occurring biological threats. *BMC Public Health, 7,* 92.

Davis, C. S., Burris, S., Kraut-Becher, J., Lynch, K. G., & Metzger, D. (2005). Effects of an intensive street-level police intervention on syringe exchange program use in Philadelphia, PA. *American Journal of Public Health, 95*(2), 233–236.

Davis, C. S., & Samuels, E. A. (2021). Continuing increased access to buprenorphine in the United States via telemedicine after COVID-19. *International Journal of Drug Policy, 93,* 102905.

Davis, F. D., & Warshaw, P. R. (1992). What do intention scales measure? *Journal of General Psychology, 119*(4), 391–407.

Davis, G. G., & National Association of Medical Examiners and American College of Medical Toxicology Expert Panel on Evaluating and Reporting Opioid Deaths (2013). Recommendations for the investigation, diagnosis, and certification of deaths related to opioid drugs. *Academic Forensic Pathology, 3*(1), 62–76.

de Bekker-Grob, E. W., Ryan, M., & Gerard, K. (2012). Discrete choice experiments in health economics: A review of the literature. *Health Economics, 21*(2), 145–172.

De Cremer, D., & Tyler, T. R. (2005). Managing group behavior: The interplay between procedural justice, sense of self, and cooperation. *Advances in Experimental Social Psychology, 37,* 151–218.

Deal, L. W., Gomby, D. S., Zippiroli, L., & Behrman, R. E. (2000). Unintentional injuries in childhood: Analysis and recommendations. *The Future of Children, 10*(1), 4–22.

Dearlove, J. V., & Glantz, S. A. (2002). Boards of health as venues for clean indoor air policy making. *American Journal of Public Health, 92*(2), 257–265.

Deaton, A. (2020). *Randomization in the tropics revisited: A theme and eleven variations.* Cambridge, MA: National Bureau of Economic Research.

Deci, E. L., & Ryan, R. M. (1985). *Intrinsic motivation and self-determination in human behavior.* New York, NY: Plenum Press.

Deflem, M. (2004). Social control and the policing of terrorism: Foundations for a sociology of counterterrorism. *The American Sociologist, 35*(2), 75–92.

Delavande, A., Goldman, D. P., & Sood, N. (2007). *Criminal prosecution and HIV-related risky behavior* (NBER Working Paper W12903). Washington, DC: National Bureau of Economic Research.

Denzin, N. K., & Lincoln, Y. S. (2005). *The Sage handbook of qualitative research* (3rd ed.). Thousand Oaks, CA: Sage.

DiClemente, R. J., Crosby, R. A., & Kegler, M. C. (Eds.) (2009). *Emerging Theories in Health Promotion Practice and Research* (2nd ed.). San Francisco: Jossey-Bass.

Flay, B. R., Snyder, F. J., & Petraitis, J. (2009). The theory of triadic influence. In R. J. DiClemente, M. C. Kegler, & R. A. Crosby (Eds.), *Emerging Theories in Health Promotion Practice and Research* (2nd ed., pp. 451–510). San Francisco: Jossey-Bass.

Dillman, D. A. (1991). The design and administration of mail surveys. *Annual Review of Sociology, 17*, 225–249.

Dillman, D. A. (2007). *Mail and Internet surveys: The tailored design method.* New York, NY: John Wiley & Sons.

Dinh-Zarr, T. B., Sleet, D. A., Shults, R. A., Zaza, S., Elder, R. W., Nichols, J. L., ... Sosin, D. M. (2001). Reviews of evidence regarding interventions to increase the use of safety belts. *American Journal of Preventive Medicine, 21*(Suppl. 4), 48–65.

Dobbin, F. (2009). *Inventing equal opportunity.* Princeton, NJ: Princeton University Press.

Dobbin, F., & Sutton, J. R. (1998). The strength of a weak state: The rights revolution and the rise of human resources management divisions. *American Journal of Sociology, 104*(2), 441–476.

Dobkin, C., & Nicosia, N. (2009). The war on drugs: Methamphetamine, public health, and crime. *American Economic Review, 99*(1), 324–349.

Dodds, C., Bourne, A., & Weait, M. (2009). Responses to criminal prosecutions for HIV transmission among gay men with HIV in England and Wales. *Reproductive Health Matters, 17*(34), 135–145.

Dodson, E. A., Fleming, C., Boehmer, T. K., Haire-Joshu, D., Luke, D. A., & Brownson, R. C. (2009). Preventing childhood obesity through state policy: Qualitative assessment of enablers and barriers. *Journal of Public Health Policy, 30*(Suppl. 1), S161–S176.

Drahos, P. (Ed.) (2017). *Regulatory theory: Foundations and applications.* Canberra, Australia: ANU Press.

Dredze, M. (2012). How social media will change public health. *IEEE Intelligent Systems, 27*(4), 81–84.

Drummond, M. F., O'Brien, B., Stoddart, G. L., & Torrance, G. W. (1998). Methods for the economic evaluation of health care programmes. *American Journal of Preventive Medicine, 14*(3), 243.

Drummond, M. F., Sculpher, M. J., Claxton, K., Stoddart, G. L., & Torrance, G. W. (2015). *Methods for the economic evaluation of health care programmes* (4th ed.). Oxford, UK: Oxford University Press.

Drummond, M. F., Sculpher, M. J., Torrance, G. W., O'Brien, B. J., & Stoddart, G. L. (2005). *Methods for the economic evaluation of health care programmes.* Oxford, UK: Oxford University Press.

Drummond, M. F., & Stoddart, G. L. (1985). Principles of economic evaluation of health programmes. *World Health Statistics Quarterly, 38*(4), 355–367.

Dubois, L., Farmer, A., Girard, M., & Peterson, K. (2007). Regular sugar-sweetened beverage consumption between meals increases risk of overweight among preschool-aged children. *Journal of the American Dietetic Association, 107*(6), 924–934.

DuBois, D. L., Flay, B. R., & Fagen, M. C. (2009). Self-esteem enhancement theory: An emerging framework for promoting health across the life-span. In R. J. DiClement, M. C. Kegler, & R. A. Crosby (Eds.), *Emerging theories in health promotion practice and research* (2nd ed.). San Francisco, CA: Jossey-Bass.

Dubowitz, T., Zenk, S. N., Ghosh-Dastidar, B., Cohen, D. A., Beckman, R., Hunter, G., ... Collins, R. L. (2015). Healthy food access for urban food desert residents: Examination of the food environment, food purchasing practices, diet and BMI. *Public Health Nutrition, 18*(12), 2220–2230.

Duncan, O. D. (1966). *Path analysis: Sociological examples.* Indianapolis, IN: Bobbs-Merrill.

Durkheim, E. (1951). *Suicide: A study in sociology.* Glencoe, IL: Free Press.

Durlauf, S. N., & Nagin, D. S. (2011). Imprisonment and crime: Can both be reduced? *Criminology & Public Policy, 10*(1), 13–54.

Dusseldorp, E., Klein Velderman, M., Paulussen, T. W., Junger, M., van Nieuwenhuijzen, M., & Reijneveld, S. A. (2014). Targets for primary prevention: Cultural, social and intrapersonal factors associated with co-occurring health-related behaviours. *Psychology & Health, 29*(5), 598–611.

Easton, D. (1965). *A systems analysis of political life.* New York, NY: John Wiley & Sons.

Easton, D. (1975). A re-assessment of the concept of political support. *British Journal of Political Science, 5*(4), 435–457.

Eccles, M. P., & Mittman, B. S. (2006). Welcome to implementation science. *Implementation Science, 1*(1), 1–3.

Eckel, C. C., & Grossman, P. J. (2008). Men, women and risk aversion: Experimental evidence. *Handbook of Experimental Economics Results, 1,* 1061–1073.

Edelman, L., & Suchman, M. C. (1997). Legal ambiguity and symbolic structures: Organizational mediation of civil rights law. *American Journal of Sociology, 97,* 1531–1576.

Edelman, L. B. (1992). Legal ambiguity and symbolic structures: Organizational mediation of civil rights law. *American Journal of Sociology, 97*(6), 199–205.

Edelman, L. B. (2005). Law at work: The endogenous construction of civil rights law. In L. B. Nielsen & R. L. Nelson (Eds.), *Handbook of employment discrimination research: Rights and realities* (pp. 337–352). Dordrecht, the Netherlands: Springer.

Edelman, L. B. (2016). *Working law: Courts, corporations, and symbolic civil rights.* Chicago, IL; London, UK: The University of Chicago Press.

Edelman, L. B., Erlanger, H. S., & Lande, J. (1993). Internal dispute resolution: The transformation of civil rights in the workplace. *Law and Society Review, 27*(3), 497–534.

Edelman, L. B., Krieger, L. H., Eliason, S. R., Albiston, C. R., & Mellema, V. (2011). When organizations rule: Judicial deference to institutionalized employment structures. *American Journal of Sociology, 117*(3), 888–954.

Edelman, L. B., & Stryker, R. (2005). A sociological approach to law and the economy. In N. Smelser & R. Swedberg (Eds.), *Handbook of economic sociology* (pp. 527–551). Princeton, NJ: Princeton University Press.

Edwards, J. R., & Lambert, L. S. (2007). Methods for integrating moderation and mediation: A general analytical framework using moderated path analysis. *Psychological Methods, 12*(1), 1–22.

Egerter, S., Braveman, P., Sadegh-Nobari, T., Grossman-Kahn, R., & Dekker, M. (2009). *Education matters for health*. Princeton, NJ: Robert Wood Johnson Foundation.

Eib, C., Bernhard-Oettel, C., Magnusson Hanson, L. L., & Leineweber, C. (2018). Organizational justice and health: Studying mental preoccupation with work and social support as mediators for lagged and reversed relationships. *Journal of Occupational Health Psychology, 23*(4), 553–567.

Ein-Dor, T., & Hirschberger, G. (2016). Rethinking attachment theory: From a theory of relationships to a theory of individual and group survival. *Current Directions in Psychological Science, 25*(4), 223–227.

Ellermann, C. R., Kataoka-Yahiro, M. R., & Wong, L. C. (2006). Logic models used to enhance critical thinking. *The Journal of Nursing Education, 45*(6), 220–227.

Elovainio, M., Kivimäki, M., Eccles, M., & Sinervo, T. (2002). Team climate and procedural justice as predictors of occupational strain. *Journal of Applied Social Psychology, 32*(2), 359–372.

Eman, K. E., Mercer, J., Moreau, M., Grava-Gubins, I., Buckeridge, D., & Jonker, E. (2011). Physician privacy concerns when disclosing patient data for public health purposes during a pandemic influenza out-break. *BMC Public Health, 11*, 454.

Emerson, R. M., Fretz, R. I., & Shaw, L. L. (1995). *Writing ethnographic fieldnotes*. Chicago, IL: University of Chicago Press.

Emmons, K. M., & Chambers, D. A. (2021). Policy implementation science—An unexplored strategy to address social determinants of health. *Ethnicity & Disease, 31*(1), 133–138.

Engel, D. M., & Munger, F. W. (1996). Rights, remembrance, and the reconciliation of difference. *Law and Society Review, 30*(1), 7–54.

Engel, D. M., & Munger, F. W. (2003). *Rights of inclusion: Law and identity in the life stories of Americans with disabilities*. Chicago, IL: University of Chicago Press.

Environmental Protection Agency (2012). *Mortality Risk Valuation*. Retrieved from https://www.epa.gov/environmental-economics/mortality-risk-valuation.

Epstein, F. H. (1996). Cardiovascular disease epidemiology: A journey from the past into the future. *Circulation, 93*, 1755–1764.

Epstein, L. H., Dearing, K. K., Roba, L. G., & Finkelstein, E. (2010). The influence of taxes and subsidies on energy purchased in an experimental purchasing study. *Psychological Science, 21*(3), 406–414.

Epstein, R. A. (2003). Let the shoemaker stick to his last: A defense of the "old" public health. *Perspectives in Biology and Medicine, 46*(Suppl. 3), S138–S159.

Erickson, D. L., Gostin, L. O., Street, J., & Mills, S. P. (2002). The power to act: Two model state statutes. *The Journal of Law, Medicine & Ethics, 30*(3), 57–62.

Eriksson, P., & Kovalainen, A. (2008). *Qualitative methods in business research.* Los Angeles, CA; London, UK: Sage.

Erwin, P. C. (2008). The performance of local health departments: A review of the literature. *Journal of Public Health Management and Practice, 14*(2), E9–E18.

Estabrooks, P. A., Brownson, R. C., & Pronk, N. P. (2018). Dissemination and implementation science for public health professionals: An overview and call to action. *Preventing Chronic Disease, 15*, E162–E162.

Estin, A. L. (2010). Sharing governance: Family law in Congress and the states. *Cornell Journal of Law and Public Policy, 18*(2), 267–335.

Evans, A. S. (1978). Causation and disease: A chronological journey. The Thomas Parran Lecture. *American Journal of Epidemiology, 108*(4), 249–258.

Evans, W. N., & Garthwaite, C. L. (2010). *Giving mom a break: The impact of higher EITC payments on maternal health.* Cambridge, MA: National Bureau of Economic Research.

Ewick, P., & Silbey, S. (1998). *The common place of law: Stories from everyday life.* Chicago, IL: University of Chicago Press.

Eyler, A. A., Chriqui, J. F., Moreland-Russell, S., & Brownson, R. C. (2015). *Prevention, policy, and public health.* New York, NY: Oxford University Press.

Facione, P., & Facione, N. (1992). *The California critical thinking dispositions inventory test manual.* Millbrae, CA: California Academic Press.

Faherty, L. J., Kranz, A. M., Russell-Fritch, J., Patrick, S. W., Cantor, J., & Stein, B. D. (2019). Association of punitive and reporting state policies related to substance use in pregnancy with rates of neonatal abstinence syndrome. *JAMA Network Open, 2*(11), –e1914078.

Fan, D., Zhu, C. J., Timming, A. R., Su, Y., Huang, X., & Lu, Y. (2020). Using the past to map out the future of occupational health and safety research: Where do we go from here? *International Journal of Human Resource Management, 31*(1), 90–127.

Feather, N. T. (1982). *Expectations and actions: Expectancy-value models in psychology.* Hillsdale, NJ: Lawrence Erlbaum Associates.

Feder, K. A., Letourneau, E. J., & Brook, J. (2019). Children in the opioid epidemic: Addressing the next generation's public health crisis. *Pediatrics, 143*(1), e20181656.

Feldman, Y., & Tyler, T. R. (2010). *Mandated justice: The potential promise and possible pitfalls of mandating procedural justice in the workplace.* Unpublished manuscript. Bar-Ilan University.

Feldstein, A. C., & Glasgow, R. E. (2008). A practical, robust implementation and sustainability model (PRISM) for integrating research findings into practice. *Joint Commission Journal on Quality and Patient Safety, 34*(4), 228–243.

Feldstein, P. J. (2012). *Health care economics* (7th ed.). Cengage Learning.

Fell, J. C., Fisher, D. A., Voas, R. B., Blackman, K., & Tippetts, A. S. (2009). Changes in alcohol-involved fatal crashes associated with tougher state alcohol legislation. *Alcoholism, Clinical and Experimental Research, 33*(7), 1208–1219.

Feng, W., & Martin, E. G. (2020). Fighting obesity at the local level? An analysis of predictors of loal health departments' policy involvement. *Preventive Medicine, 133*, 106006.

Fernández-Viña, M. H., Prood, N. E., Herpolsheimer, A., Waimberg, J., & Burris, S. (2020). State laws governing syringe services programs and participant syringe possession, 2014–2019. *Public Health Reports, 135*(1_suppl), 128S–137S.

Fichtenberg, C. M., & Glantz, S. A. (2002). Effect of smoke-free workplaces on smoking behaviour: Systematic review. *British Medical Journal, 325*(7357), 188–190.

Fidler, D. (2004). Constitutional outlines of public health's "new world order". *Temple Law Review, 77*, 247–289.

Finkelstein, A., Hendren, N., & Luttmer, E. F. (2019). The value of Medicaid: Interpreting results from the Oregon health insurance experiment. *Journal of Political Economy, 127*(6), 2836–2874.

Finkelstein, A., Taubman, S., Wright, B., Mira Bernstein, Jonathan Gruber, Joseph P Newhouse, Heidi Allen, Katherine Baicker (2011). *The Oregon health insurance experiment: Evidence from the first year* (NBER Working Paper 17190). Stanford, CA: National Bureau of Economic Research.

Finkelstein, A., Zhou, A., Taubman, S., & Doyle, J. (2020). Health care hotspotting—A randomized, controlled trial. *The New England Journal of Medicine, 382*(2), 152–162.

Finkelstein, A. N., Taubman, S. L., Allen, H. L., Wright, B. J., & Baicker, K. (2016). Effect of medicaid coverage on ED use—Further evidence from Oregon's experiment. *The New England Journal of Medicine, 375*(16), 1505–1507.

Fishbein, M., & Ajzen, I. (1975). *Belief, attitude, intention, and behavior: An introduction to theory and research*. Reading, MA: Addison-Wesley.

Fishbein, M., Triandis, H. C., Kanfer, F. H., Becker, M., & Middlestadt, S. (2001). Factors influencing behavior and behavior change. In A. Baum, T. A. Revison, & J. E. Singer (Eds.), *Handbook of health psychology* (pp. 3–17). Mahwah, NJ: Lawrence Erlbaum Associates.

Fishburn, P. C. (1981). Subjective expected utility: A review of normative theories. *Theory and Decision, 13*(2), 139–199.

Fisher, R. A. (1935). *The design of experiments*. Edinburgh, Scotland; London, UK: Oliver and Boyd.

Fitzpatrick, B. (2007). *National cultural values survey: America—A nation in moral and spiritual confusion*. Alexandria, VA: Culture and Media Institute.

Fitzpatrick, P., & Hunt, A. (1987). Critical legal studies: Introduction. *Journal of Law and Society, 14*(1), 1–3.

Fixsen, D. L., Naoom, S. F., Blase, K. A., Friedman, R. M., & Wallace, F. (2005). *Implementation research: A synthesis of the literature (FMHI Publication #231)*. Tampa, FL: University of South Florida, Louis de La Parte Florida Mental Health Institute.

Flay, B. R., & Petraitis, J. (1994). The theory of triadic influence: A new theory of health behavior with implications for preventive interventions. *Advances in Medical Sociology, 4*, 19–44.

Flay, B. R., Snyder, F. J., & Petraitis, J. (2009). The theory of triadic influence. In R. J. DiClemente, M. C. Kegler, & R. A. Crosby (Eds.), *Emerging theories in health promotion practice and research* (2nd ed., pp. 451–510). San Francisco, CA: Jossey-Bass.

Folland, S., Goodman, A. C., & Stano, M. (2016). *The economics of health and health care: Pearson New International Edition*. New York, NY: Routledge.

Folmer, C. R., Kuiper, M., Olthuis, E., Kooistra, E. B., de Bruji, A. L., Brownlee, M., ... van Rooij, B. (2021). Compliance in the 1.5 meter society: Longitudinal analysis of citizens' adherence to COVID-19 mitigation measures in a representative sample in the Netherlands. *PsyArXiv*. doi:10.31234/osf.io/dr9q3

Fong, G. T., Cummings, K. M., Borland, R., Hastings, G., Hyland, A., Giovino, G. A., ... Thompson, M. E. (2006). The conceptual framework of the international tobacco control (itc) policy evaluation project. *Tobacco Control, 15*(Suppl. 3), iii3–iii11.

Fong, G. T., Hammond, D., Laux, F. L., Zanna, M. P., Cummings, K. M., Borland, R., & Ross, H. (2004). The near-universal experience of regret among smokers in four countries: Findings from the International Tobacco Control Policy Evaluation Survey. *Nicotine & Tobacco Research, 6*, 341–351.

Foss, R. D., Feaganes, J. R., & Rodgman, E. A. (2001). Initial effects of graduated driver licensing on 16-year-old driver crashes in North Carolina. *Journal of the American Medical Association, 286*(13), 1588–1592.

Fox, K. J. (2017). Contextualizing the policy and pragmatics of reintegrating sex offenders. *Sexual Abuse, 29*, 28–50.

Fox, S. (2011). *The social life of health information, 2011*. California Healthcare Foundation.

Frakt, A. (2010). A little bit more about the RAND health insurance experiment. Retrieved from https://theincidentaleconomist.com/wordpress/a-little-bit-more-about-the-rand-health-insurance-experiment-2/.

Fraser, M., Castrucci, B., & Harper, E. (2017). Public health leadership and management in the era of public health 3.0. *Journal of Public Health Management and Practice, 23*(1), 90–92.

Frattaroli, S., & Teret, S. P. (2006). Understanding and informing policy implementation: A case study of the domestic violence provisions of the Maryland Gun Violence Act. *Evaluation Review, 30*(3), 347–360.

Frazer, K., Callinan, J. E., McHugh, J., van Baarsel, S., Clarke, A., Doherty, K., & Kelleher, C. (2016). Legislative smoking bans for reducing harms from secondhand smoke exposure, smoking prevalence and tobacco consumption. *Cochrane Database of Systematic Reviews, 2*, CD005992.

Freeman, J., & Watson, B. (2006). An application of Stafford and Warr's reconceptualization of deterrence to a group of recidivist drink drivers. *Accident Analysis and Prevention, 38*(3), 462–471.

Frey, B. S. (1997). *Not just for the money: An economic theory of personal motivation*. Cheltenham, UK: Edward Elgar.

Frey, B. S. (1998). Institutions and morale: The crowding-out effect. In A. B. Ner & L. Putterman (Eds.), *Economics, values, and organization*. Cambridge, UK: Cambridge University Press.

Frey, B. S., & Oberholzer-Gee, F. (1997). The cost of price incentives: An empirical analysis of motivation crowding-out. *The American Economic Review, 87*(4), 746–755.

Friedman, B. (2006). Taking law seriously. *Perspectives on Politics, 4*(2), 261–276.

Friedman, L. M. (1989). Law, lawyers, and popular culture. *The Yale Law Journal, 98*(8), 1579–1606.

Friedman, L. M. (2005). Coming of age: Law and society enters an exclusive club. *Annual Review of Law and Social Science, 1*(1), 1–16.

Friedman, S. R., Cooper, H. L., Tempalski, B., Keem, M., Friedman, R., Flom, P. L., & Des Jarlais, D. C. (2006). Relationships of deterrence and law enforcement to drug-related harms among drug injectors in U.S. metropolitan areas. *AIDS, 20*(1), 93–99.

Fulmer, E. B., Barbero, C., Gilchrist, S., Shantharam, S. S., Bhuiya, A. R., Taylor, L. N., & Jones, C. D. (2020). Translating workforce development policy interventions for community health workers: Application of a policy research continuum. *Journal of Public Health Management and Practice, 26 Suppl 2, Advancing Legal Epidemiology*, S10–S18.

Gadzella, B. M., Stacks, J., Stephens, R. C., & Masten, W. G. (2005). Watson-Glaser critical thinking appraisal, form S for education majors. *Journal of Instructional Psychology, 32*(1), 9–12.

Galanter, M. (1974). Why the "haves" come out ahead: Speculations on the limits of legal change. *Law and Society Review, 9*(1), 95–160.

Galea, S. (2013). An argument for a consequentialist epidemiology. *American Journal of Epidemiology, 178*(8), 1185–1191.

Galenianos, M., Pacula, R. L., & Persico, N. (2012). A search-theoretic model of the retail market for illicit drugs. *The Review of Economic Studies, 79*(3), 1239–1269.

Galletly, C. L., DiFranceisco, W., & Pinkerton, S. D. (2008). HIV-positive persons' awareness and understanding of their state's criminal HIV disclosure law. *AIDS and Behavior, 13*, 1262–1269.

Galletly, C. L., & Pinkerton, S. D. (2004). Toward rational criminal HIV exposure laws. *The Journal of Law, Medicine & Ethics, 32*(Summer), 327–337.

Galletly, C. L., & Pinkerton, S. D. (2008). Preventing HIV transmission via HIV exposure laws: Applying logic and mathematical modeling to compare statutory approaches to penalizing undisclosed exposure to HIV. *The Journal of Law, Medicine & Ethics, 36*(3), 577–584.

Gassman-Pines, A., & Hill, Z. (2013). How social safety net programs affect family economic well-being, family functioning, and children's development. *Child Development Perspectives, 7*(3), 172–181.

Gebbie, K., Rosenstock, L., & Hernandez, L. M. (Eds.) (2003). *Who will keep the public healthy? Educating public health professionals for the 21st century*. Washington, DC: National Academies Press.

Gebbie, K. M., Hodge, J. G., Jr., Meier, B. M., Barrett, D. H., Keith, P., Koo, D., … Winget, P. (2008). Improving competencies for public health emergency legal preparedness. *The Journal of Law, Medicine & Ethics, 36*(1 Suppl), 52–56.

Gee, G., & Walsemann, K. (2009). Does health predict the reporting of racial discrimination or do reports of discrimination predict health? Findings from the National Longitudinal Study of Youth. *Social Science and Medicine, 68*(9), 1676–1684.

Geller, A., & Fagan, J. (2010). Pot as pretext: Marijuana, race, and the new disorder in New York City street policing. *Journal of Empirical Legal Studies, 7*(4), 591–633.

General Accounting Office (1993). *Developing and using questionnaires (GAO/PEMD-10.1.7)*. Washington, DC: Government Printing Office.

Genn, H. G., Partington, M., Wheeler, S., & Nuffield Foundation. (2006). Law in the real world improving our understanding of how law works: Final report and recommendations. *The Nuffield Inquiry on Empirical Legal Research*. Retrieved from www.ucl.ac.uk/laws/socio-legal/empirical/docs/inquiry_report.pdf.

George, D. R., Rovniak, L. S., & Kraschnewski, J. L. (2013). Dangers and opportunities for social media in medicine. *Clinical Obstetrics and Gynecology, 56*(3), 453–462.

Ghimire, K. M., & Maclean, J. C. (2020). Medical marijuana and workers' compensation claiming. *Health Economics, 29*(4), 419–434.

Gibbins, K., & Walker, I. (1993). Multiple interpretations of the Rokeach value survey. *The Journal of Social Psychology, 133*(6), 797–805.

Givel, M. (2005). Oklahoma tobacco policy-making. *The Journal of the Oklahoma State Medical Association, 98*(3), 89–94.

Glanz, K., & Yarock, A. L. (2004). Strategies for increasing fruit and vegetable intake in grocery stores and communities: Policy, pricing and environmental change. *Preventive Medicine, 39*(Suppl. 2), 75–80.

Glaser, B. G., & Strauss, A. L. (1967). *The discovery of grounded theory: Strategies for qualitative research*. Chicago, IL: Aldine.

Glasgow, R. E., Harden, S. M., Gaglio, B., Rabin, B., Smith, M. L., Porter, G. C., … Estabrooks, P. A. (2019). RE-AIM planning and evaluation framework: Adapting to new science and practice with a 20-year review. *Frontiers in Public Health, 7*, 64.

Glasgow, R. E., Vogt, T. M., & Boles, S. M. (1999). Evaluating the public health impact of health promotion interventions: The RE-AIM framework. *American Journal of Public Health, 89*(9), 1322–1327.

Glass, G. V., Wilson, V. L., & Gottman, J. M. (1975). *Design and analysis of time-series experiments*. Boulder, CO: Colorado Associated University Press.

Glass, T. A., & McAtee, M. J. (2006). Behavioral science at the crossroads in public health: Extending horizons, envisioning the future. *Social Science & Medicine, 62*(7), 1650–1671.

Godin, G., & Shephard, R. J. (1986). Psychosocial factors influencing intentions to exercise of young students from grades 7 to 9. *Research Quarterly for Exercise and Sport, 57*(1), 41–52.

Goel, S., Rao, J. M., & Shroff, R. (2016). Precinct or prejudice? Understanding racial disparities in New York City's stop-and-frisk policy. *The Annals of Applied Statistics, 10*(1), 365–394.

Gold, M. R., Siegel, J. E., Russell, L. B., & Weinstein, M. C. (1996). *Cost-effectiveness in health and medicine*. New York, NY: Oxford University Press.

Goldman, B. M., Gutek, B. A., Stein, J. H., & Lewis, K. (2006). Employment discrimination in organizations: Antecedents and consequences. *Journal of Management, 32*(6), 786–830.

Goldsmith, J., & Vermeule, A. (2002). Empirical methodology and legal scholarship. *The University of Chicago Law Review, 69*(1), 153–167.

Goode, W. J. (1970). *World revolution and family patterns* (2nd ed.). New York, NY: Free Press.

Goode, W. J. (Ed.) (1971). *The contemporary American family*. Chicago, IL: Quadrangle Books.

Gostin, L. O. (2000). Public health law in a new century, part I: Law as a tool to advance the community's health. *Journal of the American Medical Association, 283*(21), 2837–2841.

Gostin, L. O. (2008). *Public Health Law: Power, Duty, Restraint*. Berkeley: University of California Press.

Gostin, L. O., Burris, S., & Lazzarini, Z. (1999). The law and the public's health: A study of infectious disease law in the United States. *Columbia Law Review, 99*(1), 59–128.

Gostin, L. O., Lazzarini, Z., Neslund, V. S., & Osterholm, M. T. (1996). The public health information infrastructure: A national review of the law on health information privacy. *Journal of the American Medical Association, 275*(24), 1921–1927.

Gostin, L. O., Parmet, W. E., & Rosenbaum, S. (2022). The US supreme court's rulings on large business and health care worker vaccine mandates: Ramifications for the COVID-19 response and the future of federal public health protection. *JAMA, 327*(8), 713–714.

Gostin, L. O., & Wiley, L. F. (2016). *Public health law: Power, duty, restraint* (3rd ed.). Berkeley, CA: University of California Press.

Gottfredson, D. C., Najaka, S. S., & Kearley, B. (2003). Effectiveness of drug treatment courts: Evidence from a randomized trial. *Criminology & Public Policy, 2*(2), 171–196.

Gottfredson, M. R., & Hirschi, T. (1990). *A general theory of crime*. Stanford, CA: Stanford University Press.

Grad, F. P. (2005). *Public health law manual* (3rd ed.). Washington, DC: American Public Health Association.

Graham, H. (2004). Social determinants and their unequal distribution: Clarifying policy understandings. *The Milbank Quarterly, 82*(1), 101–124.

Granovetter, M. (1978). Threshold models of collective behavior. *American Journal of Sociology, 83*(6), 1420–1443.

Green, C., & Gerard, K. (2009). Exploring the social value of health-care interventions: A stated preference discrete choice experiment. *Health Economics, 18*(8), 951–976.

Greenbaum, R. T., & Landers, J. (2009). Why are state policy-makers still proponents of enterprise zones? What explains their action in the face of a preponderance of the research? *International Regional Science Review, 32*(4), 466–479.

Greenland, S., & Brumback, B. (2002). An overview of relations among causal modelling methods. *International Journal of Epidemiology, 31*(5), 1030–1037.

Grinshteyn, E., & Hemenway, D. (2019). Violent death rates in the US compared to those of the other high-income countries, 2015. *Preventive Medicine, 123*, 20–26.

Grogger, J., & Wilils, M. (2000). The emergence of crack cocaine and the rise in Urban crime rates. *Review of Economics and Statistics, 82*(4), 519–529.

Gropas, R. (2021). Gender, anti-discrimination and diversity: The EU's role in promoting equality. In F. Levrau & N. Clycq (Eds.), *Equality: Multidisciplinary perspectives* (pp. 231–264). Cham: Springer International Publishing.

Grossman, M. (1972). On the concept of health capital and the demand for health. *Journal of Political Economy, 80*(2), 223–255.

Grossman, M. (2000). The human capital model. In A. J. Culyer & J. P. Newhouse (Eds.), *Handbook of health economics* (Vol. 1A, pp. 347–408). Amsterdam, the Netherlands: Elsevier.

Gruber, J., & Koszegi, B. (2008). *A modern economic view of tobacco taxation.* Paris, France: International Union Against Tuberculosis and Lung Disease.

Gruber, J., & Sommers, B. D. (2019). The Affordable Care Act's effects on patients, providers, and the economy: What we've learned so far. *Journal of Policy Analysis and Management, 38*(4), 1028–1052.

Gruber, J. H., & Mullainathan, S. (2005). Do cigarette taxes make smokers happier. *The BE Journal of Economic Analysis & Policy, 5*(1), 0000101515153806371412. doi:10.1515/1538-0637.1412

Guest, G., & MacQueen, K. M. (Eds.) (2008). *Handbook for team-based qualitative research.* Lanham, MD: AltaMira Press.

Gunningham, N. (2007). Corporate environmental responsibility: Law and the limits of voluntarism. In D. J. McBarnet, A. Voiculescu, & T. Campbell (Eds.), *The new corporate accountability: Corporate social responsibility and the law.* New York, NY: Cambridge University Press.

Gunningham, N. (2009a). Environment law, regulation and governance: Shifting architectures. *Journal of Environmental Law, 21*(2), 179–212.

Gunningham, N. (2009b). The new collaborative environmental governance: The localization of regulation. *Journal of Law and Society, 36*(1), 145–166.

Gupta, S., Cantor, J., Simon, K. I., Bento, A. I., Wing, C., & Whaley, C. M. (2021). Vaccinations against COVID-19 may have averted up to 140,000 deaths in the United States: Study examines role of COVID-19 vaccines and deaths averted in the United States. *Health Affairs, 40*(9), 1465–1472.

Guyatt, G. H., DiCenso, A., Farewell, V., Willan, A., & Griffith, L. (2000). Randomized trials versus observational studies in adolescent pregnancy prevention. *Journal of Clinical Epidemiology, 53*(2), 167–174.

Haacker, M., Hallett, T. B., & Atun, R. (2020). On discount rates for economic evaluations in global health. *Health Policy and Planning, 35*(1), 107–114.

Haar, C. M., Sawyer, J. P., Jr., & Cummings, S. J. (1977). Computer power and legal reasoning: A case study of judicial decision prediction in zoning amendment cases. *American Bar Foundation Research Journal, 2*(3), 651–768.

Hadland, S. E., Xuan, Z., Sarda, V., Blanchette, J., Swahn, M. H., Heeren, T. C., … Naimi, T. S. (2017). Alcohol policies and alcohol-related motor vehicle crash fatalities among young people in the US. *Pediatrics, 139*, e20163037.

Hale, T., Angrist, N., Goldszmidt, R., Kira, B., Petherick, A., Phillips, T., … Tatlow, H. (2021). A global panel database of pandemic policies (Oxford COVID-19 Government Response Tracker). *Nature Human Behaviour, 5*(4), 529–538.

Hall, J. R. (2010). *The smoking-material fire problem.* Quincy, MA: National Fire Protection Association.

Hall, M. A., Rust Smith, T., Naughton, M., & Ebbers, A. (1996). Judicial protection of managed care consumers: An empirical study of insurance coverage disputes. *Seton Hall Law Review, 26*, 1055–1068.

Hall, M. A., & Wright, R. F. (2008). Systematic content analysis of judicial opinions. *California Law Review, 96*, 63–122.

Hall, W., Leung, J., & Lynskey, M. (2020). The effects of cannabis use on the development of adolescents and young adults. *Annual Review of Developmental Psychology, 2*, 461–483.

Hall, W., & Lynskey, M. (2020). Assessing the public health impacts of legalizing recreational cannabis use: The US experience. *World Psychiatry, 19*(2), 179–186.

Hamer, M. K., & Mays, G. P. (2020). Public health systems and social services: Breadth and depth of cross-sector collaboration. *American Journal of Public Health, 110*(S2), S232–S234.

Hamilton, A. B., & Finley, E. P. (2019). Qualitative methods in implementation research: An introduction. *Psychiatry Research, 280*, 112516. doi:10.1016/j.psychres.2019.112516

Hamilton, E. (2020). Toward a focused conceptualization of collateral consequences among individuals who sexually offend: A systematic review. *Sexual Abuse*. doi:10.1177/1079063220981906

Hamilton, J., Bronte-Tinkew, J., & Child Trends Inc. (2007). *Logic models in out-of-school time programs: What are they and why are they important? (#2007–01)*. Washington, DC: Child Trends.

Harbison, P. A., & Whitman, M. V. (2008). Barriers associated with implementing a campus-wide smoke-free policy. *Health Education, 108*(4), 321–331.

Harrell, A., & Smith, B. E. (1996). Effects of restraining orders on domestic violence victims. In E. S. Buzawa & C. G. Buzawa (Eds.), *Do arrests and restraining orders work?* (pp. 214–242). Thousand Oaks, CA: Sage.

Harris, K. J., Stearns, J. N., Kovach, R. G., & Harrar, S. W. (2009). Enforcing an outdoor smoking ban on a college campus: Effects of a multicomponent approach. *Journal of American College Health, 58*(2), 121–126.

Harris, R. P., Helfand, M., Woolf, S. H., Lohr, K. N., Mulrow, C. D., Teutsch, S. M., ... Methods Work Group, Third U.S. Preventive Services Task Force (2001). Current methods of the US Preventive Services Task Force: A review of the process. *American Journal of Preventive Medicine, 20*(3 Suppl), 21–35.

Harrison, G. W., & Rutström, E. E. (2008). Experimental evidence on the existence of hypothetical bias in value elicitation methods. *Handbook of Experimental Economics Results, 1*, 752–767.

Hartsfield, D., Moulton, A. D., & McKie, K. L. (2007). A review of model public health laws. *American Journal of Public Health, 97*(Suppl. 1), S56–S61.

Healton, C. G., Cummings, M., O'Connor, R. J., & Novotny, T. E. (2011). Butt really? The environmental impact of cigarettes. *Tobacco Control, 20*, i1.

Heath, G. W., Brownson, R. C., Kruger, J., Miles, R., Powell, K. E., Ramsey, L. T., & Task Force on Community Preventive Services (2006). The effectiveness of urban design and land use policies and practices to increase physical activity: A systematic review. *Journal of Physical Activity and Health, 3*(Suppl. 1), S55–S76.

Hecht, F. M., Chesney, M. A., Lehman, J. S., Osmond, D., Vranizan, K., Colman, S., ... Bindman, A. B. (2000). Does HIV reporting by name deter testing? MESH Study Group. *AIDS, 14*(12), 1801–1808.

Heckathorn, D. D. (1997). Respondent-driven sampling: A new approach to the study of hidden populations. *Social Problems, 44*(2), 174–199.

Heckathorn, D. D. (2007). Extensions of respondent-driven sampling: Analyzing continuous variables and controlling for differential recruitment. *Sociological Methodology, 37*(1), 151–207.

Heckathorn, D. D. (2008). Respondent-driven sampling (RDS). In P. J. Lavrakas (Ed.), *Encyclopedia of survey research methods* (pp. 741–743). Thousand Oaks, CA: Sage.

Heckman, J. J., & Smith, J. A. (1995). Assessing the case for social experiments. *Journal of Economic Perspectives, 9*, 85–110.

Heimer, C. A. (1999). Competing institutions: Law, medicine, and family in neonatal intensive care. *Law and Society Review, 33*(1), 17–66.

Heimer, K., & Matsueda, R. L. (1994). Role-taking, role commitment, and delinquency: A theory of differential social control. *American Sociological Review, 59*(3), 365–390.

Hein, W., Burris, S., & Shearing, C. (2009). Conceptual models for global health governance. In K. Buse, W. Hein, & N. Drager (Eds.), *Making sense of global health governance: A policy perspective* (pp. 72–98). Houndsmills, UK: Palgrave MacMillan.

Heller, S. B., Shah, A. K., Guryan, J., Ludwig, J., Mullainathan, S., & Pollack, H. A. (2017). Thinking, fast and slow? Some field experiments to reduce crime and dropout in Chicago. *Quarterly Journal of Economics, 132*(1), 1–54.

Heloma, A., & Jaakkola, M. S. (2003). Four-year follow-up of smoke exposure, attittudes and smoking behaviour following enactment of Finland's national smoke-free workplace law. *Addiction, 98*, 1111–1117.

Hemenway, D. (2009). *While we were sleeping: Success stories in injury and violence prevention*. Berkeley, CA: University of California Press.

Henrichson, C., & Rinaldi, J. (2014). *Cost-benefit analysis and justice policy toolkit*. New York: NY: Vera Institute of Justice.

Heponiemi, T., Kouvonen, A., Vèanskèa, J., Halila, H., Sinervo, T., Kivimäki, M., & Elovainio, M. (2008). Health, psychosocial factors and retirement intentions among Finnish physicians. *Occupational Medicine, 58*(6), 406–412.

Herek, G. M. (1988). An epidemic of stigma: Public reactions to AIDS. *American Psychologist, 43*(11), 886–891.

Herek, G. M. (1993). Public reactions to AIDS in the United States: A second decade of stigma. *American Journal of Public Health, 83*(4), 574–577.

Herek, G. M., Capitanio, J., & Widaman, K. (2002). HIV-related stigma and knowledge in the United States: Prevalence and trends, 1991–1999. *American Journal of Public Health, 92*(3), 371–377.

Hernán, M. A. (2018). The c-word: Scientific euphemisms do not improve causal inference from observational data. *American Journal of Public Health, 108*(5), 616–619.

Heron, M. (2021). Deaths: Leading causes for 2019 *national vital statistics reports: From the Centers for Disease Control and Prevention, National Center for Health Statistics. National Vital Statistics System, 70*(9), 1–114.

Herrnstein, R. J., Loewenstein, G. F., Prelec, D., & Vaughan, W., Jr. (1993). Utility maximization and melioration: Internalities in individual choice. *Journal of Behavioral Decision Making, 6*(3), 149–185.

Hesse-Biber, S. N., & Leavy, P. (2006). *The practice of qualitative research.* Thousand Oaks, CA: Sage.

Higgins, S. T., Bernstein, I. M., Washio, Y., Heil, S. H., Badger, G. J., Skelly, J. M., … Solomon, L. J. (2010). Effects of smoking cessation with voucher-based contingency management on birth outcomes. *Addiction, 105*(11), 2023–2030. doi:10.1111/j.1360-0443.2010.03073.x

Higgins, S. T., Heil, S. H., Badger, G. J., Skelly, J. M., Solomon, L. J., & Bernstein, I. M. (2009). Educational disadvantage and cigarette smoking during pregnancy. *Drug and Alcohol Dependence, 104*(Suppl 1), S100–S105.

Hill, A. B. (1965). The environment and disease: Association or causation? *Proceedings of the Royal Society of Medicine, 58*, 295–300.

Hillestad, R., Bigelow, J., Bower, A., Girosi, F., Meili, R., Scoville, R., & Taylor, R. (2005). Can electronic medical record systems transform health care? Potential health benefits, savings, and costs. *Health Affairs, 24*(5), 1103–1117.

Hirsch, B. T. (2008). Sluggish institutions in a dynamic world: Can unions and industrial competion co-exist? *Journal of Economic Perspectives, 22*(1), 153–176.

Hirschhorn, L., Smith, J. D., Frisch, M. F., & Binagwaho, A. (2020). Integrating implementation science into covid-19 response and recovery. *British Medical Journal (Clinical Research Edition), 369*, m1888.

Hirschi, T. (2002). *Causes of delinquency.* New Brunswick, NJ: Transaction.

Hirth, R. A., Chernew, M. E., Miller, E., Fendrick, A. M., & Weissert, W. G. (2000). Willingness to pay for a quality-adjusted life year: In search of a standard. *Medical Decision Making, 20*(3), 332–342.

Ho, D. E., & Rubin, D. B. (2011). Credible causal inference for empirical legal studies. *Annual Review of Law and Social Science, 7*(1), 17–40.

Ho, L. (2021). High level of (passive) compliance in a low-trust society: Hong Kong citizens' response toward the COVID-19 lockdown. *Policing, 15*, 1046–1061.

Hoagwood, K. E., Purtle, J., Spandorfer, J., Peth-Pierce, R., & Horwitz, S. M. (2020). Aligning dissemination and implementation science with health policies to improve children's mental health. *The American Psychologist, 75*(8), 1130–1145.

Hodge, J. G., Jr., Lant, T., Arias, J., & Jehn, M. (2011). Building evidence for legal decision making in real time: Legal triage in public health emergencies. *Disaster Medicine and Public Health Preparedness, 5*(Suppl. 2), S242–S251.

Hodge, J. G., Jr., Pulver, A., Hogben, M., Bhattacharya, D., & Brown, E. F. (2008). Expedited partner therapy for sexually transmitted diseases: Assessing the legal environment. *American Journal of Public Health, 98*(2), 238–243.

Hoffman, D. A., Izenman, A. J., & Lidicker, J. R. (2007). Docketology, district courts, and doctrine. *Washington University Law Review, 85*(4), 681–752.

Hoffman, S. J., Poirier, M. J. P., Rogers Van Katwyk, S., Baral, P., & Sritharan, L. (2019). Impact of the WHO Framework Convention on Tobacco Control on global cigarette consumption: Quasi-experimental evaluations using interrupted time series analysis and in-sample forecast event modelling. *BMJ, 365*, l2287.

Holmes, W. M. (2014). *Using propensity scores in quasi-experimental designs.* Los Angeles, CA: Sage.

Holtrop, J. S., Estabrooks, P. A., Gaglio, B., Harden, S. M., Kessler, R. S., King, D. K., ... Glasgow, R. E. (2021). Understanding and applying the RE-AIM framework: Clarifications and resources. *Journal of Clinical and Translational Science, 5*(1), e126.

Homans, G. C. (1958). Social behavior as exchange. *American Journal of Sociology, 63*(6), 597–606.

Hoppe, T., McClelland, A., & Pass, K. (2022). Beyond criminalization: Reconsidering HIV criminalization in an era of reform. *Current Opinion in HIV and AIDS.* doi:10.1097/coh.0000000000000715

Horlick, G. A., Beeler, S. F., & Linkins, R. W. (2001). A review of state legislation related to immunization registries. *American Journal of Preventive Medicine, 20*(3), 208–213.

Horton, H., Birkhead, G. S., Bump, C., Burris, S., Cahill, K., Goodman, R. A., ... Vernick, J. S. (2002). The dimensions of public health law research. *The Journal of Law, Medicine & Ethics, 30*(3), 197–201.

Horvath, K. J., Weinmeyer, R., & Rosser, S. (2010). Should it be illegal for HIV-positive persons to have unprotected sex without disclosure? An examination of attitudes among U.S. men who have sex with men and the impact of state law. *AIDS Care, 22*(10), 1221–1228.

Horwitz, J. R., Davis, C., McClelland, L., Fordon, R., & Meara, E. (2021). The importance of data source in prescription drug monitoring program research. *Health Services Research, 56*(2), 268–274.

Hotz, V. J. (2003). The earned income tax credit. In R. A. Moffit (Ed.), *Means-tested transfer programs in the United States.* Chicago, IL: University of Chicago Press.

House, J. S. (2015). *Beyond Obamacare: Life, death, and social policy.* New York, NY: Russell Sage Foundation.

House, J. S., Kessler, R. C., & Herzog, A. R. (1990). Age, socioeconomic status, and health. *The Milbank Quarterly, 68*(3), 383–411.

Househ, M. (2013). The use of social media in healthcare: Organizational, clinical, and patient perspectives. In *Enabling health and healthcare through ICT: Available, tailored and closer* (Vol. 183, pp. 244–248). Amsterdam, the Netherlands: IOS Press.

Houston, A. (1997). *Survey handbook (TQLO Publication Number 97-06).* Washington, DC: Department of the Navy.

Houston, D. J., & Richardson, L. E., Jr. (2005). Getting Americans to buckle up: The efficacy of state seat belt laws. *Accident Analysis & Prevention, 37*(6), 1114–1120.

Howard, K. A., Ribisl, K. M., Howard-Pitney, B., Norman, G. J., & Rohrbach, L. A. (2001). What factors are associated with local enforcement of laws banning illegal tobacco sales to minors? A study of 182 law enforcement agencies in California. *Preventive Medicine, 33*(2 Pt. 1), 63–70.

Howe, E. S., & Brandau, C. J. (1988). Additive effects of certainty, severity, and celerity of punishment on judgments of crime deterrence scale value. *Journal of Applied Social Psychology, 18*(9), 796–812.

Howe, E. S., & Loftus, T. C. (1996). Integration of certainty, severity, and celerity information in judged deterrence value: Further evidence and methodological equivalence. *Journal of Applied Social Psychology, 26*(3), 226–242.

Howell, B. L., Deb, P., Ma, S., Reid, R. O., Levy, J., Riley, G. F., ... Shrank, W. H. (2017). Encouraging medicare advantage enrollees to switch to higher quality plans: Assessing the effectiveness of a "Nudge" letter. *Medical Decision Making Policy & Practice.* doi:10.1177/2381468317707206

Huang, J., Fisher, B. T., Tam, V., Wang, Z., Song, L., Shi, J., ... Rubin, D. M. (2022). the effectiveness of government masking mandates on COVID-19 county-level case incidence across the United States, 2020. *Health Affairs, 41*(3), 445–453.

Huesmann, L. R., & Guerra, N. G. (1997). Children's normative beliefs about aggression and aggressive behavior. *Journal of Personality and Social Psychology, 72*, 408–419.

Hull, K. E. (2003). The cultural power of law and the cultural enactment of legality: The case of same-sex marriage. *Law & Social Inquiry, 28*(3), 629–657.

Hung, D. Y., Rundall, T. G., Tallia, A. F., Cohen, D. J., Halpin, H. A., & Crabtree, B. F. (2007). Rethinking prevention in primary care: Applying the chronic care model to address health risk behaviors. *The Milbank Quarterly, 85*(1), 69–91.

Hupert, N., Mushlin, A. I., & Callahan, M. A. (2002). Modeling the public health response to bioterrorism: Using discrete event simulation to design antibiotic distribution centers. *Medical Decision Making, 22*(Suppl. 5), S17–S25.

Hyde, J. K., & Shortell, S. M. (2012). The structure and organization of local and state public health agencies in the U.S.: A systematic review. *American Journal of Preventive Medicine, 42*(5 Suppl. 1), S29–S41.

Ibrahim, J. K., Anderson, E. D., Burris, S. C., & Wagenaar, A. C. (2011). State laws restricting driver use of mobile communications devices: "Distracted-driving" provisions, 1992–2010. *American Journal of Preventive Medicine, 40*(6), 659–665.

Ibrahim, J. K., & Glantz, S. A. (2006). Tobacco industry litigation strategies to oppose tobacco control media campaigns. *Tobacco Control, 15*(1), 50–58.

Ibrahim, J. K., Sorensen, A. A., Grunwald, H., & Burris, S. (2017). Supporting a culture of evidence-based policy: Federal funding for public health law evaluation research, 1985-2014. *Journal of Public Health Management and Practice, 23*(6), 658–666.

Ibrahim, J. K., Tsoukalas, T. H., & Glantz, S. A. (2004). Public health foundations and the tobacco industry: Lessons from Minnesota. *Tobacco Control, 13*(3), 228–236.

Immordino, G., & Russo, F. F. (2015). Regulating prostitutes: A health risk approach. *Journal of Public Economics, 121*, 14–31.

Innvaer, S., Vist, G., Trommald, M., & Oxman, A. (2002). Health policy-makers' perceptions of their use of evidence: A systematic review. *Journal of Health Services Research & Policy, 7*, 239–244.

Insel, T. R., & Gogtay, N. (2014). National Institute of Mental Health clinical trials: New opportunities, new expectations. *JAMA Psychiatry, 71*(7), 745–746.

Institute of Medicine (1988). *The future of public health.* Washington, DC: National Academies Press.

Institute of Medicine (2002). *The future of the public's health in the 21st century.* Washington, DC: National Academies Press.

Institute of Medicine (2011). *For the public's health: Revitalizing law and policy to meet new challenges*. Washington, DC: The National Academies Press.

Institute of Medicine Committee on the Assessment of the U.S. Drug Safety System, Baciu, A., Stratton, K. R., & Burke, S. P. (2007). *The future of drug safety promoting and protecting the health of the public*. Washington, DC: National Academies Press.

International Agency for Research on Cancer (IARC), & World Health Organization (2009). *IARC handbooks of cancer prevention tobacco control: Evaluating the effectiveness of smoke-free policies* (Vol. 13). Lyon, France: International Agency for Research on Cancer.

International Agency for Research on Cancer (IARC), & World Health Organization (2011). *IARC handbooks of cancer prevention tobacco control: Effectiveness of tax and price policies in tobacco control* (Vol. 14). Lyon, France: International Agency for Research on Cancer.

International Tobacco Control Policy Evaluation Project (ITCPEP) (2009). *FTC Article 11 tobacco warning labels: Evidence and recommendations from the ITC*. Waterloo, Canada: University of Waterloo.

Isaacs, K. R., Atreyapurapu, S., Alyusuf, A. H., Ledgerwood, D. M., Finnegan, L. P., Chang, K. H. K., ... Washio, Y. (2021). Neonatal outcomes after combined opioid and nicotine exposure in Utero: A scoping review. *International Journal of Environmental Research and Public Health, 18*(19), 10215.

Jabbari, D. (1998). Is there a proper subject matter for "socio-legal studies"? *Oxford Journal of Legal Studies, 18*(4), 707–728.

Jacobson, N., Butterill, D., & Goering, P. (2005). Consulting as a strategy for knowledge transfer. *The Milbank Quarterly, 83*(2), 299–321.

Jacobson, P. D., & Soliman, S. (2002). Litigation as public health policy: Theory or reality? *The Journal of Law, Medicine & Ethics, 30*(2), 224–238.

Jacobson, P. D., & Warner, K. E. (1999). Litigation and public health policy making: The case of tobacco control. *Journal of Health Politics, Policy and Law, 24*(4), 769–804.

Jacobson, P. D., & Wasserman, J. (1999). The implementation and enforcement of tobacco control laws: Policy implications for activists and the industry. *Journal of Health Politics, Policy and Law, 24*(3), 567–598.

Jacobson, P. D., Wasserman, J., Botoseneanu, A., Silverstein, A., & Wu, H. W. (2012). The role of law in public health preparedness: Opportunities and challenges. *Journal of Health Politics, Policy and Law, 37*(2), 297–328.

Janesick, V. J. (2004). *"Stretching" exercises for qualitative researchers* (2nd ed.). Thousand Oaks, CA: Sage.

Jenkins, P. H. (1997). School delinquency and the school social bond. *Journal of Research in Crime and Delinquency, 34*(3), 337–367.

Jepsen, C., & Rivkin, S. (2009). Class size reduction and student achievement: The potential tradeoff between teacher quality and class size. *Journal of Human Resources, 44*(1), 223–250.

Jewell, C. A., & Bero, L. A. (2008). Developing good taste in evidence: Facilitators of and hindrances to evidence-informed health policymaking in state government. *The Milbank Quarterly, 86*(2), 177–208.

Jha, P., Musgrove, P., Chaloupka, F. J., & Yurekli, A. (2000). The economic rationale for intervention in the tobacco market. In P. Jha & F. J. Chaloupka (Eds.), *Tobacco control in developing countries*. Oxford, UK; New York, NY: Oxford University Press.

Johnson, A. L., Ecker, A. H., Fletcher, T. L., Hundt, N., Kauth, M. R., Martin, L. A., … Cully, J. A. (2020). Increasing the impact of randomized controlled trials: An example of a hybrid effectiveness-implementation design in psychotherapy research. *Translational Behavioral Medicine, 10*(3), 629–636.

Johnson, C. A. (1987). Law, politics, and judicial decision making: Lower federal court uses of supreme court decisions. *Law and Society Review, 21*(2), 325–340.

Johnson, F. R., Lancsar, E., Marshall, D., Kilambi, V., Mühlbacher, A., Regier, D. A., … Bridges, J. F. (2013). Constructing experimental designs for discrete-choice experiments: Report of the ISPOR conjoint analysis experimental design good research practices task force. *Value in Health, 16*(1), 3–13.

Johnson, R. B., & Onwuegbuzie, A. J. (2004). Mixed methods research: A research paradigm whose time has come. *Educational Researcher, 33*(7), 14–26.

Johnston, L. D., O'Malley, P. M., Bachman, J. G., & Schulenberg, J. E. (2011). *Monitoring the future national survey results on drug use, 1975–2010. Volume II: College students and adults ages 19–50*. Ann Arbor, MI: Institute for Social Research, University of Michigan.

Jolls, C. (2006). *Behavioral law and economics* (Yale Law School, Public Law working paper no. 130; Yale Law & Economics research paper no. 342). Retrieved from papers.ssrn.com/sol3/papers.cfm?abstract_id=959177.

Jolls, C., Sunstein, C. R., & Thaler, R. (1998). A behavioral approach to law and economics. *Stanford Law Review, 50*, 1471–1550.

Jones, B. T., Corbin, W., & Fromme, K. (2001). A review of expectancy theory and alcohol consumption. *Addiction, 96*(1), 57–72.

Jones, S. J., Jahns, L., Laraia, B. A., & Haughton, B. (2003). Lower risk of overweight in school-aged food insecure girls who participate in food assistance. *Archives of Pediatrics and Adolescent Medicine, 157*(8), 780–784.

Jordan, G. B. (2010). A theory-based logic model for innovation policy and evaluation. *Research Evaluation, 19*(4), 263–273.

Joseph, J. G., Emmons, C. A., Kessler, R. C., Wortman, C. B., O'Brien, K., Hocker, W. T., & Schaefer, C. (1984). Coping with the threat of AIDS: An approach to psychosocial assessment. *The American Psychologist, 39*(11), 1297–1302.

Jost, J. T., & Major, B. (2001). *The psychology of legitimacy: Emerging perspectives on ideology, justice, and intergroup relations*. New York, NY: Cambridge University Press.

Joyce, M., Sklenar, E., & Weatherby, G. (2019). Decriminalizing drug addiction: The effects of the label. *MOJ Research Review, 2*, 83–91.

Kaestner, R. (2012). Mortality and access to care after Medicaid expansions. *New England Journal of Medicine, 367*(25), 2453–2454.

Kaestner, R., & Ziedan, E. (2019). *Mortality and socioeconomic consequences of prescription opioids: Evidence from state policies* (National Bureau of Economic Research Working Paper W26135) (August, 2019).

Kagan, R. A., & Skolnick, J. H. (1993). Banning smoking: Compliance without enforcement. In R. L. Rabin & S. D. Sugerman (Eds.), *Smoking policy: Law, politics and culture* (pp. 69–94). New York, NY: Oxford University Press.

Kahn, L. M. (2000). Wage inequality, collective bargaining, and relative employment from 1985 to 1994: Evidence from fifteen OECD countries. *The Review of Economics and Statistics, 82*(4), 564–579.

Kahneman, D. (1999). Objective happiness in well being: The foundations of hedonic psychology. In D. Kahneman, E. Diener, & N. Schwarz (Eds.), *Well-being: Foundations of hedonic psychology*. New York, NY: Russell Sage Foundation.

Kahneman, D., Fredrickson, B. L., Schreiber, C. A., & Redelmeier, D. A. (1993). When more pain is preferred to less. *Psychological Science, 4*(6), 401–405.

Kahneman, D., & Tversky, A. (1979). Prospect theory: An analysis of decision under risk. *Econometrica, 47*(2), 263–292.

Kahneman, D. (2011). *Thinking, fast and slow*. New York, NY: Macmillan.

Kahnemann, D., Slovic, P., & Tversky, A. (Eds.) (1982). *Judgment under uncertainty: Heuristics and biases*. Cambridge, UK: Cambridge University Press.

Kalev, A., Dobbin, F., & Kelly, E. (2006). Best practices or best guesses? Assessing the efficacy of corporate affirmative action and diversity policies. *American Sociological Review, 71*(4), 589–617.

Kaplan, G. A. (2004). What's wrong with social epidemiology, and how can we make it better? *Epidemiologic Reviews, 26*(1), 124–135.

Karoly, L. A. (2012). Toward standardization of benefit-cost analysis of early childhood interventions. *Journal of Benefit-Cost Analysis, 3*(1), 1–45.

Kaufman, J. A., Salas-Hernández, L. K., Komro, K. A., & Livingston, M. D. (2020). Effects of increased minimum wages by unemployment rate on suicide in the USA. *Journal of Epidemiology and Community Health, 74*(3), 219–224.

Kaufman, N. J., Castrucci, B. C., Pearsol, J., Leider, J. P., Sellers, K., Kaufman, I. R., ... Sprague, J. B. (2014). Thinking beyond the silos: Emerging priorities in workforce development for state and local government public health agencies. *Journal of Public Health Management and Practice, 20*(6), 557–565.

Kavanagh, M. M. (2016). The right to health: Institutional effects of constitutional provisions on health outcomes. *Studies in Comparative International Development, 51*(3), 328–364.

Kavanagh, M. M., Meier, B. M., Pillinger, M., Huffstetler, H., & Burris, S. (2020). Global policy surveillance: Creating and using comparative national data on health law and policy. *American Journal of Public Health, 110*(12), 1805–1810.

Kellogg, K. C. (2011). *Challenging operations: Medical reform and resistance in surgery*. Chicago, IL: University of Chicago Press.

Kelly, E. L., Moen, P., & Tranby, E. (2011). Changing workplaces to reduce work-family conflict: Schedule control in a white-collar organization. *American Sociological Review, 76*(2), 265–290.

Kelly, M. P., McDaid, D., Ludbrook, A., & Powell, J. (2005). *Economic appraisal of public health interventions*. London, UK: Health Development Agency.

Kemp, C. G., Wagenaar, B. H., & Haroz, E. E. (2019). Expanding hybrid studies for implementation research: Intervention, implementation strategy, and context. *Frontiers in Public Health, 7,* 325.

Kesler, M. A., Kaul, R., Loutfy, M., Myers, T., Brunetta, J., Remis, R. S., & Gesink, D. (2018). Prosecution of non-disclosure of HIV status: Potential impact on HIV testing and transmission among HIV-negative men who have sex with men. *PLoS One, 13*(2), e0193269.

Keyes, K. M., & Galea, S. (2014). *Epidemiology matters: A new introduction to methodological foundations.* New York, NY: Oxford University Press.

Khan, M., Wohl, D., Weir, S., Adimora, A. A., Moseley, C., Norcott, K., ... Miller, W. C. (2008). Incarceration and risky sexual partnerships in a southern U.S. city. *Journal of Urban Health, 85*(1), 100–113.

Kidd, P. S., & Parshall, M. B. (2000). Getting the focus and the group: Enhancing analytical rigor in focus group research. *Qualitative Health Research, 10*(3), 293–308.

Kilmer, B., Burgdorf, J. R., D'amico, E. J., Miles, J., & Tucker, J. (2011). Multisite cost analysis of a school-based voluntary alcohol and drug prevention program. *Journal of Studies on Alcohol and Drugs, 72*(5), 823–831.

Kilmer, B., Caulkins, J. P., Pacula, R. L., MacCoun, R. J., & Reuter, P. (2010). *Altered state?: Assessing how marijuana legalization in California could influence marijuana consumption and public budgets.* Santa Monica, CA: RAND.

Kim, B. (2021). Must-access prescription drug monitoring programs and the opioid overdose epidemic: The unintended consequences. *Journal of Health Economics, 75,* 102408.

Kimball, A. M., Moore, M., French, H. M., Arima, Y., Ungchusak, K., Wibulpolprasert, S., ... Leventhal, A. (2008). Regional infectious disease surveillance networks and their potential to facilitate the implementation of the international health regulations. *Medical Clinics of North America, 92*(6), 1459–1471.

King, E. B., Dawson, J. F., Kravitz, D. A., & Gulick, L. M. (2012). A multilevel study of the relationships between diversity training, ethnic discrimination and satisfaction in organizations. *Journal of Organizational Behavior, 33*(1), 5–20.

Kinney, E. D. (2002). Administrative law and the public's health. *The Journal of Law, Medicine & Ethics, 30*(2), 212–223.

Kirzinger, A., Sparks, G., Kearney, A., Stokes, M., Hamel, L., & Brodie, M. (2021). *KFF COVID-19 vaccine monitor: November 2021.* Retrieved from https://www.kff.org/coronavirus-covid-19/poll-finding/kff-covid-19-vaccine-monitor-november-2021/.

Kitzinger, J. (1994). The methodology of focus groups: The importance of interaction between research participants. *Sociology of Health & Illness, 16*(1), 103–121.

Kivimäki, M., Elovainio, M., Vahtera, J., Virtanen, M., & Stansfeld, S. A. (2003). Association between organizational inequity and incidence of psychiatric disorders in female employees. *Psychological Medicine, 33*(2), 319–326.

Kivimäki, M., Ferrie, J. E., Brunner, E., Head, J., Shipley, M. J., Vahtera, J., & Marmot, M. G. (2005). Justice at work and reduced risk of coronary heart disease among employees. *Archives of Internal Medicine, 165*(19), 2245–2251.

Kivimäki, M., Ferrie, J. E., Head, J., Shipley, M. J., Vahtera, J., & Marmot, M. G. (2004). Organisational justice and change in justice as predictors of employee health. *Journal of Epidemiology and Community Health, 58*(11), 931–937.

Klepeis, N. E., Ott, W. R., & Switzer, P. (2007). Real-time measurement of outdoor tobacco smoke particles. *Journal of the Air & Waste Management Association, 57*, 522–534.

Klepper, S., & Nagin, D. S. (1989). Certainty and severity of punishment revisited. *Criminology, 27*(4), 721–746.

Klitzman, R., Kirshenbaum, S., Kittel, L., Morin, S., Daya, S., Mastrogiacomo, M., & Rotheram-Borus, M. J. (2004). Naming names: Perceptions of name-based HIV reporting, partner notification, and criminalization of non-disclosure among persons living with HIV. *Sexuality Research & Social Policy, 1*(3), 38–57.

Ko, N. Y., Lee, H. C., Hung, C. C., Chang, J.-L., Lee, N.-Y., Chang, C.-M., ... Ko, W.-C. (2009). Effects of structural intervention on increasing condom availability and reducing risky sexual behaviours in gay bath-house attendees. *AIDS Care, 21*(12), 1499–1507.

Komro, K. A. (2020). The centrality of law for prevention. *Prevention Science, 21*(7), 1001–1006.

Komro, K. A., Dunlap, P., Sroczynski, N., Livingston, M. D., Kelly, M. A., Pepin, D., ... Wagenaar, A. C. (2020). Anti-poverty policy and health: Attributes and diffusion of state earned income tax credits across U.S. states from 1980 to 2020. *PLoS One, 15*(11), e0242514.

Komro, K. A., Flay, B. R., Biglan, A., & the Promise Neighborhoods Research Consortium (2011). Creating nurturing environments: A science-based framework for promoting child health and development within high-poverty neighborhoods. *Clinical Child and Family Psychology Review, 14*(2), 111–134.

Komro, K. A., Livingston, M. D., Markowitz, S., & Wagenaar, A. C. (2016). The effect of an increased minimum wage on infant mortality and birth weight. *American Journal of Public Health, 106*(8), 1514–1516.

Komro, K. A., Markowitz, S., Livingston, M. D., & Wagenaar, A. C. (2019). Effects of state-level earned income tax credit laws on birth outcomes by race and ethnicity. *Health Equity, 3*(1), 61–67.

Kooistra, E. B., Folmer, C. R., Kuiper, M. E., Olthuis, E., Brownlee, M., Fine, A., & van Rooij, B. (2021). Mitigating COVID-19 in a nationally representative UK sample: Personal abilities and obligation to obey the law shape compliance with mitigation measures. *PsyArXiv*. doi:10.31234/osf.io/zuc23

Korda, H., & Itani, Z. (2013). Harnessing social media for health promotion and behavior change. *Health Promotion Practice, 14*(1), 15–23.

Korfmacher, K. (2019). *Bridging silos: Collaborating for health and justice in urban communities.* Cambridge, MA: MIT Press.

Kouvonen, A., Kivimäki, M., Elovainio, M., Väänänen, A., De Vogli, R., Heponiemi, T., ... Vahtera, J. (2008). Low organisational justice and heavy drinking: A prospective cohort study. *Occupational and Environmental Medicine, 65*(1), 44–50.

Kouvonen, A., Vahtera, J., Elovainio, M., Cox, S. J., Cox, T., Linna, A., ... Kivimäki, M. (2007). Organisational justice and smoking: The Finnish public sector study. *Journal of Epidemiology and Community Health, 61*(5), 427–433.

Kramer, M. S., & Shapiro, S. H. (1984). Scientific challenges in the application of randomized trials. *JAMA, 252*(19), 2739–2745. doi:10.1001/jama.1984.03350190041017

Kratochwill, T. R., Hitchcock, J., Horner, R. H., … Shadish, W. R. (2010). *Single-case designs technical documentation.* Washington, DC: U.S. Department of Education, Institute of Education Sciences, National Center for Education Evaluation and Regional Assistance, What Works Clearinghouse. Retrieved from chrome-extension://efaidnbmnnnibpcajpcglclefindmkaj/viewer.html?pdfurl=https%3A%2F%2Fies.ed.gov%2Fncee%2Fwwc%2Fdocs%2Freferenceresources%2Fwwc_scd.pdf&chunk=true.

Krieger, J. W., Chan, N. L., Saelens, B. E., Ta, M. L., Solet, D., & Fleming, D. W. (2013). Menu labeling regulations and calories purchased at chain restaurants. *American Journal of Preventive Medicine, 44*(6), 595–604.

Krieger, N., Chen, J. T., Waterman, P. D., Rehkopf, D. H., & Subramanian, S. V. (2005). Painting a truer picture of U.S. socioeconomic and racial/ethnic health inequalities: The public health disparities geocoding project. *American Journal of Public Health, 95*(2), 312–323.

Krieger, N., & Davey Smith, G. (2016). The tale wagged by the DAG: Broadening the scope of causal inference and explanation for epidemiology. *International Journal of Epidemiology, 45*(6), 1787–1808.

Krippendorff, K. (1980). *Content analysis: An introduction to its methodology.* London, UK: Sage.

Krippendorff, K. (2004). *Content analysis: An introduction to its methodology* (2nd ed.). Thousand Oaks, CA: Sage.

Krislov, S., Boyum, K. O., Clark, J. N., Shaefer, R. C., & White, S. O. (1966). *Compliance and the law: A multi-disciplinary approach.* Beverly Hills, CA: Sage.

Kromm, J. N., Frattaroli, S., Vernick, J. S., & Teret, S. P. (2009). Public health advocacy in the courts: Opportunities for public health professionals. *Public Health Reports, 124*(6), 889–894.

Lacey, A., & Luff, D. (2001). *Trent focus for research and development in primary health care: An introduction to qualitative data analysis.* Nottingham, UK: Trent Focus.

LaFond, C., Toomey, T. L., Rothstein, C., Wagenaar, A. C., & Manning, W. (2000). Policy evaluation research: Measuring the independent variables. *Evaluation Review, 24*(1), 92–101.

Lakey, B. (2010). Social support: Basic research and new strategies for intervention. In J. E. Maddux & J. P. Tangney (Eds.), *Social psychological foundations of clinical psychology* (pp. 177–194). New York, NY: Guildford.

Lally, J. R., Mangoine, P. L., & Honig, A. S. (1987). *The Syracuse University Family Development Research program: Long-range impact of an early intervention with low-income children and their families.* New York, NY: Grant (W.T.) Foundation.

LaLonde, R. J. (1986). Evaluating the econometric evaluations of training programs with experimental data. *American Economic Review, 76*(4), 604–620.

Lamberty, G., Pachter, L. M., & Crnic, K. (2000). *Social stratification: Implications for understanding racial, ethnic and class disparities in child health and development.* Paper presented at the Role of Partnerships: Second Annual Meeting of Child Health Services Researchers, Rockville, Maryland, June 27, 2000.

Lamont, M., & White, P. (2005). *Workshop on interdisciplinary standards for systematic qualitative research*. National Science Foundation supported workshop. Retrieved from www.nsf.gov/sbe/ses/soc/ISSQR_workshop_rpt.pdf.

Lancsar, E., & Louviere, J. (2008). Conducting discrete choice experiments to inform healthcare decision making. *PharmacoEconomics, 26*(8), 661–677.

Land, K. C. (1969). Principles of path analysis. *Sociological Methodology, 1*, 3–37.

Landes, S. J., McBain, S. A., & Curran, G. M. (2019). An introduction to effectiveness-implementation hybrid designs. *Psychiatry Research, 280*, 112513.

Larkin, M. A., & McGowan, A. K. (2008). Introduction: Strengthening public health. *The Journal of Law, Medicine & Ethics, 36*(Suppl. 3), 4–5.

Larsen, L. L., & Berry, J. A. (2003). The regulation of dietary supplements. *Journal of the American Academy of Nurse Practitioners, 15*(9), 410–414.

Larson, N. I., Story, M., & Nelson, M. C. (2009). Neighborhood environments: Disparities in access to healthy foods in the U.S. *American Journal of Preventive Medicine, 36*(1), 74–81.

Latané, B. (1981). The psychology of social impact. *American Psychologist, 36*(4), 343–356.

Lavis, J., Oxman, A., Moynihan, R., & Paulsen, E. (2008). Evidence-informed health policy 1—Synthesis of findings from a multi-method study of organizations that support the use of research evidence. *Implementation Science, 3*(1), 53.

Law, D. S. (2005). Strategic judicial lawmaking: Ideology, publication, and asylum law in the Ninth Circuit. *University of Cincinnati Law Review, 73*(3), 817–866.

Lawson, J., & Xu, F. (2007). SARS in Canada and China: Two approaches to emergency health policy. *Governance, 20*(2), 209–232.

Lazzarini, Z., Bray, S., & Burris, S. (2002). Evaluating the impact of criminal laws on HIV risk behavior. *The Journal of Law, Medicine & Ethics, 30*(2), 239–253.

Lazzarini, Z., & Rosales, L. (2002). Legal issues concerning public health efforts to reduce perinatal HIV transmission. *Yale Journal of Health Law, Policy, and Ethics, 3*(1), 67–98.

Leary, W. E. (1996, October 18). Questions on ethics lead to review of needle-exchange study. *New York Times*. Retrieved from https://www.nytimes.com/1996/10/18/us/questions-on-ethics-lead-to-review-of-needle-exchange-study.html.

Leatherdale, S. T. (2019). Natural experiment methodology for research: A review of how different methods can support real-world research. *International Journal of Social Research Methodology, 22*(1), 19–35.

Ledderer, L., Kjær, M., Madsen, E. K., Busch, J., & Fage-Butler, A. (2020). Nudging in public health lifestyle interventions: A systematic literature review and metasynthesis. *Health Education & Behavior, 47*(5), 749–764.

Lee, K., Ingram, A., Lock, K., & McInnes, C. (2007). Bridging health and foreign policy: The role of health impact assessments. *Bulletin of the World Health Organization, 85*(3), 207–211.

Lehmkuhl, D. (2008). Control modes in the age of transnational governance. *Law & Policy, 30*(3), 336–363.

Leigh, J. P., Leigh, W. A., & Du, J. (2019). Minimum wages and public health: A literature review. *Preventive Medicine, 118*, 122–134.

Leischow, S. J., Best, A., Trochim, W. M., Clark, P. I., Gallagher, R. S., Marcus, S. E., & Matthews, E. (2008). Systems thinking to improve the public's health. *American Journal of Preventive Medicine, 35*(2), S196–S203.

Lemert, E. M. (1951). *Social pathology.* New York, NY: McGraw-Hill.

Lemert, E. M. (1967). *Human deviance, social problems, and social control.* Englewood Cliffs, NJ: Prentice-Hall.

Levin, H. M., McEwan, P. J., Belfield, C. R., Bowden, A. B., & Shand, R. D. (2017). *Economic evaluation in education: Cost-effectiveness and benefit-cost analysis* (3rd ed.). Los Angeles, CA: Sage.

Levy, D. T., Yuan, Z., Luo, Y., & Mays, D. (2018). Seven years of progress in tobacco control: An evaluation of the effect of nations meeting the highest level MPOWER measures between 2007 and 2014. *Tobacco Control, 27*(1), 50–57.

Lewandowska, M., Wieckowska, B., Sztorc, L., & Sajdak, S. (2020). Smoking and smoking cessation in the risk for fetal growth restriction and low birth weight and additive effect of maternal obesity. *Journal of Clinical Medicine, 9*(11), 3504.

Lewin, K. (1952). *Field theory in social science: Selected theoretical papers.* New York, NY: Harper & Brothers.

Lewis, C. C., Klasnja, P., Powell, B. J., Lyon, A. R., Tuzzio, L., Jones, S., … Weiner, B. (2018). From classification to causality: Advancing understanding of mechanisms of change in implementation science. *Frontiers in Public Health, 6*, 136.

Lewis, C. C., Scott, K., & Marriott, B. R. (2018). A methodology for generating a tailored implementation blueprint: An exemplar from a youth residential setting. *Implementation Science, 13*(1), 68.

Lewis, J. (1985). Lead poisoning: A historical perspective. *EPA Journal, 11*(4), 15–18.

Lewis, K. M., Schure, M. B., Bavarian, N. B., DuBois, D. L., Day, J., Ji, P., … Flay, B. R. (2013). Problem behavior and urban, low-income youth: A randomized controlled trial of Positive Action in Chicago. *American Journal of Preventive Medicine, 44*(6), 622–630. https://doi.org/10.1016/j.amepre.2013.01.030

Li, H., & Sakamoto, Y. (2014). Social impacts in social media: An examination of perceived truthfulness and sharing of information. *Computers in Human Behavior, 41*, 278–287.

Liang, T. J., & Ward, J. W. (2018). Hepatitis C in injection-drug users—A hidden danger of the opioid epidemic. *New England Journal of Medicine, 378*(13), 1169–1171.

Libbey, H. P. (2004). Measuring student relationships to school: Attachment, bonding, connectedness, and engagement. *Journal of School Health, 74*(7), 274–283.

Lichtveld, M., Hodge, J. G., Jr., Gebbie, K., Thompson, F. E., Jr., & Loos, D. I. (2002). Preparedness on the frontline: What's law got to do with it? *Journal of Law Medicine & Ethics, 30*(Suppl. 3), 184–188.

Liljegren, M., & Ekberg, K. (2009). The associations between perceived distributive, procedural, and interactional organizational justice, self-rated health and burnout. *Work, 33*(1), 43–51.

Lin, H.-x., Liu, Z., & Chang, C. (2020). The effects of smoke-free workplace policies on individual smoking behaviors in China. *Nicotine & Tobacco Research, 22*(12), 2158–2163.

Lincoln, Y. S., & Guba, E. G. (1985). *Naturalistic inquiry*. Beverly Hills, CA: Sage.

Lind, E. A., & Tyler, T. R. (1988). *The social psychology of procedural justice*. New York, NY: Plenum Press.

Link, B. G., & Phelan, J. (1995). Social conditions as fundamental causes of disease. *Journal of Health and Social Behavior, 35*, 80–94.

Lipschultz, J. H. (2020). *Social media communication: Concepts, practices, data, law and ethics*. Routledge.

Lobel, O. (2004). The renew deal: The fall of regulation and the rise of governance in contemporary legal thought. *Minnesota Law Review, 89*, 342–471.

Lobel, O., & Amir, O. (2009). Stumble, predict, nudge: How behavioral economics informs law and policy. *Columbia Law Review, 108*, 2098–2138.

Lochner, K. A., Kawachi, I., Brennan, R. T., & Buka, S. L. (2003). Social capital and neighborhood mortality rates in Chicago. *Social Science & Medicine, 56*, 1797–1805.

Loevinger, L. (1961). Jurimetrics: Science and prediction in the field of law. *Minnesota Law Review, 46*, 255–275.

Logan, W. A. (2009). *Knowledge as power: Criminal registration and community notification laws in America*. Palo Alto, CA: Stanford University Press.

Lombard, M., Snyder-Duch, J., & Campanella Bracken, C. (2005). *Practical resources for assessing and reporting intercoder reliability in content analysis research projects*. Retrieved from www.temple.edu/mmc/reliability/.

Lorch, S. A., Rogowski, J., Profit, J., & Phibbs, C. S. (2021). Access to risk-appropriate hospital care and disparities in neonatal outcomes in racial/ethnic groups and rural-urban populations. *Seminars in Perinatology, 45*(4), 151409.

Ludwig, J., & Cook, P. J. (2000). Homicide and suicide rates associated with implementation of the Brady Handgun Violence Prevention Act. *Journal of the American Medical Association, 284*(5), 585–591.

Ludwig, J., Kling, J. R., & Mullainathan, S. (2011). Mechanism experiments and policy evaluations. *Journal of Economic Perspectives, 25*(3), 17–38.

Ludwig, J., Sanbonmatsu, L., Gennetian, L., Adam, E., Duncan, G. J., Katz, L. F., … McDade, T. W. (2011). Neighborhoods, obesity, and diabetes: A randomized social experiment. *New England Journal of Medicine, 365*(16), 1509–1519.

Lurie, N., Wasserman, J., Stoto, M., Myers, S., Namkung, P., Fielding, J., & Valdez, R. B. (2004). Local variation in public health preparedness: Lessons from California. *Health Affairs, Web Exclusive*, W4341–W4353.

Lutfey, K., & Freese, J. (2005). Toward some fundamentals of fundamental causality: Socioeconomic status and health in the routine clinic visit for diabetes. *American Journal of Sociology, 110*(5), 1326–1372.

Maantay, J. (2002). Zoning law, health, and environmental justice: What's the connection? *The Journal of Law, Medicine & Ethics, 30*(4), 572–593.

MacCoun, R. J. (1993). Drugs and the law: A psychological analysis of drug prohibition. *Psychological Bulletin, 113*(3), 497–512.

Macdonald, H. R., & Glantz, S. A. (1997). Political realities of statewide smoking legislation: The passage of California's Assembly Bill 13. *Tobacco Control, 6*(1), 41–54.

Macinko, J., & Silver, D. (2015). Diffusion of impaired driving laws among US states. *American Journal of Public Health, 105*(9), 1893–1900.

Maclean, J. C., Mallatt, J., Ruhm, C. J., & Simon, K. (2021). Economic studies on the opioid crisis: costs, causes, and policy responses. In *Oxford Research Encyclopedia of Economics and Finance*. Oxford: Oxford University Press. Retrieved from https://oxfordre.com/economics/display/10.1093/acrefore/9780190625979.001.0001/acrefore-9780190625979-e-283?rskey = FMFQld&result = 1.

Magnusson, R. S. (2007). Mapping the scope and opportunities for public health law in liberal democracies. *The Journal of Law, Medicine & Ethics, 35*(4), 571–587.

Magnusson, R. S. (2009). Rethinking global health challenges: Towards a "global compact" for reducing the burden of chronic disease. *Public Health, 123*(3), 265–274.

Mamudu, H. M., & Glantz, S. A. (2009). Civil society and the negotiation of the Framework Convention on Tobacco Control. *Global Public Heatlh, 4*(2), 150–168.

Manning, W. G. (1991). *The costs of poor health habits*. Cambridge, MA: Harvard University Press.

Manning, W. G., Newhouse, J. P., Duan, N., Keeler, E. B., Leibowitz, A., & Marquis, M. S. (1987). Health insurance and the demand for medical care: Evidence from a randomized experiment. *The American Economic Review, 77*(3), 251–277.

Marie, O., & Zölitz, U. (2017). "High" achievers? Cannabis access and academic performance. *The Review of Economic Studies, 84*(3), 1210–1237.

Markowitz, S., Komro, K. A., Livingston, M. D., Lenhart, O., & Wagenaar, A. C. (2017). Effects of state-level Earned Income Tax Credit laws in the U.S. on maternal health behaviors and infant health outcomes. *Social Science & Medicine, 194*, 67–75.

Marks, M., Wood, J., Ali, F., Walsh, T., & Witbooi, A. (2010). Worlds apart? On the possibilities of police/academic collaborations. *Policing: A Journal of Policy and Practice, 4*(2), 112–118.

Marmot, M. (2005). Social determinants of health inequalities. *Lancet, 365*, 1099–1104.

Marsh, K., Phillips, C. J., Fordham, R., Bertranou, E., & Hale, J. (2012). Estimating cost-effectiveness in public health: A summary of modelling and valuation methods. *Health Economics Review, 2*(17), 1–6.

Martin, R., Conseil, A., Longstaff, A., Kodo, J., Siegert, J., Duguet, A.-M., … Coker, R. (2010). Pandemic influenza control in Europe and the constraints resulting from incoherent public health laws. *BMC Public Health, 10*(1), 532.

Masse, L. N., & Barnett, W. S. (2002). *A benefit cost analysis of the Abecedarian Early Childhood Intervention*. New Brunswick, NJ: National Institute for Early Education Research.

Matjasko, J. L., Cawley, J. H., Baker-Goering, M. M., & Yokum, D. V. (2016). Applying behavioral economics to public health policy: Illustrative examples and promising directions. *American Journal of Preventive Medicine, 50*(5), S13–S19.

Matsueda, R. L. (1988). The current state of differential association theory. *Crime & Delinquency, 34*(3), 277–306.

Mayne, S. L., Widome, R., Carroll, A. J., Schreiner, P. J., Gordon-Larsen, P., Jacobs, D. R., & Kershaw, K. N. (2018). Longitudinal Associations of smoke-free policies and incident cardiovascular disease. *Circulation, 138*(6), 557–566.

Mays, G., Beitsch, L. M., Corso, L., Chang, C., & Brewer, R. (2007). States gathering momentum: Promising strategies for accreditation and assessment activities in multi-state learning collaborative applicant states. *Journal of Public Health Management and Practice, 13*(4), 364–373.

Mays, G. P., Halverson, P. K., & Scutchfield, F. D. (2004). Making public health improvement real: The vital role of systems research. *Journal of Public Health Management and Practice, 10*(3), 183–185.

Mays, G. P., & Scutchfield, F. D. (2012). Advancing the science of delivery: Public health services and systems research. *Journal of Public Health Management and Practice, 18*(6), 481–484.

Mays, G. P., Scutchfield, F. D., Bhandari, M. W., & Smith, S. A. (2010). Understanding the organization of public health delivery systems: An empirical typology. *Milbank Quarterly, 88*(1), 81–111.

McAlinden, A. M. (2006). Managing risk: From regulation to the reintegration of sex offenders. *Criminology and Criminal Justice, 6*(2), 197–218.

McBarnet, D. J., Voiculescu, A., & Campbell, T. (Eds.) (2007). *The new corporate accountability: Corporate social responsibility and the law.* Cambridge, UK: Cambridge University Press.

McCann, M. W. (1994). *Rights at work: Pay equity reform and the politics of legal mobilization.* Chicago, IL: University of Chicago Press.

McCann, P. J. C. (2009). Agency discretion and public health service delivery. *Health Services Research, 44*(5), 1897–1908.

McCarthy, M., Murphy, K., Sargeant, E., & Williamson, H. (2021). Policing COVID-19 physical distancing measures: Managing defiance and fostering compliance among individuals least likely to comply. *Policing and Society, 31*, 601–620.

McChesney, F. S. (1993). Doctrinal analysis and statistical modeling in law: The case of defective incorporation. *Washington University Law Quarterly, 71*(3), 493–534.

McCluskey, J. D. (2003). *Police requests for compliance: Coercive and procedurally just tactics.* New York, NY: LFB Scholarly.

McCoy, D., & Hilson, M. (2009). Civil society, its organizations, and global health governance. In K. Buse, W. Hein, & N. Drager (Eds.), *Making sense of global health governance* (pp. 209–231). London, UK: Palgrave MacMillan.

McDougall, G. (1997). Direct legislation: Determinants of legislator support for voter initiatives. *Public Finance Review, 25*(3), 327–343.

McGuire, K. T., Vanberg, G., Smith, C. E., & Caldeira, G. A. (2009). Measuring policy content on the U.S. Supreme Court. *The Journal of Politics, 71*(4), 1305–1321.

McMillen, R. C., Winickoff, J. P., Klein, J. D., & Weitzman, M. (2003). U.S. adult attitudes and practices regarding smoking restrictions and child exposure to environmental tobacco smoke: Changes in the social climate from 2000–2001. *Pediatrics, 112*(1), e55–e60.

McNeill, L. H., Kreuter, M. W., & Subramanian, S. V. (2006). Social environment and physical activity: A review of concepts and evidence. *Social Science and Medicine, 63*(4), 1011–1022.

McNeill, W. (1977). *Plagues and peoples.* Garden City, NJ: Anchor Press.

Mead, G. H. (1934). *Mind, self, & society: From the standpoint of a social behaviorist* (Vol. 1). Chicago, IL: University of Chicago Press.

Meier, B. M., Hodge, J. G., Jr., & Gebbie, K. M. (2009). Transitions in state public health law: Comparative analysis of state public health law reform following the Turning Point Model State Public Health Act. *American Journal of Public Health, 99*(3), 423–430.

Meier, B. M., Merrill, J., & Gebbie, K. M. (2009). Modernizing state public health enabling statutes to reflect the mission and essential services of public health. *Journal of Public Health Management and Practice, 15*(4), 284–291.

Meier, B. M., Tureski, K., Bockh, E., Carr, D., Ayala, A., Roberts, A., ... Burris, S. (2017). Examining national public health law to realize the Global Health Security Agenda. *Medical Law Review, 25*(2), 240–269.

Meier, L. L., Semmer, N. K., & Hupfeld, J. (2009). The impact of unfair treatment on depressive mood: The moderating role of self-esteem level and self-esteem instability. *Personality and Social Psychology Bulletin, 35*(5), 643–655.

Mello, M., & Brennan, T. (2002). Deterrence of medical errors: Theory and evidence for malpractice reform. *Texas Law Review, 80*, 1595–1638.

Mello, M. M., Pomeranz, J., & Moran, P. (2008). The interplay of public health law and industry self-regulation: The case of sugar-sweetened beverage sales in schools. *American Journal of Public Health, 98*(4), 595–604.

Mello, M. M., Powlowski, M., Nañagas, J. M. P., & Bossert, T. (2006). The role of law in public health: The case of family planning in the Philippines. *Social Science & Medicine, 63*(2), 384–396.

Mello, M. M., & Zeiler, K. (2008). Empirical health law scholarship: The state of the field. *Georgetown Law Journal, 96*(2), 649–702.

Melnick, R. S. (1983). *Regulation and the courts: The case of the Clean Air Act.* Washington, DC: Brookings Institution.

Melton, G. B. (Ed.) (1986). *The law as a behavioral instrument: Nebraska Symposium on Motivation, 1985.* Volume 33 in the series *Current Theory and Research in Motivation.* Lincoln, NE: University of Nebraska Press.

Mentovich, A., Rhee, E., & Tyler, T. R. (2014). My life for a voice: The influence of voice on health-care decisions. *Social Justice Research, 27*(1), 99–117.

Merrill, J., Keeling, J., Meier, B. M., Gebbie, K. M., & Jia, H. (2009). Examination of the relationship between public health statute modernization and local public health system performance. *Journal of Public Health Management and Practice, 15*(4), 292–298.

Merry, S. E. (1990). *Getting justice and getting even: Legal consciousness among working-class Americans.* Chicago, IL: University of Chicago Press.

Mertz, K. J., & Weiss, H. B. (2008). Changes in motorcycle-related head injury deaths, hospitalizations, and hospital charges following repeal of Pennsylvania's mandatory motorcycle helmet law. *American Journal of Public Health, 98*(8), 1464–1467.

Metcalfe, J. J., Ellison, B., Hamdi, N., Richardson, R., & Prescott, M. P. (2020). A systematic review of school meal nudge interventions to improve youth food behaviors. *International Journal of Behavioral Nutrition and Physical Activity, 17*(1), 77.

Meyers, D. G., Neuberger, J. S., & He, J. (2009). Cardiovascular effect of bans on smoking in public places. *Journal of the American College of Cardiology, 54*(15), 1249–1255.

Midgette, G., Kilmer, B., Nicosia, N., & Heaton, P. (2021). A natural experiment to test the effect of sanction certainty and celerity on substance-impaired driving: North Dakota's 24/7 Sobriety program. *Journal of Quantitative Criminology, 37*(3), 647–670.

Miech, R., Johnston, L., O'Malley, P. M., Bachman, J. G., & Patrick, M. E. (2019). Trends in adolescent vaping, 2017–2019. *New England Journal of Medicine, 381*(15), 1490–1491.

Miech, R., Leventhal, A., Johnston, L., O'Malley, P. M., Patrick, M. E., & Barrington-Trimis, J. (2021). Trends in use and perceptions of nicotine vaping among US youth from 2017 to 2020. *JAMA Pediatrics, 175*(2), 185–190.

Miech, R. A., Patrick, M. E., O'Malley, P. M., Johnston, L. D., & Bachman, J. G. (2020). Trends in reported marijuana vaping among US adolescents, 2017-2019. *JAMA, 323*(5), 475–476.

Miller, H. V., Barnes, J., & Beaver, K. M. (2011). Self-control and health outcomes in a nationally representative sample. *American Journal of Health Behavior, 35*(1), 15–27.

Miller, M., Azrael, D., & Hemenway, D. (2002). Rates of household firearm ownership and homicide across U.S. regions and states. *American Journal of Public Health, 92*(12), 1988–1993.

Miller, S., Johnson, N., & Wherry, L. R. (2021). Medicaid and mortality: New evidence from linked survey and administrative data. *Quarterly Journal of Economics, 136*(3), 1783–1829.

Miller, W. L., & Crabtree, B. F. (2004). Depth interviewing. In S. N. Hesse-Biber & P. Leavy (Eds.), *Approaches to qualitative research: A reader on theory and practice* (pp. 185–202). New York, NY: Oxford University Press.

Milmo, D., & Paul, K. (2021, September 30). Facebook disputes its own research showing harmful effects of Instagram on teens' mental health. *The Guardian*.

Mindell, J., Sheridan, L., Joffe, M., Samson-Barry, H., & Atkinson, S. (2004). Health impact assessment as an agent of policy change: Improving the health impacts of the mayor of London's draft transport strategy. *Journal of Epidemiology and Community Health, 58*(3), 169–174.

Mir, I., & Zaheer, A. (2012). Verification of social impact theory claims in social media context. *Journal of Internet Banking and Commerce, 17*(1), 1.

Misue, K., Eades, P., Lai, W., & Sugiyama, K. (1995). Layout adjustment and the mental map. *Journal of Visual Languages and Computing, 6*(2), 183–210.

Mitchell, R. C., & Carson, R. T. (2013). *Using surveys to value public goods: The contingent valuation method*. RFF Press.

Moen, P., Kelly, E. L., Huang, Q., & Tranby, E. (2011). Changing work, changing health: Can real work-time flexibility promote health behaviors and well-being? *Journal of Health and Social Behavior, 52*(4), 404–429.

Moerman, J. W., & Potts, G. E. (2011). Analysis of metals leached from smoked cigarette litter. *Tobacco Control, 20*, i30–i35.

Mokdad, A. H., Ballestros, K., Echko, M., Glenn, S., Olsen, H. E., Mullany, E., ... US Burden of Disease Collaborators (2018). The state of US health, 1990–2016: Burden of diseases, injuries, and risk factors among US states. *JAMA, 319*(14), 1444–1472.

Montez, J. K., Beckfield, J., Cooney, J. K., Grumbach, J. M., Hayward, M. D., Koytak, H. Z., ... Zajacova, A. (2020). US state policies, politics, and life expectancy. *The Milbank Quarterly, 98*(3), 668–669.

Montez, J. K., Hayward, M. D., & Wolf, D. A. (2017). Do U.S. states' socioeconomic and policy contexts shape adult disability? *Social Science & Medicine, 178*, 115–126.

Montini, T., & Bero, L. (2008). Implementation of a workplace smoking ban in bars: The limits of local discretion. *BMC Public Health, 8*(1), 402.

Moor, I., Spallek, J., & Richter, M. (2017). Explaining socioeconomic inequalities in self-rated health: A systematic review of the relative contribution of material, psychosocial and behavioural factors. *Journal of Epidemiology and Community Health, 71*(6), 565–575.

Moran, M. (2002). Review article: Understanding the regulatory state. *British Journal of Political Science, 32*(2), 391–413.

Moreau, S. (2010). What is discrimination? *Philosophy and Public Affairs, 38*(2), 143–179.

Morgan, D. L. (2004). Focus groups. In S. N. Hesse-Biber & P. Leavy (Eds.), *Approaches to qualitative research: A reader on theory and practice* (pp. 263–285). New York, NY: Oxford University Press.

Morrisey, M. A., Grabowski, D. C., Dee, T. S., & Campbell, C. (2006). The strength of graduated drivers license programs and fatalities among teen drivers and passengers. *Accident Analysis and Prevention, 38*(1), 135–141.

Mosley, J., Marwell, N., & Ybarra, M. (2019). How the "what works" movement is failing human service organizations, and what social work can do to fix it. *Human Service Organizations: Management, Leadership & Governance, 43*, 1–10.

Moss, K., Burris, S., Ullman, M., Johnsen, M. C., & Swanson, J. (2001). Unfunded mandate: An empirical study of the implementation of the Americans with Disabilities Act by the Equal Employment Opportunity Commission. *Kansas Law Review, 50*(1), 1–110.

Moulton, A., Gottfried, R., Goodman, R., Murphy, A., & Rawson, R. (2003). What is public health legal preparedness? *The Journal of Law, Medicine & Ethics, 31*(4), 672–683.

Moulton, A. D., Mercer, S. L., Popovic, T., Briss, P. A., Goodman, R. A., Thombley, M. L., ... Fox, D. M. (2009). The scientific basis for law as a public health tool. *American Journal of Public Health, 99*(1), 17–24.

Moxham-Hall, V. L., & Ritter, A. (2017). Indexes as a metric for drug and alcohol policy evaluation and assessment. *World Medical & Health Policy, 9*(1), 103–126.

Mundt, M. P., Fiore, M. C., Piper, M. E., Adsit, R. T., Kobinsky, K. H., Alaniz, K. M., & Baker, T. B. (2021). Cost-effectiveness of stop smoking incentives for medicaid-enrolled pregnant women. *Preventive Medicine, 153*, 106777.

Murphy, K., Bradford, B., Sargeant, E., & Cherney, A. (2021). Building immigrants' solidarity with police: Procedural justice, identity and immigrants' willingness to cooperate with police. *British Journal of Criminology*, azab052.

Musheno, M. (1997). Legal consciousness on the margins of society: Struggles against stigmatization in the AIDS crisis. *Identities, 2*(1/2), 101.

Myers, T., Orr, K. W., Locker, D., & Jackson, E. A. (1993). Factors affecting gay and bisexual men's decisions and intentions to seek HIV testing. *American Journal of Public Health, 83*(5), 701–704.

Mykhalovskiy, E. (2011). The problem of "significant risk": Exploring the public health impact of criminalizing HIV non-disclosure. *Social Science & Medicine, 73*(5), 668–675.

Nagin, D. S. (1998). Criminal deterrence research at the outset of the twenty-first century. In M. Tonry (Ed.), *Crime and justice: A review of research* (Vol. 23, pp. 1–42). Chicago, IL: University of Chicago Press.

Nagin, D. S. (2010). Imprisonment and crime control: Building evidence-based policy. In R. Rosenfeld, K. Quinet, & C. Garcia (Eds.), *Contemporary issues in criminological theory and research: The role of social institutions*. Belmont, CA: Wadsworth.

Nagin, D. S., & Pogarsky, G. (2001). Integrating celerity, impulsivity, and extralegal sanction threats into a model of general deterrence: Theory and evidence. *Criminology, 39*(4), 865–891.

Naimi, T. S., Blanchette, J., Nelson, T. F., Nguyen, T., Oussayef, N., Heeren, T. C., ... Xuan, Z. (2014). A new scale of the U.S. alcohol policy environment and its relationship to binge drinking. *American Journal of Preventive Medicine, 46*(1), 10–16.

Nakkash, R., & Lee, K. (2009). The tobacco industry's thwarting of marketing restrictions and health warnings in Lebanon. *Tobacco Control, 18*(4), 310–316.

National Academies of Sciences, Engineering, and Medicine (2016). *Advancing the power of economic evidence to inform investments in children, youth, and families*. Washington, DC: The National Academies Press.

National Academies of Sciences, Engineering, and Medicine (2019). *A roadmap to reducing child poverty*. Washington, DC: The National Academies Press.

National Association of Local Boards of Health. (2011). *Profile of local boards of health launched*. Retrieved from www.nalboh.org/Profile.htm.

National Cancer Institute (2008). *The role of the media in promoting and reducing tobacco use* (NIH Publication No. 07–6242). Bethesda, MD: National Cancer Institute.

National Center for Health Statistics (NCHS). (2016). *Health, United States, 2015: With special feature on racial and ethnic health disparities* (Report No. 2016-1232). National Center for Health Statistics (US).

National Highway Traffic Safety Administration (2010). *Motorcycle helmet use in 2010—Overall results (DOT HS-811–419)*. Washington, DC: U.S. Department of Transportation, National Highway Traffic Safety Administration.

National Institute for Health and Care Excellence (NICE) (2014). *Developing NICE guidelines: The manual. Process and methods (PMG20)*. London, UK: Author. Retrieved from https://www.nice.org.uk/process/pmg20/chapter/incorporating-economic-evaluation

National Institute on Alcohol Abuse and Alcoholism. (2021). Underage drinking: Underage purchase of alcohol. *Alcohol Policy Information System (APIS)*. Retrieved from https://alcoholpolicy.niaaa.nih.gov/apis-policy-topics/underage-purchase-of-alcohol/43.

National Research Council & Institute of Medicine (2002). *Executive summary. Health insurance is a family matter*. Washington, DC: The National Academies Press.

Ndjaboué, R., Brisson, C., & Vézina, M. (2012). Organisational justice and mental health: A systematic review of prospective studies. *Occupational and Environmental Medicine, 69*, 694–700.

Network for Public Health Law. (2021). *Proposed limits on public health author-ity: Dangerous for public health.* Retrieved from https://www.networkforphl.org/wp-content/uploads/2021/05/Proposed-Limits-on-Public-Health-Authority-Dangerous-for-Public-Health-FINAL.pdf.

Neuendorf, K. A. (2002). *The content analysis guidebook.* Thousand Oaks, CA: Sage.

Neuendorf, K. A. (2017). *The content analysis guidebook* (2nd ed.). Los Angeles, CA: Sage.

Neumark, D., & Young, T. (2020). *Heterogeneous effects of state enterprise zone pro-grams in the shorter run and longer run.* Retrieved from https://www.nber.org/papers/w27545.

New State Ice Co. v. Liebmann, 285 U.S. 262 (1932).

New York State Office of Mental Health. (2011). *Implementation of assisted outpatient treatment.* Retrieved from www.omh.ny.gov/omhweb/Kendra_web/interimreport/implementation.htm.

Nicholas, L. H., & Maclean, J. C. (2019). The effect of medical marijuana laws on the health and labor supply of older adults: Evidence from the health and retirement study. *Journal of Policy Analysis and Management, 38*(2), 455–480.

Nighbor, T. D., Coleman, S. R. M., Bunn, J. Y., Kurti, A. N., Zvorsky, I., Orr, E. J., & Higgins, S. T. (2020). Smoking prevalence among U.S. national samples of pregnant women. *Preventive Medicine, 132*, 105994.

Nilsen, P. (2015). Making sense of implementation theories, models and frameworks. *Implementation Science, 10*, 53.

Nilsen, P., Ståhl, C., Roback, K., & Cairney, P. (2013). Never the twain shall meet?— A comparison of implementation science and policy implementation research. *Implementation Science, 8*, 63.

Nixon, M. L., Mahmoud, L., & Glantz, S. A. (2004). Tobacco industry litigation to deter local public health ordinances: The industry usually loses in court. *Tobacco Control, 13*(1), 65–73.

Noble, A., Vega, W. A., Kolody, B., Porter, P., Hwang, J., Merk, G. A., 2nd, & Bole, A. (1997). Prenatal substance abuse in California: Findings from the Perinatal Substance Exposure Study. *Journal of Psychoactive Drugs, 29*(1), 43–53.

Novak, J. D., & Cañas, A. J. (2008). *The theory underlying concept maps and how to construct and use them.* Ponta Grossa, Puerto Rico: Universidade Estadual de Ponta Grossa.

Novick, L., Morrow, C., & Mays, G. (Eds.) (2008). *Public health administration: Principles for population-based management.* Sudbury, MA: Jones and Bartlett.

Novotny, T. E., Lum, K., Smith, E., Wang, V., & Barnes, R. (2009). Cigarette butts and the case for an environmental policy on hazardous cigarette waste. *International Journal of Environmental Research and Public Health, 6*(5), 1691–1705.

Nowak, A., Szamrej, J., & Latané, B. (1990). From private attitude to public opinion: A dynamic theory of social impact. *Psychological Review, 97*(3), 362–376.

Nunez-Smith, M., Pilgrim, N., Wynia, M., Desai, M. M., Bright, C., Krumholz, H. M., & Bradley, E. H. (2009). Health care workplace discrimination and physician turnover. *Journal of the National Medical Association, 101*(12), 1274–1282.

Nunnally, J. C. (1978). *Psychometric theory* (2nd ed.). New York, NY: McGraw-Hill.

Oetting, E. R., & Beauvais, F. (1986). Peer cluster theory: Drugs and the adolescent. *Journal of Counseling and Development, 65*, 17–65.

Office of Disease Prevention and Health Promotion & U.S. Department of Health and Human Services. (2010). *Healthy people 2010*. Retrieved from www.healthypeople.gov/2010/default.htm.

Office of Disease Prevention and Health Promotion, & U.S. Department of Health and Human Services. (2011). *Healthy people 2020*. Retrieved from www.healthypeople.gov/2020/topicsobjectives2020/objectiveslist.aspx?topicid=35.

Office of Disease Prevention and Health Promotion, & U.S. Department of Health and Human Services. (2020). *Healthy people 2030: Public health infrastructure*. Healthy People 2030. Retrieved from https://health.gov/healthypeople/objectives-and-data/browse-objectives/public-health-infrastructure#: ~ :text=Healthy People 2030 focuses on,systems%2C planning%2C and partnerships.

Office of Management and Budget. (2003). *Circular A-4: Regulatory analysis*. Retrieved from https://obamawhitehouse.archives.gov/sites/default/files/omb/assets/omb/circulars/a004/a-4.pdf

Omran, A. R. (1971). The epidemiologic transition: A theory of the epidemiology of population change. *The Milbank Memorial Fund Quarterly, 49*(4), 509–538.

Orphanides, A., & Zervos, D. (1995). Rational addiction with learning and regret. *Journal of Political Economy, 103*(4), 739–758.

Osborne, D., & Gaebler, T. (1993). *Reinventing government*. New York, NY: Plume.

Ostrom, E. (2005). *Understanding institutional diversity*. Princeton, NJ: Princeton University Press.

Outterson, K. (2005). The vanishing public domain: Antibiotic resistance, pharmaceutical innovation and global public health. *University of Pittsburgh Law Review, 67*, 67–123.

Pachter, L. M., & Coll, C. G. (2009). Racism and child health: A review of the literature and future directions. *Journal of Developmental and Behavioral Pediatrics, 30*(3), 255–263.

Pacula, R. L., & Powell, D. (2018). A supply-side perspective on the opioid crisis. *Journal of Policy Analysis and Management, 37*(2), 438–446.

Pacula, R. L., Powell, D., Heaton, P., & Sevigny, E. (2015). Assessing the effects of medical marijuana laws on marijuana: The devil is in the details. *Journal of Policy Analysis and Management, 34*(1), 7–31.

Park, R. E., Fink, A., Brook, R. H., Chassin, M. R., Kahn, K. L., Merrick, N. J., … Solomon, D. H. (1986). Physician ratings of appropriate indications for six medical and surgical procedures. *American Journal of Public Health, 76*(7), 766–772.

Parker, C. (2002). *The open corporation: Effective self-regulation and democracy*. Cambridge, UK: Cambridge University Press.

Parker, C., & Braithwaite, J. (2003). Regulation. In P. Cane & M. Tushnet (Eds.), *Oxford handbook of legal studies* (pp. 119–145). Oxford, UK: Oxford University Press.

Parmet, W. (2009). *Populations, public health, and the law*. Washington, DC: Georgetown University Press.

Parmet, W. E., Burris, S., Gable, L., Guia, S. d., Levin, D. E., & Terry, N. P. (2021). COVID-19: The promise and failure of law in an inequitable nation. *American Journal of Public Health, 111*(1), 47–49.

Parmet, W. E., & Daynard, R. A. (2000). The new public health litigation. *Annual Review of Public Health, 21*, 437–454.

Parrott, S., Godfrey, C., & Raw, M. (2000). Costs of employee smoking in the workplace in Scotland. *Tobacco Control, 9*(2), 187–192.

Parsons, T. (1967). *Sociological theory and modern society*. New York, NY: Free Press.

Pascoe, E. A., & Richman, L. S. (2009). Perceived discrimination and health: A metaanalytic review. *Psychological Bulletin, 135*(4), 531–554.

Pataki, G. E., & Carpinello, S. E. (2005). *Kendra's Law: Final report on the status of assisted outpatient treatment*. Albany, NY: New York State Office of Mental Health. Retrieved from https://omh.ny.gov/omhweb/kendra_web/finalreport/program_eval.htm.

Paternoster, R., & Piquero, A. R. (1995). Reconceptualizing deterrence: An empirical test of personal and vicarious experiences. *Journal of Research in Crime and Delinquency, 32*(3), 251–286.

Patrick, S. W., Fry, C. E., Jones, T. F., & Buntin, M. B. (2016). Implementation of prescription drug monitoring programs associated with reductions in opioid-related death rates. *Health Affairs, 35*(7), 1324–1332.

Patton, C. (1990). *Inventing AIDS*. New York, NY: Routledge.

Pawson, R. (2006). *Evidence-based policy: A realist perspective*. London, UK; Thousand Oaks, CA: Sage.

Pawson, R., Greenhalgh, T., Harvey, G., & Walshe, K. (2005). Realist review—A new method of systematic review designed for complex policy interventions. *Journal of Health Services Research & Policy, 10*(1_suppl), 21–34.

Payne, K., McAllister, M., & Davies, L. M. (2013). Valuing the economic benefits of complex interventions: When maximising health is not sufficient. *Health Economics, 22*(3), 258–271.

Pedriana, N., & Abraham, A. (2006). Now you see them, now you don't: The legal field and newspaper desegregation of sex-segregated help wanted ads 1965-75. *Law & Social Inquiry, 31*(4), 905–938.

Pedriana, N., & Stryker, R. (2004). The strength of a weak agency: Enforcement of Title VII of the 1964 Civil Rights Act and the expansion of state capacity, 1965-1971. *American Journal of Sociology, 110*(3), 709–760.

Pell, J. P., Haw, S., Cobbe, S., Newby, D. E., Pell, A. C., Fischbacher, C., … Borland, W. (2008). Smoke-free legislation and hospitalizations for acute coronary syndrome. *New England Journal of Medicine, 359*(5), 482–491.

Percy, S. L. (1989). *Disability, civil rights, and public policy: The politics of implementation*. Tuscaloosa, AL: University of Alabama Press.

Percy, S. L. (2001). Challenges and dilemmas in implementing the Americans with Disabilities Act: Lessons from the first decade. *Policy Studies Journal, 29*(4), 633–640.

Perdue, W. C., Gostin, L. O., & Stone, L. A. (2003). Public health and the built environment: Historical, empirical, and theoretical foundations for an expanded role. *The Journal of Law, Medicine & Ethics, 31*(4), 557–566.

Pérez, D. J., & Larkin, M. A. (2009). Commentary: Partnership for the future of public health services and systems research. *Health Services Research, 44*(5p2), 1788–1795.

Pérez-Stable, E. J., & Webb Hooper, M. (2021). Acknowledgment of the legacy of racism and discrimination. *Ethnicity & Disease, 31*(Suppl 1), 289–292.

Persky, J. (1995). Retrospectives: The ethology of homo economicus. *The Journal of Economic Perspectives, 9*(2), 221–231.

Pessar, S. C., Boustead, A., Ge, Y., Smart, R., & Pacula, R. L. (2021). Assessment of state and federal health policies for opioid use disorder treatment during the COVID-19 pandemic and beyond. *JAMA Health Forum, 2*(11), –e213833.

Peter, A., & Ekeanyanwu, N. T. (2010). The theory of triadic influence, media literacy, adolescents and alcohol advertising in Lagos state. *International Journal of Social Sciences and Humanities Review, 1*(3), 34–39.

Petraitis, J., Flay, B. R., & Miller, T. Q. (1995). Reviewing theories of adolescent substance use: Organizing pieces in the puzzle. *Psychological Bulletin, 117*(1), 67–86.

Phelan, A. L., & Katz, R. (2019). Legal epidemiology for global health security and universal health coverage. *The Journal of Law, Medicine & Ethics, 47*(3), 427–429.

Phibbs, C. S., Baker, L. C., Caughey, A. B., Danielsen, B., Schmitt, S. K., & Phibbs, R. H. (2007). Level and volume of neonatal intensive care and mortality in very-low-birth-weight infants. *The New England Journal of Medicine, 356*(21), 2165–2175.

Phibbs, C. S., & Lorch, S. A. (2018). Choice of hospital as a source of racial/ethnic disparities in neonatal mortality and morbidity rates. *JAMA Pediatrics, 172*(3), 221–223.

Pho, M., Erzouki, F., Boodram, B., Jimenez, A. D., Pineros, J., Shuman, V., ... Pollack, H. A. (2021). Reducing Opioid Mortality in Illinois (ROMI): A case management/peer recovery coaching critical time intervention clinical trial protocol. *Journal of Substance Abuse Treatment, 128*, 108348.

Pigou, A. C. (1962). *A study in public finance* (3rd revised ed.). London, UK: Macmillan.

Pike, E., Tillson, M., Webster, J. M., & Staton, M. (2019). A mixed-methods assessment of the impact of the opioid epidemic on first responder burnout. *Drug and Alcohol Dependence, 205*, 107620.

Piquero, A. R., & Paternoster, R. (1998). An application of Stafford and Warr's reconceptualization of deterrence to drinking and driving. *Journal of Research in Crime and Delinquency, 35*(1), 3–39.

Piquero, A. R., & Pogarsky, G. (2003). Can punishment encourage offending? Investigating the "resetting" effect. *Journal of Research in Crime and Delinquency, 40*(1), 95–120.

Polaschek, D. L. L., Collie, R. M., & Walkey, F. H. (2004). Criminal attitudes to violence: Development and preliminary validation of a scale for male prisoners. *Aggressive Behavior, 30*(6), 484–503.

Polinsky, A. M., & Shavell, S. (2007). The theory of public enforcement of law. In A. M. Polinsky & S. Shavell (Eds.), *Handbook of law and economics* (Vol. 1, pp. 403–454). Amsterdam, the Netherlands: Elsevier.

Politis, C. E., Halligan, M. H., Keen, D., & Kerner, J. F. (2014). Supporting the diffusion of healthy public policy in Canada: The Prevention Policies Directory. *Online Journal of Public Health Informatics, 6*(2), e177.

Polsky, D., Glick, H. A., Willke, R., & Schulman, K. (1997). Confidence intervals for cost-effectiveness ratios: A comparison of four methods. *Health Economics, 6*(3), 243–252.

Pomeranz, J. L., Zellers, L., Bare, M., Sullivan, P. A., & Pertschuk, M. (2019). State preemption: Threat to democracy, essential regulation, and public health. *American Journal of Public Health, 109*(2), 251–252.

Popova, S., Giesbrecht, N., Bekmuradov, D., & Patra, J. (2009). Hours and days of sale and density of alcohol outlets: Impacts on alcohol consumption and damage: A systematic review. *Alcohol and Alcoholism, 44*(5), 500–516.

Powell, B. J., Beidas, R. S., Lewis, C. C., Aarons, G. A., McMillen, J. C., Proctor, E. K., & Mandell, D. S. (2017). Methods to improve the selection and tailoring of implementation strategies. *The Journal of Behavioral Health Services & Research, 44*(2), 177–194.

Powell, B. J., Waltz, T. J., Chinman, M. J., Damschroder, L. J., Smith, J. L., Matthieu, M. M., ... Kirchner, J. E. (2015). A refined compilation of implementation strategies: Results from the Expert Recommendations for Implementing Change (ERIC) project. *Implementation Science, 10*, 21.

Powell, D., Alpert, A., & Pacula, R. L. (2019). A transitioning epidemic: How the opioid epidemic is driving the rise in Hepatitis C. *Health Affairs, 38*(2), 287–294.

Powell, D., & Pacula, R. L. (2021). The evolving consequences of oxycontin reformulation on drug overdoses. *American Journal of Health Economics, 7*(1), 41–67.

Powell, D., Pacula, R. L., & Jacobson, M. (2018). Do medical marijuana laws reduce addictions and deaths related to pain killers? *Journal of Health Economics, 25*, 29–42.

Powell, L. M., Chaloupka, F. J., & Bao, Y. (2007). The availability of fast food and full-service restaurants in the United States: Associations with neighborhood characteristics. *American Journal of Preventive Medicine, 33*(Suppl. 4), S240–S245.

Powell, L. M., & Chriqui, J. F. (2011). Food taxes and subsidies: Evidence and policies for obesity prevention. In J. Crawley (Ed.), *The Oxford handbook of the social science of obesity*. New York, NY: Oxford University Press.

Powell, L. M., Han, E., & Chaloupka, F. J. (2010). Economic contextual factors, food consumption, and obesity among US adolescents. *The Journal of Nutrition, 140*(6), 1175–1180.

Powell, L. M., Schermbeck, R. M., Szczypka, G., Chaloupka, F. J., & Braunschweig, C. L. (2011). Trends in the nutritional content of television food advertisements seen by children in the United States: Analysis by age, food categories, and companies. *Archives of Pediatrics & Adolescent Medicine, 165*(12), 1078–1086.

Powell, L. M., Slater, S., Mirtcheva, D., Bao, Y., & Chaloupka, F. J. (2007). Food store availability and neighborhood characteristics in the United States. *Preventive Medicine, 44*(3), 189–195.

Power, M. (1997). *The audit society: Rituals of verification*. Oxford, UK; New York, NY: Oxford University Press.

Pratt, T. C., & Cullen, F. T. (2005). Assessing macro-level predictors and theories of crime: A meta-analysis. In M. Tonry (Ed.), *Crime and justice: A review of research* (Vol. 32, pp. 373–450). Chicago, IL: University of Chicago Press.

Pratt, T. C., Cullen, F. T., Blevins, K. R., Daigle, L. E., & Madensen, T. D. (2006). The empirical status of deterrence theory: A meta-analysis. In F. T. Cullen, J. P. Wright, & K. R. Blevins (Eds.), *Taking stock: The empirical status of criminological theory: Advances in criminological theory* (Vol. 15, pp. 367–395). New Brunswick, NJ: Transaction.

Preusser, D., & Tison, J. (2007). GDL then and now. *Journal of Safety Research, 38*(2), 159–163.

Proctor, E., Silmere, H., Raghavan, R., Hovmand, P. A., Aarons, G., Bunger, A., … Hensley, M. (2011). Outcomes for implementation research: Conceptual distinctions, measurement challenges, and research agenda. *Administration and Policy in Mental Health, 38*(2), 65–76.

Proctor, E. K., Powell, B. J., & McMillen, J. C. (2013). Implementation strategies: Recommendations for specifying and reporting. *Implementation Science, 8*, 139.

Public Health Accreditation Board. (2009). *Draft national voluntary accreditation standards for public health accreditation.* Retrieved from www.phaboard.org/index.php/beta_test/standards/.

Public Health Functions Steering Committee Office of Disease Prevention and Health Promotion (1994). *Public health in America.* Washington, DC: United States Public Health Service.

Public Health National Center for Innovation, & Public Health Accreditation Board. (2020). *Ten Essential Public Health Services: EPHS Toolkit 2020.* Retrieved from https://spark.adobe.com/page/Qy1veOhGWyeu5/.

Purtle, J., Peters, R., & Brownson, R. C. (2016). A review of policy dissemination and implementation research funded by the National Institutes of Health, 2007-2014. *Implementation Science, 11*, 1.

Pusch, N., & Holtfreter, K. (2021). Individual and organizational predictors of white-collar crime: A meta-analysis. *Journal of White Collar and Corporate Crime, 2*, 5–23.

Quadagno, J. S. (2005). *One nation, uninsured: Why the U.S. has no national health insurance.* New York, NY: Oxford University Press.

Rabin, B. A., Brownson, R. C., Haire-Joshu, D., Kreuter, M. W., & Weaver, N. (2008). A glossary for dissemination and implementation research in health. *Journal of Public Health Management and Practice, 14*(2), 117–123.

Rahkovsky, I., Lin, B. H., Lin, C. T. J., & Lee, J. Y. (2013). Effects of the Guiding Stars Program on purchases of ready-to-eat cereals with different nutritional attributes. *Food Policy, 43*, 100–107.

Rashiden, I., Ahmad Tajuddin, N. A. N. B., Yee, A., Zhen, S. T. E., & Bin Amir Nordin, A. S. (2020). The efficacy of smoking ban policy at the workplace on secondhand smoking: Systematic review and meta-analysis. *Environmental Science and Pollution Research, 27*(24), 29856–29866.

Ratcliffe, J. H., Taniguchi, T., Groff, E. R., & Wood, J. D. (2011). The Philadelphia foot patrol experiment: A randomized controlled trial of police patrol effectiveness in violent crime hotspots. *Criminology, 49*(3), 795–831.

Reason, P., & Bradbury, H. (2008). *The Sage handbook of action research: Participative inquiry and practice.* Los Angeles, CA; London, UK: Sage.

Rebonato, R. (2014). A critical assessment of libertarian paternalism. *Journal of Consumer Policy, 37*(3), 357–396.

Recker, J., Rosemann, M., Indulska, M., & Green, P. (2009). Business process modeling: A comparative analysis. *Journal of the Association of Information Systems, 10*(4), 333–363.

Reinders, F. C., Kuiper, M. E., Olthuis, E., Kooistra, E. B., de Bruijn, A. L., Brownlee, M., & van Rooij, B. (2020). Sustaining compliance with Covid-19 mitigation measures? Understanding distancing behavior in the Netherlands during June. *PsyArXiv.* doi:10.31234/osf.io/xafwp

Retting, R., & Cheung, I. (2008). Traffic speeds associated with implementation of 80 MPH speed limits on West Texas rural interstates. *Journal of Safety Research, 39*(5), 529–534.

Revesz, R. L. (1997). Environmental regulation, ideology, and the D.C. circuit. *Virginia Law Review, 83*(8), 1717–1772.

Revesz, R. L. (2001). Congressional influence on judicial behavior? An empirical examination of challenges to agency action in the D.C. circuit. *New York University Law Review, 76*, 1100–1137.

Rhodes, R. A. W. (1997). *Understanding governance: Policy networks, governance, reflexivity and accountability.* Buckingham, UK; Philadelphia, PA: Open University Press.

Robertson, C., & O'Brien, R. (2018). Health endowment at birth and variation in intergenerational economic mobility: Evidence from US county birth cohorts. *Demography, 55*(1), 249–269.

Robson, L. S. (2007). The effectiveness of occupational health and safety management system interventions: A systematic review. *Safety Science, 45*(3), 329–353.

Roche, S. P., Wilson, T., & Pickett, J. T. (2020). Perceived control, severity, certainty, and emotional fear: Testing an expanded model of deterrence. *Journal of Research in Crime and Delinquency, 57*, 493–531.

Rodgers, J., Valuev, A. V., Hswen, Y., & Subramanian, S. V. (2019). Social capital and physical health: An updated review of the literature for 2007–2018. *Social Science & Medicine, 236*, 112360.

Rokeach, M. (1973). *The nature of human values.* New York, NY: Free Press.

Rokeach, M., & Ball-Rokeach, S. J. (1989). Stability and change in American value priorities, 1968–1981. *American Psychologist, 44*(5), 775–784.

Rose, G. (1985). Sick individuals and sick populations. *International Journal of Epidemiology, 14*(1), 32–38.

Rosenbaum, M. (1980). A schedule for assessing self-control behaviors: Preliminary findings. *Behavior Therapy, 11*(1), 109–121.

Rosenberg, A., Groves, A. K., & Blankenship, K. M. (2017). Comparing Black and White drug offenders: Implications for racial disparities in criminal justice and reentry policy and programming. *Journal of Drug Issues, 47*, 132–142.

Rosenberg, G. N. (1991). *The hollow hope: Can courts bring about social change?* Chicago, IL: University of Chicago Press.

Rosenfeld, M. J. (2005). A critique of exchange theory in mate selection. *American Journal of Sociology, 110*(5), 1284–1325.

Rosenquist, N. A., Cook, D. M., Ehntholt, A., Omaye, A., Muennig, P., & Pabayo, R. (2020). Differential relationship between state-level minimum wage and infant mortality risk among US infants born to white and black mothers. *Journal of Epidemiology and Community Health, 74*(1), 14–19.

Ross, H. L. (1982). Interrupted time series studies of deterrence and drinking and driving. In J. Hagan (Ed.), *Deterrence reconsidered: Methodological innovations* (pp. 89–100). Beverly Hills, CA: Sage.

Rothman, K. J., Adami, H. O., & Trichopoulos, D. (1998). Should the mission of epidemiology include the eradication of poverty? *Lancet, 352*(9130), 810–813.

Rothman, K. J., & Greenland, S. (2005). Causation and causal inference in epidemiology. *American Journal of Public Health, 95*, S144–S150.

Rubin, D. (1974). Estimating causal effects of treatments in randomized and non-randomized studies. *Journal of Educational Psychology, 66*(5), 688–701.

Ruger, J. P. (2006). Toward a theory of a right to health: Capability and incompletely theorized agreements. *Yale Journal of Law & the Humanities, 18*, 273–326.

Ruhl, S., Stephens, M., & Locke, P. (2003). The role of non-governmental organizations (NGOs) in public health law. *The Journal of Law, Medicine & Ethics, 31*(Suppl. 4), 76–77.

Ruhm, C. J. (2016). Drug poisoning deaths in the United States, 1999–2012: A statistical adjustment analysis. *Population Health Metrics, 14*(1), 1–12.

Ruhm, C. J. (2017). Geographic variation in opioid and heroin involved drug poisoning mortality rates. *American Journal of Preventive Medicine, 53*(6), 745–753.

Rutkow, L., & Teret, S. P. (2010). Role of state attorneys general in health policy. *Journal of the American Medical Association, 304*(12), 1377–1378.

Ryan, M., Gerard, K., & Amaya-Amaya, M. (2008). *Using discrete choice experiments to value health and health care.* New York, NY: Springer, Berlin Heidelberg New York Ed.

Ryan, R. M., & Deci, E. L. (2000). Self-determination theory and the facilitation of intrinsic motivation, social development, and well-being. *American Psychologist, 55*(1), 68–78.

Sage, W. M. (2008). Relationship duties, regulatory duties, and the widening gap between health law and collective health policy. *Georgetown Law Journal, 96*(2), 497–522.

Salganik, M. J., & Heckathorn, D. D. (2004). Sampling and estimation in hidden populations using respondent-driven sampling. *Sociological Methodology, 34*(1), 193–240.

Saltz, R. F., Paschall, M. J., & O'Hara, S. E. (2021). Effects of a community-level intervention on alcohol-related motor vehicle crashes in California cities: A randomized trial. *American Journal of Preventive Medicine, 60*(1), 38–46.

Sampson, R. J., Morenoff, J., & Gannon-Rowley, T. (2002). Assessing "neighborhood effects": Social processes and new directions in research. *Annual Review of Sociology, 28*, 443–478.

Sampson, R. J., Raudenbush, S. W., & Earles, F. (1997). Neighborhoods and violent crime: A multilevel study of collective efficacy. *Science, 277*, 918–924.

Sanbonmatsu, L., Katz, L. F., Ludwig, J., Gennetian, L. A., Duncan, G. J., Kessler, R. C., … Lindau, S. T. (2011). *Moving to opportunity for fair housing demonstration program: Final impacts evaluation.* US Department of Housing and Urban Development.

Sandler, J. C., Freeman, N. J., & Socia, K. M. (2008). Does a watched pot boil? A time series analysis of New York State's sex offender registration and notification law. *Psychology, Public Policy, and Law, 14*(4), 284–302.

Sanner, L., Grant, S., Walter-McCabe, H., & Silverman, R. D. (2021). The challenges of conducting intrastate policy surveillance: A methods note on county and city laws in Indiana. *American Journal of Public Health, 111*(6), 1095–1098.

Sarat, A. (1990). "… The law is all over": Power, resistance and the legal consciousness of the welfare poor. *Yale Journal of Law & the Humanities, 2*, 343–379.

Saunders, R. P., Pate, R. R., Felton, G., Dowda, M., Weinrich, M. C., Ward, D. S., … Baranowski, T. (1997). Development of questionnaires to measure psychosocial influences on children's physical activity. *Preventive Medicine, 26*(2), 241–247.

Savage, L. J. (1954). *Foundations of statistics.* New York, NY: John Wiley & Sons.

Scheingold, S. A. (2004). *The politics of rights: Lawyers, public policy, and political change* (2nd ed.). Ann Arbor, MI: University of Michigan Press.

Schensul, J. J. (1999). Organizing community research partnerships in the struggle against AIDS. *Health Education & Behavior, 26*(2), 266–283.

Schilling, J., & Linton, L. S. (2005). The public health roots of zoning: In search of active living's legal genealogy. *American Journal of Preventive Medicine, 28*(Suppl. 2), 96–104.

Schmelz, K. (2021). Enforcement may crowd out voluntary support for COVID-19 policies, especially where trust in government is weak and in a liberal society. *Proceedings of the National Academy of Science, 118*, 2016385118.

Schmitt, M., & Dorfel, M. (1999). Procedural injustice at work, justice sensitivity, job satisfaction and psychosomatic well-being. *European Journal of Social Psychology, 29*(4), 443–453.

Schnake-Mahl, A. S., O'Leary, G., Mullachery, P. H., Vaidya, V., Connor, G., Rollins, H., … Bilal, U. (2022). The impact of keeping indoor dining closed on COVID-19 rates among large UScities: A quasi-experimental design. *Epidemiology, 33*(2), 200–208.

Schneider, J. E., Peterson, N. A., Kiss, N., Ebeid, O., & Doyle, A. S. (2011). Tobacco litter costs and public policy: A framework and methodology for considering the use of fees to offset abatement costs. *Tobacco Control, 20*(Suppl. 1), i36–i41.

Schnittker, J., & McLeod, J. D. (2005). The social psychology of health disparities. *Annual Review of Sociology, 31*, 75.

Schramm, D. D., & Milloy, C. D. (1995). *Community notification: A study of offender characteristics and recidivism (95-10-1101).* Seattle, WA: Urban Policy Research.

Scobie, H. M., Johnson, A. G., Suthar, A. B., Severson, R., Alden, N. B., Balter, S., ... Silk, B. J. (2021). Monitoring incidence of covid-19 cases, hospitalizations, and deaths, by vaccination status—13 US jurisdictions, April 4–July 17, 2021. *Morbidity and Mortality Weekly Report, 70*(37), 1284.

Scollo, M., Lal, A., Hyland, A., & Glantz, S. A. (2003). Review of the quality of studies on the economic effects of smoke-free policies on the hospitality industry. *Tobacco Control, 12*(1), 13–20.

Scott, C. (2001). Analysing regulatory space: Fragmented resources and institutional design. *Public Law, 2001*(Summer), 329–353.

Scott, C. (2002). Private regulation of the public sector: A neglected facet of contemporary governance. *Journal of Law and Society, 29*(1), 56–76.

Scott, W. R., Ruef, M., Mendel, P. J., & Caronna, C. A. (Eds.) (2000). *Institutional change and healthcare organizations: From professional dominance to managed care.* Chicago, IL: University of Chicago Press.

Scutchfield, F. D. (2009). Foreword. *Health Services Research, 44*(5p2), 1773–1774.

Scutchfield, F. D., Marks, J. S., Perez, D. J., & Mays, G. P. (2007). Public health services and systems research. *American Journal of Preventive Medicine, 33*(2), 169–171.

Scutchfield, F. D., Mays, G. P., & Lurie, N. (2009). Applying health services research to public health practice: An emerging priority. *Health Services Research, 44*(5p2), 1775–1187.

Scutchfield, F. D., & Patrick, K. (2007). Public health systems research: The new kid on the block. *American Journal of Preventive Medicine, 32*(2), 173–174.

Seeman, T. E., & Crimmins, E. (2001). Social environment effects on health and aging: Integrating epidemiologic and demographic approaches and perspectives. *Annals of the New York Academy of Sciences, 954*, 88–117.

Selznick, P., Nonet, P., & Vollmer, H. M. (1969). *Law, society, and industrial justice.* New York, NY: Russell Sage Foundation.

Sen, A. (1969). Quasi-transitivity, rational choice and collective decisions. *The Review of Economic Studies, 36*(3), 381–393.

Sen, A., Sen, M. A., Foster, J. E., Amartya, S., & Foster, J. E. (1997). *On economic inequality.* Oxford, UK: Oxford University Press.

Shadish, W. R., Cook, T. D., & Campbell, D. T. (2002). *Experimental and quasi-experimental designs for generalized causal inference.* Boston, MA: Houghton–Mifflin.

Shah, G. H., Sotnikov, S., Leep, C. J., Ye, J., & Van Wave, T. W. (2017). Creating a taxonomy of local boards of health based on local health departments' perspectives. *American Journal of Public Health, 107*(1), 7280.

Shamir, R. (2008). Corporate social responsibility: Towards a new market-embedded morality? *Theoretical Inquiries in Law, 9*(2), 371–394.

Shattuck, L. (1850). *Report of a general plan for the promotion of public and personal health.* Boston, MA: Dutton & Wentworth.

Shaw, F. E., McKie, K. L., Liveoak, C. A., & Goodman, R. A. (2007). Legal tools for preparedness and response: Variation in quarantine powers among the 10 most populous U.S. states in 2004. *American Journal of Public Health, 97*(Suppl. 1), S38–S43.

Sheffer, C., Stitzer, M., & Wheeler, G. J. (2009). Smoke-free medical facility campus legislation: Support, resistance, difficulties and cost. *International Journal of Environmental Research and Public Health, 6*(1), 246–258.

Shekelle, P. G., Kahan, J. P., Bernstein, S. J., Leape, L. L., Kamberg, C. J., & Park, R. E. (1998). The reproducibility of a method to identify the overuse and underuse of medical procedures. *New England Journal of Medicine, 338*(26), 1888–1895.

Shelton, R. C., Adsul, P., & Oh, A. (2021). Recommendations for addressing structural racism in implementation science: A call to the field. *Ethnicity & Disease, 31*(Suppl 1), 357–364.

Shelton, R. C., Chambers, D. A., & Glasgow, R. E. (2020). An extension of RE-AIM to enhance sustainability: Addressing dynamic context and promoting health equity over time. *Frontiers in Public Health, 8*, 134.

Shelton, R. C., Cooper, B. R., & Stirman, S. W. (2018). The sustainability of evidence-based interventions and practices in public health and health care. *Annual Review of Public Health, 39*, 55–76.

Sherman, A., DeBot, B., & Huang, C. C. (2016). Boosting low-income children's opportunities to succeed through direct income support. *Academic Pediatrics, 16*(3 Suppl), S90–S97.

Sherman, L. W., & Strang, H. (2004). Experimental ethnography: The marriage of qualitative and quantitative research. *The Annals of the American Academy of Political and Social Science, 595*(1), 204–222.

Siegler, A. J., Komro, K. A., & Wagenaar, A. C. (2020). Law everywhere: A causal framework for law and infectious disease. *Public Health Reports, 135*(1 Suppl)), 25S–31S.

Silbey, S. (2002). The law and society movement. In H. Kritzer (Ed.), *Legal systems of the world: A political social and cultural encyclopedia* (Vol. 2, pp. 860–863). Santa Barbara, CA: ABC-CLIO.

Silbey, S. S. (2005). After legal consciousness. *Annual Review of Law and Social Science, 1*(1), 323–368.

Simon, H. A. (1959). Theories of decision-making in economics and behavioral science. *The American Economic Review, 49*(3), 253–283.

Skov, L. R., Lourenco, S., Hansen, G. L., Mikkelsen, B. E., & Schofield, C. (2013). Choice architecture as a means to change eating behaviour in self-service settings: A systematic review. *Obesity Reviews, 14*(3), 187–196.

Slaughter, E., Gersberg, R. M., Watanabe, K., Rudolph, J., Stransky, C., & Novotny, T. E. (2011). Toxicity of cigarette butts, and their chemical components, to marine and freshwater fish. *Tobacco Control, 20*(Suppl. 1), i25–i29.

Smart, R., Pardo, B., & Davis, C. S. (2021). Systematic review of the emerging literature on the effectiveness of naloxone access laws in the United States. *Addiction, 116*(1), 6–17.

Smit, L. A., & Heederik, D. (2017). Impacts of intensive livestock production on human health in densely populated regions. *GeoHealth, 1*(7), 272–277.

Smith, A. (1776). *An inquiry into the nature and causes of the wealth of nations.* Dublin, Ireland: Whitestone.

Smith, H. J., Tyler, T. R., Huo, Y. J., Ortiz, D. J., & Lind, E. A. (1998). The self-relevant implications of the group-value model: Group membership, self-worth, and procedural justice. *Journal of Experimental Social Psychology, 34*, 470–493.

Smith, J. D., & Hasan, M. (2020). Quantitative approaches for the evaluation of implementation research studies. *Psychiatry Research, 283*, 112521. doi:10.1016/j.psychres.2019.112521

Smith, T. A. (2005). *The web of law*. San Diego Legal Studies research paper no. 06-11. Retrieved from https://papers.ssrn.com/sol3/papers.cfm?abstract_id=642863.

Snell-Rood, C., Jaramillo, E. T., Hamilton, A. B., Raskin, S. E., Nicosia, F. M., & Willging, C. (2021). Advancing health equity through a theoretically critical implementation science. *Translational Behavioral Medicine, 11*(8), 1617–1625.

Snowdon, C. (2010). *The spirit level delusion: Fact-checking the left's new theory of everything*. Ripton, North Yorkshire: Little Dice.

Sobeyko, J., Leszczyszyn-Pynka, M., Duklas, T., Parczewski, M., Bejnarowicz, P., Burris, S., ... Chintalova-Dallas, R. (2006). *Bridging the gaps between needs and services in the health and criminal justice systems: Szczecin RPAR final report and recommendations*. Szczecin, Poland: RPAR. Retrieved from https://papers.ssrn.com/sol3/papers.cfm?abstract_id = 1276335.

Solar, O., & Irwin, A. (2010). *A conceptual framework for action on social determinants of health*. Social Determinants of Health Discussion Paper 2 (Policy and Practice). Retrieved from http://www.who.int/sdhconference/resources/ConceptualframeworkforactiononSDH_eng.pdf.

Sonfield, A., & Gold, R. B. (2001). States' implementation of the Section 510 abstinence education program, FY 1999. *Family Planning Perspectives, 33*(4), 166–171.

Sosin, D. M., & Sacks, J. J. (1992). Motorcycle helmet-use laws and head injury prevention. *Journal of the American Medical Association, 267*(12), 1649–1651.

Sox, H. C., & Greenfield, S. (2009). Comparative effectiveness research: A report from the Institute of Medicine. *Annals of Internal Medicine, 151*(3), 203–205.

Spackman, M. (2020). Social discounting and the cost of public funds: A practitioner's perspective. *Journal of Benefit-Cost Analysis, 11*(2), 244–271.

Spencer, J. H. (2007). Neighborhood economic development effects of the earned income tax credit in Los Angeles. *Urban Affairs Review, 42*(6), 851–873.

Spencer, R. A., & Komro, K. A. (2017). Family economic security policies and child and family health. *Clinical Child and Family Psychology Review, 20*(1), 45–63.

Spencer, R. A., Livingston, M. D., Woods-Jaeger, B., Rentmeester, S. T., Sroczynski, N., & Komro, K. A. (2020). The impact of temporary assistance for needy families, minimum wage, and Earned Income Tax Credit on Women's well-being and intimate partner violence victimization. *Social Science & Medicine, 266*, 113355.

Sperling, D. (2010). Food law, ethics, and food safety regulation: Roles, justifications, and expected limits. *Journal of Agricultural and Environmental Ethics, 23*(3), 267–278.

Stafford, M., & Warr, M. (1993). A reconceptualization of general and specific deterrence. *Journal of Research in Crime and Delinquency, 30*(2), 123–135.

Stake, R. E. (2005). Qualitative case studies. In N. K. Denzin & Y. S. Lincoln (Eds.), *The Sage handbook of qualitative research* (3rd ed., pp. 443–466). Thousand Oaks, CA: Sage.

Starmer, C. (2000). Developments in non-expected utility theory: The hunt for a descriptive theory of choice under risk. *Journal of Economic Literature, 38*(2), 332–382.

Stein, M. A. (2004). Under the empirical radar: An initial expressive law analysis of the ADA. *Virginia Law Review, 90*(4), 1151–1191.

Sterman, J. D. (2006). Learning from evidence in a complex world. *American Journal of Public Health, 96*(3), 505–514.

Stern, A. M., & Markel, H. (2005). The history of vaccines and immunization: Familiar patterns, new challenges. *Health Affairs, 24*(3), 611–621.

Stier, D. D., Thombley, M. L., Kohn, M. A., & Jesada, R. A. (2012). The status of legal authority for injury prevention practice in state health departments. *American Journal of Public Health, 102*(6), 1067–1078.

Stigler, G. J. (1950). The development of utility theory. *The Journal of Political Economy, 58*(4), 307–327.

Stringer, E. T. (2007). *Action research* (3rd ed.). Thousand Oaks, CA: Sage.

Strully, K. W., Rehkopf, D. H., & Xuan, Z. (2010). Effects of prenatal poverty on infant health: State earned income tax credits and birth weight. *American Sociological Review, 75*(4), 534–562.

Stryker, R. (1994). Rules, resources, and legitimacy processes: Some implications for social conflict, order, and change. *American Journal of Sociology, 99*(4), 847–910.

Stryker, R. (2000). Legitimacy processes as institutional politics: Implications for theory and research in the sociology of organizations. In M. Lounsbury (Ed.), *Research in the sociology of organizations* (Vol. 17, pp. 179–223). Bingley, UK: Emerald Group.

Stryker, R. (2007). Half empty, half full, or neither: Law, inequality, and social change in capitalist democracies. *Annual Review of Law and Social Science, 3*(1), 69–97.

Stryker, R., Docka-Filipek, D., & Wald, P. (2011). Employment discrimination law and industrial psychology: Social science as social authority and the co-production of law and science. *Law & Social Inquiry.* doi:10.1111/j.1747-4469.2011.01277.x

Stryker, S., & Serpe, R. T. (1982). Commitment, identity salience and role behavior. In W. Ickes & E. S. Knowles (Eds.), *Personality, roles and social behavior* (pp. 199–218). New York, NY: Springer-Verlag.

Studdert, D. M., Mello, M. M., Gawande, A. A., Brennan, T. A., & Wang, Y. C. (2007). Disclosure of medical injury to patients: An improbable risk management strategy. *Health Affairs, 26*(1), 215–226.

Suchman, M. (2010). *Sharing is (s)caring on the digital frontier: The challenges of IT governance in health care organizations.* Retrieved from https://sites.google.com/brown.edu/hits/the-big-picture?authuser=0#h.e2mpg6ofwgec.

Sunshine, J., & Tyler, T. R. (2003a). The role of procedural justice and legitimacy in shaping public support for policing. *Law and Society Review, 37*(3), 513–548.

Sunshine, J., & Tyler, T. R. (2003b). Moral solidarity, identification with the community, and the importance of procedural justice: The police as prototypical representatives of a group's moral values. *Social*

Susser, M. (1991). What is a cause and how do we know one? A grammar for pragmatic epidemiology. *American Journal of Epidemiology, 133*(7), 635–648.

Sutherland, E. H. (1942). Development of the theory. In K. Schuessier & H. Edwin (Eds.), *On analyzing crime* (pp. 13–29). Chicago, IL: University of Chicago Press.

Sutton, J. R., Dobbin, F., Meyer, J. W., & Scott, W. R. (1994). The legalization of the workplace. *American Journal of Sociology, 99*(4), 944–971.

Suurd, C. D. (2009). *A test of the relationships among justice facets, overall justice, strain and turnover intention in a military context.* Ottawa, Canada: Defence Research & Development Canada.

Swanson, J. W., Burris, S. C., Moss, K., Ullman, M. D., & Ranney, L. M. (2006). Justice disparities: Does the ADA enforcement system treat people with psychiatric disabilities fairly? *Maryland Law Review, 66*, 94–139.

Swanson, J. W., McCrary, S. V., Swartz, M. S., Elbogen, E. B., & Van Dorn, R. A. (2006). Superseding psychiatric advance directives: Ethical and legal considerations. *The Journal of the American Academy of Psychiatry and the Law, 34*(3), 385–394.

Swanson, J. W., Tong, G., Robertson, A. G., & Swartz, M. S. (2020). Gun-related and other violent crime after involuntary commitment and short-term emergency holds. *Journal of the American Academy of Psychiatry and the Law,* 200082-200020.

Swartz, M. S., Swanson, J. W., Kim, M., & Petrila, J. (2006). Use of outpatient commitment or related civil court treatment orders in five U.S. communities. *Psychiatric Services, 57*(3), 343–349.

Syme, S. L. (2004). Social determinants of health: The community as an empowered partner. *Preventing Chronic Disease, 1*(1), 1–5.

Talukder, M., & Quazi, A. (2011). The impact of social influence on individuals' adoption of innovation. *Journal of Organizational Computing and Electronic Commerce, 21*(2), 111–135.

Tapp, J. L., & Levine, F. J. (1977). *Law, justice, and the individual in society: Psychological and legal issues.* New York, NY: Holt, Rinehart and Winston.

ISPOR Task Force (2013). Consolidated Health Economic Evaluation Reporting Standards (CHEERS)—Explanation and elaboration: A report of the ISPOR health economic evaluation publication guidelines good reporting practices task force. *Value in Health, 16*(2), 231–250.

Tasnim, S., Hossain, M. M., & Mazumder, H. (2020). Impact of rumors and misinformation on COVID-19 in social media. *Journal of Preventive Medicine and Public Health, 53*(3), 171–174.

Taubman, S. L., Allen, H. L., Wright, B. J., Baicker, K., & Finkelstein, A. N. (2014). Medicaid increases emergency-department use: Evidence from Oregon's Health Insurance Experiment. *Science, 343*(6168), 263–268.

Temple University, Beasley School of Law. (2004). *Rapid Policy Assessment and Response: Module 1: Project Planning and Community Action Boards.* Retrieved from www.temple.edu/lawschool/phrhcs/rpar/index.html.

Tenforde, M. W., Self, W. H., Adams, K., Gaglani, M., Ginde, A. A., McNeal, T., ... Network, I. a. O. V. i. t. A. I. I. (2021). Association between mRNA vaccination and COVID-19 hospitalization and disease severity. *JAMA, 326*(20), 2043–2054.

Teret, S. P., Wells, J. K., Williams, A. F., & Jones, A. S. (1986). Child restraint laws: An analysis of gaps in coverage. *American Journal of Public Health, 76*(1), 31–34.

Terry, K. J., & Ackerman, A. R. (2009). A brief history of major sex offender laws. In R. G. Wright (Ed.), *Sex offender laws: Failed policies, new directions* (pp. 65–98). New York, NY: Springer.

Terry-McElrath, Y. M., O'Malley, P. M., & Johnston, L. D. (2020). Changes in the order of cigarette and marijuana initiation and associations with cigarette use, nicotine vaping, and marijuana use: US 12th grade students, 2000–2019. *Prevention Science, 21*(7), 960–971.

Tesoriero, J. M., Battles, H. B., Heavner, K., Leung, S.-Y. J., Nemeth, C., Pulver, W., & Birkhead, G. S. (2008). The effect of name-based reporting and partner notification on HIV testing in New York State. *American Journal of Public Health, 98*(4), 728–735.

Teubner, G. (1987). Juridification: Concepts, aspects, limits, solutions. In G. Teubner (Ed.), *Juridification of social spheres: A comparative analysis in the areas of labor, corporate, antitrust and social and welfare law* (pp. 3–48). Berlin, Germany: De Gruyter.

Tewksbury, R. (2005). Collateral consequences of sex offender registration. *Journal of Contemporary Criminal Justice, 21*(1), 67–81.

Tewksbury, R., & Jennings, W. G. (2010). Assessing the impact of sex offender registration and community notification on sex offending trajectories. *Criminal Justice and Behavior, 37*(5), 570–582.

Thaler, R. H., & Sunstein, C. R. (2009). *Nudge: Improving decisions about health, wealth, and happiness*. London: Penguin.

The Community Guide. (2009). *Community guide 101: Using evidence for public health decision making*. Retrieved from www.thecommunityguide.org/about/cg_101.html.

Thoits, P. A. (1986). Multiple identities: Examining gender and marital status differences in distress. *American Sociological Review, 51*(2), 259–272.

Thomas, R., & Perera, R. (2006). Are school-based programmes effective in the long term in preventing uptake of smoking? *Cochrane Database of Systematic Reviews, 3*, CD001293.

Thomas, W. I., & Thomas, D. S. (1928). *The child in America: Behavior problems and programs*. New York, NY: Alfred A. Knopf.

Thompson, O. (2014). Genetic mechanisms in the intergenerational transmission of health. *Journal of Health Economics, 35*, 132–146.

Thorpe, L. E., & Gourevitch, M. N. (2022). Data dashboards for advancing health and equity: Proving their promise? *American Journal of Public Health, 112*(6), 889–892.

Tidwell, J. E., & Doyle, D. (1995). Driver and pedestrian comprehension of pedestrian law and traffic control devices. *Transportation Research Record, 1502*, 119–128.

Titus, A. R., Kalousova, L., Meza, R., Levy, D. T., Thrasher, J. F., Elliott, M. R., ... Fleischer, N. L. (2019). Smoke-free policies and smoking cessation in the United States, 2003–2015. *International Journal of Environmental Research and Public Health, 16*(17), 3200.

Tobey, J. (1939). *Public health law: A manual of law for sanitarians* (2nd ed.). New York, NY: Commonwealth Press.

Tonry, M. (1994). Racial politics, racial disparities, and the war on crime. *Crime & Delinquency, 40*(4), 475–494.

Torres, C., Ogbu-Nwobodo, L., Alsan, M., Stanford, F. C., Banerjee, A., Breza, E., ... Group, C.-W. (2021). effect of physician-delivered COVID-19 public health messages and messages acknowledging racial inequity on black and white adults' knowledge, beliefs, and practices related to COVID-19: A Randomized Clinical Trial. *JAMA Network Open, 4*(7), e2117115.

Tremper, C., Thomas, S., & Wagenaar, A. C. (2010). Measuring law for evaluation research. *Evaluation Review, 34*(3), 242–266.

Trivedi, A. N., Zaslavsky, A. M., Schneider, E. C., & Ayanian, J. Z. (2006). Relationship between quality of care and racial disparities in Medicare health plans. *JAMA, 296*(16), 1998–2004.

Trochim, W. M. K. (2005). *Research methods: The concise knowledge base*. Cincinnati, OH: Atomic Dog.

Trubek, L. (2006). New governance and soft law in health care reform. *Indiana Health Law Review, 2006*(4), 139–169.

Tsoukalas, T., & Glantz, S. A. (2003). The Duluth clean indoor air ordinance: Problems and success in fighting the tobacco industry at the local level in the 21st century. *American Journal of Public Health, 93*(8), 1214–1221.

Tuller, D. (2017). The health effects of legalizing same-sex marriage. *Health Affairs, 36*(6), 978–981.

Tversky, A., & Kahneman, D. (1974). Judgment under uncertainty: Heuristics and biases. *Science, 185*(4157), 1124–1131.

Tyler, T. R. (1990). *Why people obey the law*. New Haven, CT: Yale University Press.

Tyler, T. R. (1999). Why people cooperate with organizations: An identity-based perspective. *Research in Organizational Behavior, 21*, 201–246.

Tyler, T. R. (2000). Social justice: Outcome and procedure. *International Journal of Psychology, 35*(2), 117–125.

Tyler, T. R. (2003). Procedural justice, legitimacy, and the effective rule of law. In M. H. Tonry (Ed.), *Crime and justice: A review of research* (Vol. 30, pp. 431–505). Chicago, IL; London, UK: University of Chicago Press.

Tyler, T. R. (2006a). *Why people obey the law*. Princeton, NJ: Princeton University Press.

Tyler, T. R. (2006b). Psychological perspectives on legitimacy and legitimation. *Annual Review of Psychology, 57*(1), 375–400.

Tyler, T. R. (2007). *Psychology and the design of legal institutions*. Nijmegen, the Netherlands: Wolf Legal Publishers.

Tyler, T. R. (2008). Psychology and institutional design. *Review of Law & Economics, 4*(3), 801–887.

Tyler, T. R. (2009). Tom Tyler and why people obey the law. In S. Halliday & P. D. Schmidt (Eds.), *Conducting law and society research: Reflections on methods and practices* (pp. 141–151). Cambridge, UK; New York, NY: Cambridge University Press.

Tyler, T. R., & Blader, S. L. (2000). *Cooperation in groups: Procedural justice, social identity, and behavioral engagement*. Philadelphia, PA: Psychology Press.

Tyler, T. R., & Fagan, J. (2008). Legitimacy and cooperation: Why do people help the police fight crime in their communities? *Ohio State Journal of Criminal Law, 6*(1), 231–275.

Tyler, T. R., & Fagan, J. (2010). Legitimacy and cooperation. In *Race, ethnicity, and policing* (pp. 84–117). New York, NY: New York University Press.

Tyler, T. R., & Huo, Y. J. (2002). *Trust in the law: Encouraging public cooperation with the police and courts*. New York, NY: Russell Sage Foundation.

Tyler, T. R., Lind, E. A., Ohbuchi, K., Sugawara, I., & Huo, Y. J. (1998). Conflict with outsiders: Disputing within and across cultural boundaries. *Personality and Social Psychology Bulletin, 24*, 137–146.

Tyler, T. R., & Markell, D. L. (2008). Using empirical research to explore ways to enhance citizen roles in environmental compliance and enforcement. *University of Kansas Law Review, 57*, 1–38.

Tyler, T. R., Mentovich, T., & Satyavada, S. (2011). *Accepting health care recommendations: Assessing the role of procedural justice*. Unpublished manuscript. New York University.

Tyler, T. R., Sherman, L., Strang, H., Barnes, G. C., & Woods, D. (2007). Reintegrative shaming, procedural justice, and recidivism: The engagement of offenders' psychological mechanisms in the Canberra RISE drinking-and-driving experiment. *Law and Society Review, 41*(3), 553–586.

U.S. Bureau of Justice. (2011). *Criminal justice system flowchart*. Retrieved from bjs.ojp.usdoj.gov/content/largechart.cfm#prosecution.

U.S. Department of Health and Human Services (U.S. HHS) (2004). *The health consequences of smoking: A report of the Surgeon General*. Washington, DC: U.S. DHHS, Centers for Disease Control and Prevention, National Center for Chronic Disease Prevention and Health Promotion, Office on Smoking and Health.

U.S. Department of Health and Human Services (U.S. HHS) (2006). *Healthy People 2010 midcourse review*. Washington, DC: Author.

U.S. Department of Health and Human Services (U.S. HHS) (2012). *Preventing tobacco use among youth and young adults: A report of the surgeon general*. Washington, DC: U.S. Department of Health and Human Services, Centers for Disease Control and Prevention, National Center for Chronic Disease Prevention and Health Promotion, Office on Smoking and Health.

U.S. Department of Health and Human Services (U.S. HHS) (2021). *Appendix D: Updating value per statistical life (VSL) estimates for inflation and charges in real income. A SUPPLEMENT to the U.S. HHS 2016 guidelines for regulatory impact analysis*. Retrieved from https://aspe.hhs.gov/sites/default/files/2021-07/hhs-guidelines-appendix-d-vsl-update.pdf.

Uchino, B. (2009). Understanding the links between social support and physical health: A life-span perspective with emphasis on the separability of perceived and received support. *Perspectives on Psychological Science, 4*(3), 236–255.

Ulmer, R. G., & Preusser, D. F. (2003). *Evaluation of the repeal of motorcycle helmet laws in Kentucky and Louisiana (HS-809 530)*. Washington, DC: U.S. Department of Transportation.

Unger, J. B., Cruz, T., Baezconde-Garbanati, L., Shields, A., Baezconde-Garbanati, L., Palmer, P., … Johnson, C. A. (2003). Exploring the cultural context of tobacco use: A transdisciplinary framework. *Nicotine & Tobacco Research, 5*(Suppl. 1), S101–S117.

Unger, R. M. (1983). The critical legal studies movement. *Harvard Law Review, 96*(3), 561–675.

United States Department of Transportation (DOT). (2016). *Revised Department Guidance 2016: Treatment of the value of Preventing Fatalities and Injuries in Preparing Economic Analyses.* Office of the Secretary of Transportation. Retrieved from https://www.transportation.gov/sites/dot.gov/files/docs/2016%20Revised%20Value%20of%20a%20Statistical%20Life%20Guidance.pdf.

Upenieks, L., Sendroiu, I., Levi, R., & Hagan, J. (2021). Beliefs about legality and benefits for mental health. *Journal of Health and Social Behavior.* doi:10.1177/00221465211046359

van der Heijden, J. (2019a). *Risk governance and risk-based regulation: A review of the international academic literature.* Retrieved from http://researcharchive.vuw.ac.nz/xmlui/bitstream/handle/10063/8357/Research%20paper.pdf?sequence=1.

van der Heijden, J. (2019b). *Behavioural insights and regulatory practice: A review of the international academic literature.* Retrieved from https://papers.ssrn.com/sol3/Papers.cfm?abstract_id=3332699.

van der Heijden, J. (2020a). *Responsive regulation in practice: A review of the international academic literature.* Retrieved from https://www.wgtn.ac.nz/__data/assets/pdf_file/0005/1873103/2020-State-of-the-Art-in-Regulatory-Governance-06-Responsive-regulation-in-practice.pdf.

van der Heijden, J. (2020b). Urban climate governance informed by behavioural insights: A commentary and research agenda. *Urban Studies, 57*(9), 1994–2007.

van der Heijden, J., Kuhlmann, J., Lindquist, E., & Wellstead, A. (2021). Have policy process scholars embraced causal mechanisms? A review of five popular frameworks. *Public Policy and Administration, 36*(2), 163–186.

Van Dyke, M. E., Komro, K. A., Shah, M. P., Livingston, M. D., & Kramer, M. R. (2018). State-level minimum wage and heart disease death rates in the United States, 1980–2015: A novel application of marginal structural modeling. *Preventive Medicine, 112*, 97–103.

van Panhuis, W. G., Paul, P., Emerson, C., Grefenstette, J., Wilder, R., Herbst, A. J., ... Burke, D. S. (2014). A systematic review of barriers to data sharing in public health. *BMC Public Health, 14*(1), 1144.

Van Rooij, B., de Bruijn, A. L., Reinders Folmer, C. P., Kooistra, E., Kuiper, M. E., Brownlee, M., & Fine, A. (2021). Compliance with COVID-19 Mitigation measures in the United States. *PsyArXiv.* doi:10.2139/ssrn.3582626

Vasquez, B. E., Maddan, S., & Walker, J. T. (2008). The influence of sex offender registration and notification laws in the United States: A time-series analysis. *Crime & Delinquency, 54*(2), 175–192.

Vega, W. A., Kolody, B., Hwang, J., & Noble, A. (1993). Prevalence and magnitude of perinatal substance exposures in California. *The New England Journal of Medicine, 329*(12), 850–854.

Ventola, C. L. (2014). Social media and health care professionals: Benefits, risks, and best practices. *Pharmacy and Therapeutics, 39*(7), 491–499, 520.

Vermunt, R., & Steensma, H. (2003). Physiological relaxation: Stress reduction through fair treatment. *Social Justice Research, 16*(2), 135–149.

Vernick, J. S., & Teret, S. P. (2000). A public health approach to regulating firearms as consumer products. *University of Pennsylvania Law Review, 148*(4), 1193–1211.

Victor, R. G., Ravenell, J. E., Freeman, A., Leonard, D., Bhat, D. G., Shafiq, M., ... Haley, R. W. (2011). Effectiveness of a barber-based intervention for improving hypertension control in black men: The BARBER-1 study: A cluster randomized trial. *Archives of Internal Medicine, 171*(4), 342–350.

Vining, A., & Weimer, D. L. (2010). An assessment of important issues concerning the application of benefit-cost analysis to social policy. *Journal of Benefit-Cost Analysis, 1*(1), 1–40.

Vining, A. R., & Weimer, D. L. (2006). Efficiency and cost-benefit analysis. *Handbook of Public Policy,* 417–432.

Viscusi, W. K. (2010). The heterogeneity of the value of statistical life: Introduction and overview. *Journal of Risk and Uncertainty, 40*(1), 1–13.

Viscusi, W. K., & Aldy, J. E. (2003). The value of a statistical life: A critical review of market estimates throughout the world. *Journal of Risk and Uncertainty, 27*(1), 5–76.

Viscusi, W. K., & Masterman, C. (2017). Anchoring biases in international estimates of the value of a statistical life. *Journal of Risk and Uncertainty, 54*(2), 103–128.

Voas, R., Tippetts, A. S., & Fell, J. C. (2003). Assessing the effectiveness of minimum legal drinking age and zero tolerance laws in the United States. *Accident Analysis and Prevention, 35*(4), 579–587.

von Tigerstrom, B., Larre, T., & Sauder, J. (2011). Using the tax system to promote physical activity: Critical analysis of Canadian initiatives. *American Journal of Public Health, 101*(8), e10–e16.

Vyshemirskaya, I., Osipenko, V., Koss, A., Burkhanova, O., Lazzarini, Z., Burris, S., ... Chintalova-Dallas, R. (2008). *HIV and drug policy in Kaliningrad: Risk, silence and the gap between human needs and health services.* Kaliningrad, Russia: RPAR.

W. K. Kellogg Foundation (2004). *Logic model development guide: Using logic models to bring together planning, evaluation.* Battle Creek, MI: Author.

Wagenaar, A., & Burris, S. (2013). *Public health law research: Theory and methods.* San Francisco, CA: Jossey-Bass.

Wagenaar, A. C. (1983a). *Alcohol, young drivers, and traffic accidents: Effects of minimum age laws.* Lexington, MA: Lexington Books.

Wagenaar, A. C. (1983b). Raising the legal drinking age in Maine: Impact on traffic accidents among young drivers. *International Journal of the Addictions, 18*(3), 365–377.

Wagenaar, A. C. (2007). Deterring sales and marketing of alcohol to youth: The role of litigation. In J. E. Henningfield, P. B. Santora, & W. K. Bickel (Eds.), *Addiction treatment: Science and the policy for the twenty-first century* (pp. 177–183). Baltimore, MA: Johns Hopkins University Press.

Wagenaar, A. C., Erickson, D. J., Harwood, E. M., & O'Malley, P. M. (2006). Effects of state coalitions to reduce underage drinking: A national evaluation. *American Journal of Preventive Medicine, 31*(4), 307–315.

Wagenaar, A. C., Finnegan, J. R., Wolfson, M., Anstine, P. S., Williams, C. L., & Perry, C. L. (1993). Where and how adolescents obtain alcoholic beverages. *Public Health Reports, 108*(4), 459–464.

Wagenaar, A. C., & Maldonado-Molina, M. M. (2007). Effects of drivers' license suspension policies on alcohol-related crash involvement: Long-term follow-up in forty-six states. *Alcoholism, Clinical and Experimental Research, 31*(8), 1399–1406.

Wagenaar, A. C., Maldonado-Molina, M. M., Erickson, D. J., Ma, L., Tobler, A. L., & Komro, K. A. (2007). General deterrence effects of U.S. statutory DUI fine and jail penalties: Long-term follow-up in 32 states. *Accident Analysis & Prevention, 39*(5), 982–994.

Wagenaar, A. C., & Perry, C. L. (1994). Community strategies for the reduction of youth drinking: Theory and application. *Journal of Research on Adolescence, 4*(2), 319–345.

Wagenaar, A. C., Salois, M. J., & Komro, K. A. (2009). Effects of beverage alcohol price and tax levels on drinking: A meta-analysis of 1003 estimates from 112 studies. *Addiction, 104*(2), 179–190.

Wagenaar, A. C., Tobler, A. L., & Komro, K. A. (2010). Effects of alcohol tax and price policies on morbidity and mortality: A systematic review. *American Journal of Public Health, 100*(11), 2270–2278.

Wagenaar, A. C., & Wolfson, M. (1994). Enforcement of the legal minimum drinking age in the United States. *Journal of Public Health Policy, 15*(1), 37–53.

Wahlbeck, P. J., Spriggs, J. F., & Sigelman, L. (2002). Ghostwriters on the court? *American Politics Research, 30*(2), 166–192.

Wang, J.-C., & Chiang, M.-J. (2009). Social interaction and continuance intention in online auctions: A social capital perspective. *Decision Support Systems, 47*(4), 466–476.

Wang, Y., McKee, M., Torbica, A., & Stuckler, D. (2019). Systematic literature review on the spread of health-related misinformation on social media. *Social Science & Medicine, 240*, 112552.

Ward, A. (2009). Causal criteria and the problem of complex causation. *Medicine, Health Care and Philosophy, 12*(3), 333–343.

Ward, H. (2007). Prevention strategies for sexually transmitted infections: Importance of sexual network structure and epidemic phase. *Sexually Transmitted Infections, 83*(Suppl. 1), i43–i49.

Waters, M., & Moore, W. J. (1990). The theory of economic regulation and public choice and the determinants of public sector bargaining legislation. *Public Choice, 66*(2), 161–175.

Watson, G., & Glaser, E. M. (1980). *Manual for the Watson Glaser critical thinking appraisal.* Cleveland, OH: Psychological Corporation.

Weait, M. (2007). *Intimacy and responsibility: The criminalisation of HIV transmission.* Abingdon, UK: Routledge-Cavendish.

Weatherly, H., Drummond, M., Claxton, K., Cookson, R., Ferguson, B., Godfrey, C., ... Sowden, A. (2009). Methods for assessing the cost-effectiveness of public health interventions: Key challenges and recommendations. *Health Policy, 93*(2–3), 85–92.

Weber, M. (1968). *Economy and society.* Berkeley, CA: University of California Press.

Weimer, D. L., & Vining, A. R. (Eds.) (2009). *Investing in the disadvantaged: Assessing the benefits and costs of social policies.* Washington, DC: Georgetown University Press.

Weinberger, A. H., Zhu, J., Lee, J., Xu, S., & Goodwin, R. D. (2021). Cannabis use and the onset of cigarette and e-cigarette use: A prospective, longitudinal study among youth in the United States. *Nicotine & Tobacco Research, 23*(3), 609–613.

Wells, J. K., Williams, A. F., & Fields, M. (1989). Coverage gaps in seat belt use laws. *American Journal of Public Health, 79*(3), 332–333.

Whitman, M. V., & Harbison, P. A. (2010). Examining general hospitals' smoke-free policies. *Health Education, 110*(2), 98–108.

Wiese, S. L., Vallacher, R. R., & Strawinska, U. (2010). Dynamical social psychology: Complexity and coherence in human experience. *Social and Personality Psychology Compass, 4*(11), 1018–1030.

Wigfield, A. (1994). Expectancy-value theory of achievement motivation: A developmental perspective. *Educational Psychology Review, 6*(1), 49–78.

Wigfield, A., & Eccles, J. S. (2000). Expectancy-value theory of achievement motivation. *Contemporary Educational Psychology, 25*(1), 68–81.

Wilkinson, R., & Pickett, K. (2009). *The spirit level: Why greater equality makes societies stronger*. London, UK: Bloomsbury Press.

Wilkinson, T., Chalkidou, K., Walker, D., Lopert, R., Teerawattananon, Y., Chantarastapornchit, V., ... Briggs, A. (2019). The international decision support initiative (iDSI) reference case for health economic evaluation. *F1000Research, 8*(841), –841.

Wilkinson, T., Sculpher, M. J., Claxton, K., Revill, P., Briggs, A., Cairns, J. A., ... Walker, D. G. (2016). The international decision support initiative reference case for economic evaluation: An aid to thought. *Value in Health, 19*(8), 921–928.

Williams, D. M.; Bohlen, L. C., Motivation for exercise: Reflective desire versus hedonic dread. Chapter 19 363–385. In Anshel, M. H., Petruzzello, S. J., & Labbé, E. E. (Eds.). (2019). *APA Handbook of Sport and Exercise Psychology, Vol. 2. Exercise Psychology*. American Psychological Association. https://doi.org/10.1037/0000124-000.

Williams, D. R., & Collins, C. (1995). U.S. socioeconomic and racial differences in health: Patterns and explanations. *Annual Review of Sociology, 21*, 349–386.

Williams, D. R., & Collins, C. (2001). Racial residential segregation: A fundamental cause of racial disparities in health. *Public Health Reports, 116*, 404–416.

Williams, D. R., Costa, M. V., Odunlami, A. O., & Mohammed, S. A. (2008). Moving upstream: How interventions that address the social determinants of health can improve health and reduce disparities. *Journal of Public Health Management and Practice, 14*(Suppl. 6), S8–S17.

Williams, D. R., & Mohammed, S. A. (2009). Discrimination and racial disparities in health: Evidence and needed research. *Journal of Behavioral Medicine, 32*(1), 20–47.

Williams, K., & Hawkins, R. (1986). Perceptual research on general deterrence: A critical overview. *Law and Society Review, 20*(4), 545–572.

Williams, K. D., & Williams, K. B. (1989). Impact of source strength on two compliance techniques. *Basic and Applied Social Psychology, 10*(2), 149–159.

Willis, J. W. (2007). *Foundations of qualitative research: Interpretive and critical approaches*. Thousand Oaks, CA: Sage.

Wilson, J. W. (2009). Toward a framework for understanding forces that contribute to or reinforce racial inequality. *Race and Social Problems, 1*, 3–11.

Winston, G. C. (1980). Addiction and backsliding: A theory of compulsive consumption. *Journal of Economic Behavior & Organization, 1*(4), 295–324.

Wisdom, J. P., Michael, Y. L., Ramsey, K., & Berline, M. (2008). Women's health policies associated with obesity, diabetes, high blood pressure, and smoking: A follow-up on the Women's Health Report Card. *Women and Health, 48*(4), 103–122.

Wolf, D. A., Monnat, S. M., & Montez, J. K. (2021). Effects of US state preemption laws on infant mortality. *Preventive Medicine, 145*, 106417.

Wolf, L. E., & Vezina, R. (2004). Crime and punishment: Is there a role for criminal law in HIV prevention policy? *Whittier Law Review, 25*(Summer), 821–887.

Wood, J. (2004). Cultural change in the governance of security. *Policing and Society, 14*(1), 31–48.

Wood, J. D. (2019). Private policing and public health: A neglected relationship. *Journal of Contemporary Criminal Justice, 36*(1), 19–38.

Woodruff, S. I., Pichon, L. C., Hoerster, K. D., Forster, J. L., Gilmer, T., & Mayer, J. A. (2007). Measuring the stringency of states' indoor tanning regulations: Instrument development and outcomes. *Journal of the American Academy of Dermatology, 56*(5), 774–780.

Woods, W. J., Binson, D., Pollack, L. M., Wohlfeiler, D., Stall, R. D., & Catania, J. A. (2003). Public policy regulating private and public space in gay bathhouses. *Journal of Acquired Immune Deficiency Syndromes, 32*, 417–423.

Woods, W. J., Euren, J., Pollack, L. M., & Binson, D. (2010). HIV prevention in gay bathhouses and sex clubs across the United States. *Journal of Acquired Immune Deficiency Syndromes, 55*(Suppl 2), S88–S90.

World Health Organization (WHO) (2006). In G. Hutton & E. Rehfuess (Eds.), *Guidelines for conducting cost-benefit analysis of household energy and health interventions.* Geneva, Switzerland: Author.

World Health Organization, United Nations Office on Drugs and Crime, & UNAIDS (2007). *Interventions to address HIV in prisons: Comprehensive review.* Geneva, Switzerland: World Health Organization.

Wright, R. F., & Huck, P. (2002). Counting cases about milk, our "most nearly perfect" food, 1860–1940. *Law and Society Review, 36*(1), 51–112.

Wright, S. (1934). The method of path coefficients. *Annals of Mathematical Statistics, 5*, 161–215.

Xiong, L., Bruck, D., & Ball, M. (2017). Unintentional residential fires caused by smoking-related materials: Who is at risk? *Fire Safety Journal, 90*, 148–155.

Xu, X., & Chaloupka, F. J. (2011). The effects of prices on alcohol use and its consequences. *Alcohol Research and Health, 34*(2), 236–245.

Xuan, Z., Chaloupka, F. J., Blanchette, J. G., Nguyen, T. H., Heeren, T. C., Nelson, T. F., & Naimi, T. S. (2015). The relationship between alcohol taxes and binge drinking: Evaluating new tax measures incorporating multiple tax and beverage types. *Addiction, 110*(3), 441–450.

Yang, I., & Hall, L. (2019). Factors related to prenatal smoking among socioeconomically disadvantaged women. *Women & Health, 59*(9), 1026–1074.

Yang, I., Hall, L. A., Ashford, K., Paul, S., Polivka, B., & Ridner, S. L. (2017). Pathways from socioeconomic status to prenatal smoking: A test of the reserve capacity model. *Nursing Research, 66*(1), 2–11.

Yates, B. T. (2018). Commentary on "standards of evidence for conducting economic evaluations in prevention science". *Prevention Science, 19*, 396–401.

Yates, B. T., & Marra, M. (2017). Introduction: Social return on investment (SROI). *Evaluation and Program Planning, 64*, 95–97.

Yeager, P. C. (1990). *The limits of law: The public regulation of private pollution.* Cambridge, UK; New York, NY: Cambridge University Press.

Yearby, R. (2018). Racial disparities in health status and access to healthcare: The continuation of inequality in the United States due to structural racism. *American Journal of Economics and Sociology, 77*(3–4), 1113–1152.

Yearby, R., & Mohapatra, S. (2020). Law, structural racism, and the COVID-19 pandemic. *Journal of Law and the Biosciences, 7*(1). doi:10.1093/jlb/lsaa036

Yngvesson, B. (1988). Making law at the doorway: The clerk, the court, and the construction of community in a New England town. *Law and Society Review, 22*(3), 409–448.

Zelditch, M., Jr. (2001). Theories of legitimacy. In J. T. Jost & B. Major (Eds.), *The psychology of legitimacy* (pp. 33–53). Cambridge, UK: Cambridge University Press.

Zgoba, K., Veysey, B., & Dalessandro, M. (2010). An analysis of the effectiveness of community notification and registration: Do the best intentions predict the best practices? *Justice Quarterly, 27*(5), 667–691.

Zimring, F., Jennings, W. G., Piquero, A. R., & Hays, S. (2009). Investigating the continuity of sex offending: Evidence from the second Philadelphia birth cohort. *Justice Quarterly, 26*(1), 58–76.

Zimring, F., Piquero, A. R., & Jennings, W. G. (2007). Sexual delinquency in Racine: Does early sex offending predict later sex offending in youth and adulthood? *Criminology & Public Policy, 6*(3), 507–534.